2010
YEAR BOOK OF
OPHTHALMOLOGY®

The 2010 Year Book Series

Year Book of Anesthesiology and Pain Management™: Drs Chestnut, Abram, Black, Gravlee, Lien, Mathru and Roizen

Year Book of Cardiology®: Drs Gersh, Cheitlin, Elliott, Gold, Graham, and Suri

Year Book of Critical Care Medicine®: Drs Dellinger, Parrillo, Balk, Dorman, Dries, and Zanotti-Cavazzoni

Year Book of Dermatology and Dermatologic Surgery™: Dr Del Rosso

Year Book of Diagnostic Radiology®: Drs Osborn, Abbara, Birdwell, Elster, Manaster, Oestreich, Offiah, Rosado de Christenson, and Walker

Year Book of Emergency Medicine®: Drs Hamilton, Bruno, Handly, Mullin, Quintana, and Ramoska

Year Book of Endocrinology®: Drs Schott, Apovian, Clarke, Eugster, Ludlam, Meikle, Ovalle, Schinner, Schteingart, and Toth

Year Book of Gastroenterology™: Drs Talley, Dempsey, Harnois, Lange, Pearson, Picco, Rombeau, and Scolapio

Year Book of Hand and Upper Limb Surgery®: Drs Yao and Steinmann

Year Book of Medicine®: Drs Barker, Berney, Garrick, Gersh, Khardori, LeRoith, Talley, and Thigpen

Year Book of Neonatal and Perinatal Medicine®: Drs Fanaroff, Benitz, Donn, Neu, and Papile

Year Book of Neurology and Neurosurgery®: Drs Klimo and Rabinstein

Year Book of Obstetrics, Gynecology, and Women's Health®: Drs Dungan and Shulman

Year Book of Oncology®: Drs Thigpen, Arceci, Bauer, Byhardt, Gordon, and Lawton

Year Book of Ophthalmology®: Drs Rapuano, Cohen, Flanders, Hammersmith, Milman, Myers, Nelson, Penne, Pyfer, Sergott, Shields, and Vander

Year Book of Orthopedics®: Drs Morrey, Beauchamp, Huddleston, Swiontkowski, and Trigg

Year Book of Otolaryngology-Head and Neck Surgery®: Drs Sindwani, Balough, Franco, Gapany, and Mitchell

Year Book of Pathology and Laboratory Medicine®: Drs Raab, Parwani, Bejarano, and Bissell

Year Book of Pediatrics®: Dr Stockman

Year Book of Plastic and Aesthetic Surgery™: Drs Miller, Gosain, Gurtner, Gutowski, Ruberg, Salisbury, and Smith

Year Book of Psychiatry and Applied Mental Health®: Drs Talbott, Ballenger, Buckley, Frances, Krupnick, and Mack

Year Book of Pulmonary Disease®: Drs Barker, Jones, Maurer, Raza, Tanoue, and Willsie

Year Book of Sports Medicine®: Drs Shephard, Cantu, Feldman, Jankowski, Khan, Lebrun, Nieman, Pierrynowski, and Rowland

Year Book of Surgery®: Drs Copeland, Behrns, Daly, Eberlein, Fahey, Huber, Mozingo, and Pruett

Year Book of Urology®: Drs Andriole and Coplen

Year Book of Vascular Surgery®: Drs Moneta, Gillespie, Starnes, and Watkins

2010

The Year Book of OPHTHALMOLOGY®

Editor-in-Chief

Christopher J. Rapuano, MD

Professor of Ophthalmology, Jefferson Medical College of Thomas Jefferson University; Director, Cornea Service; Co-Director, Refractive Surgery Department, Wills Eye Institute, Philadelphia, Pennsylvania

Wills Eye®

ELSEVIER
MOSBY

ELSEVIER
MOSBY

Vice President, Continuity: Kimberly Murphy
Associate Developmental Editor: Yonah Korngold
Production Supervisor: Donna M. Skelton
Electronic Article Manager: Emily Ogle
Illustrations and Permissions Coordinator: Dawn Vohsen

2010 EDITION

Printed in the United States of America
Composition by TnQ Books and Journals Pvt Ltd, India
Printing/binding by Sheridan Books, Inc.

Editorial Office:
Elsevier
1600 John F. Kennedy Blvd.
Suite 1800
Philadelphia, PA 19103-2899

International Standard Serial Number: 0084-392X
International Standard Book Number: 978-0-323-06838-3

Editorial Board

Table of Contents

Journals Represented

Journals represented in this YEAR BOOK are listed below.

Acta Ophthalmologica
American Journal of Neuroradiology
American Journal of Ophthalmology
Annals of Neurology
Archives of Neurology
Archives of Ophthalmology
Archives of Pathology & Laboratory Medicine
Archives of Physical Medicine and Rehabilitation
British Journal of Cancer
British Journal of Ophthalmology
British Journal of Radiology
British Medical Journal
Canadian Journal of Ophthalmology
Clinics in Dermatology
Cornea
Emerging Infectious Diseases
Eye
Eye & Contact Lens
Family Medicine
Journal of American Association for Pediatric Ophthalmology and Strabismus
Journal of Cataract & Refractive Surgery
Journal of Clinical Endocrinology & Metabolism
Journal of Clinical Microbiology
Journal of Pediatric Ophthalmology & Strabismus
Journal of Refractive Surgery
Journal of the American Medical Association
Journal of the Neurological Sciences
Medicine and Science in Sports and Exercise
Nature
Neurology
New England Journal of Medicine
Ophthalmic Plastic and Reconstructive Surgery
Ophthalmic Surgery, Lasers & Imaging
Ophthalmology
Radiology
Retina
Stroke
Transplantation

STANDARD ABBREVIATIONS

The following terms are abbreviated in this edition: acquired immunodeficiency syndrome (AIDS), cardiopulmonary resuscitation (CPR), central nervous system (CNS), cerebrospinal fluid (CSF), computed tomography (CT), deoxyribonucleic acid (DNA), diopter (D), electrocardiography (ECG), health maintenance organization (HMO), human immunodeficiency virus (HIV), intensive care unit (ICU), intramuscular (IM), intravenous (IV), magnetic resonance (MR) imaging (MRI), ribonucleic acid (RNA), ultrasound (US), and ultraviolet (UV).

Note

The Year Book of Ophthalmology® is a literature survey service providing abstracts of articles published in the professional literature. Every effort is made to assure the accuracy of the information presented in these pages. Neither the editors nor the publisher of the Year Book of Ophthalmology® can be responsible for errors in the original materials. The editors' comments are their own opinions. Mention of specific products within this publication does not constitute endorsement.

To facilitate the use of theYear Book of Ophthalmology® as a reference tool, all illustrations and tables included in this publication are now identified as they appear in the original article. This change is meant to help the reader recognize that any illustration or table appearing in the Year Book of Ophthalmology® may be only one of many in the original article. For this reason, figure and table numbers will often appear to be out of sequence within the Year Book of Ophthalmology®.

Foreword

I am again very pleased that my Editorial team has done such an outstanding job with the 2010 edition of the YEAR BOOK OF OPHTHALMOLOGY! The goal of the YEAR BOOK continues to be to provide a concise summary of the most important peer-reviewed journal articles covering the span of ophthalmic subspecialties from the previous year. The summary is accompanied by brief discussion of the relevance (or irrelevance) of the paper to practicing ophthalmologists. I believe it does just that.

While the phrase "information overload" (popularized by Alvin Toffler, well-known futurist and author of *Future Shock*) is not new, it seems especially relevant in the world of medicine these days. I think it is getting harder and harder to not only keep up with the latest developments in ophthalmology but also to sift through the literature to find what is noteworthy. The YEAR BOOK OF OPHTHALMOLOGY accomplishes that task *and* puts it into perspective. For those of us with hardly enough time to review the important literature in our own subspecialties, the YEAR BOOK can't be beat for keeping us abreast of the significant issues in other subspecialties.

I encourage readers to contact me (via e-mail is the best, at cjrapuano@willseye.org) with comments, criticisms and suggestions. Your input continues to help mold the YEAR BOOK into what is most useful for our readers. I look forward to hearing from you.

Christopher J. Rapuano, MD

1 Cataract Surgery

Dissatisfaction after multifocal intraocular lens implantation

Woodward MA, Randleman JB, Stulting RD (Emory Eye Ctr and Emory Vision, Atlanta, GA)

J Cataract Refract Surg 35:992-997, 2009

Purpose.—To analyze the reasons for patient dissatisfaction after phacoemulsification with multifocal intraocular lens (IOL) implantation and the outcomes after intervention.

Setting.—Emory Eye Center, Atlanta, Georgia, USA.

Methods.—This retrospective review comprised eyes of patients dissatisfied with visual outcomes after multifocal IOL implantation. Outcomes analyzed included type of visual complaint, treatment modality for each complaint, and degree of clinical improvement after intervention.

Results.—Thirty-two patients (43 eyes) reported unwanted visual symptoms after multifocal IOL implantation, including in 28 eyes (65%) with an AcrySof ReSTOR IOL and 15 (35%) with a ReZoom IOL. Thirty patients (41 eyes) reported blurred vision, 15 (18 eyes) reported photic phenomena, and 13 (16 eyes) reported both. Causes of blurred vision included ametropia (12 eyes, 29%), dry eye syndrome (6 eyes, 15%), posterior capsule opacification (PCO) (22 eyes, 54%), and unexplained etiology (1 eye, 2%). Causes of photic phenomena included IOL decentration (2 eyes, 12%), retained lens fragment (1 eye, 6%), PCO (12 eyes, 66%), dry-eye syndrome (1 eye, 2%), and unexplained etiology (2 eyes, 11%). Photic phenomena attributed to PCO also caused blurred vision. Thirty-five eyes (81%) had improvement with conservative treatment. Five eyes (12%) did not have improvement despite treatment combinations. Three eyes (7%) required IOL exchange.

Conclusions.—Complaints of blurred vision and photic phenomena after multifocal IOL implantation were effectively managed with appropriate treatment. Few eyes (7%) required IOL exchange. Neodymium:YAG capsulotomy should be delayed until it has been determined that IOL exchange will not be necessary.

▶ This article examines a series of patients who presented to a tertiary referral center and were dissatisfied with their initial visual outcome after multifocal intraocular lens (MFIOL) implantation. In this study, 81% of patients had satisfactory resolution of symptoms after additional intervention without intraocular lens (IOL) exchange. Only 7% of patients ultimately required IOL exchange, but

12% remained dissatisfied despite treatment, including one who underwent IOL exchange.

The authors developed a stepwise treatment algorithm for 2 of the most common complaints, blurred vision and unwanted photic phenomena. They support the now common consensus recommendation that neodymium:YAG (Nd:YAG) laser capsulotomy be delayed until the surgeon is reasonably certain that IOL exchange will not be necessary. This makes sense in that IOL exchange surgery is much more difficult in the setting of an open posterior capsule. This point is supported by another recent article examining the outcomes of IOL exchange surgery[1] in which the rate of vitreous loss was 49% in eyes with prior Nd:YAG capsulotomy, and only 10% in those with an intact posterior capsule.

Surgeons should advise patients who elect to receive a MFIOL that further intervention, including IOL exchange, may be necessary. Patients and surgeons can be reassured that in the large majority of cases, those interventions are ultimately successful.

M. F. Pyfer, MD

Reference

1. Leysen I, Bartholomeeusen E, Coeckelbergh T, Tassignon MJ. Surgical outcome of intraocular lens exchange: five year study. *J Cataract Refract Surg*. 2009;35: 1013-1018.

Intraocular lens exchange in patients with negative dysphotopsia symptoms

Vámosi P, Csákány B, Németh J (Semmelweis Univ, Budapest, Hungary)
J Cataract Refract Surg 36:418-424, 2010

Purpose.—To evaluate the results of intraocular lens (IOL) exchange in cases of severe negative dysphotopsia and to measure the distance between the iris and the IOL optic using ultrasound biomicroscopy (UBM).

Setting.—Szent Rókus Hospital and Eye Clinic, Semmelweis University, Budapest, Hungary.

Methods.—Data of patients with major negative dysphotopsia symptoms after phacoemulsification with IOL implantation were reviewed retrospectively. In cases in which IOL exchange was performed to diminish the symptoms, the distance between the iris and the anterior surface of the IOL optic was measured by UBM and compared with that in a group of nonsymptomatic pseudophakic patients (control group).

Results.—In 3806 cataract procedures, 5 eyes (4 patients) had severe negative dysphotopsia symptoms. Intraocular lens exchange was performed in 3 cases. In 1 case, the secondary IOL was implanted in the reopened capsular bag and the symptoms persisted. In 2 cases, the secondary IOL was implanted in the ciliary sulcus and the symptoms resolved. On UBM, the mean iris–optic distance was 0.45 mm ± 0.07 (SD) in the symptomatic group, 0.59 ± 0.29 mm in the control group (n = 21) (P =.353), and 0.00 mm in the sulcus-fixated group.

Conclusions.—The iris–optic distance was not statistically significantly different between eyes with severe negative dysphotopsia symptoms and nonsymptomatic eyes. However, when IOL exchange reduced the iris–IOL distance, the severe negative dysphotopsia symptoms resolved.

▶ This article presents 5 cases of persistent negative dysphotopsia after cataract extraction. The authors provide a concise review of the current literature regarding the etiology and the treatment of this phenomenon. All patients described the common triad of a persistent temporal dark crescent-shaped shadow, worse under photopic conditions, and accentuated by nasal rotation of the symptomatic eye. Similar to several other recent reports of this phenomenon, at least 1 patient was motivated to create a drawing of his visual perception, which is reproduced in the article.

Several authors have postulated that negative dysphotopsia is at least partially related to a large space between the iris and the intraocular lens (IOL) optic and to the presence of a temporal beveled corneal incision. The novel contribution of this report is that ultrasound biomicroscopy (UBM) was used to measure the iris-IOL distance both in symptomatic patients and asymptomatic controls. No significant difference was found; in fact, the iris-IOL distance was slightly larger in the asymptomatic controls. However, in 2 cases when the IOL was exchanged for a sulcus-fixated IOL and postoperative UBM showed the iris-IOL distance was reduced to zero, the patients' symptoms resolved. Also, 3 of the 5 cases in this report had superior corneal incisions, indicating that the temporal corneal incision is not solely responsible for persistent negative dysphotopsia.

The troublesome phenomenon of persistent negative dysphotopsia is most likely multifactorial in nature, a combined effect of a prominent globe and/or shallow orbit, space between a darker colored iris and capsule-fixated IOL, clear peripheral capsule, and accentuated by a temporal corneal incision. Fortunately, in most patients this phenomenon decreases over time and does not require intervention. Further study is needed to help identify those patients most at risk for persistent symptoms and to elucidate surgical maneuvers or IOL design modifications to eliminate the problem.

M. F. Pyfer, MD

Intraocular Lens Power Selection in the Second Eye of Patients Undergoing Bilateral, Sequential Cataract Extraction

Covert DJ, Henry CR, Koenig SB (The Eye Inst, Milwaukee, WI)
Ophthalmology 117:49-54, 2010

Purpose.—To determine if the 1-month postoperative error of predicted refraction of the first eye can be used to alter intraocular lens (IOL) power selection and improve refractive results for the second eye in patients undergoing bilateral, sequential phacoemulsification with IOL implantation (phaco/IOL).

Design.—Retrospective, consecutive, case series.

Participants.—Three hundred consecutive patients who underwent uncomplicated bilateral, sequential phaco/IOL between January 1, 2006, and December 31, 2007, by a single surgeon using a single IOL platform.

Methods.—The observed second eye 1-month postoperative spherical equivalent refractive error was compared with calculations of the hypothetic 1-month postoperative spherical equivalent refractive error if the first eye error had been fully or partially incorporated into the choice of IOL power for the second eye. The optimal amount of partial adjustment was determined.

Main Outcome Measures.—The error of predicted refraction: the difference between the actual or hypothetic spherical equivalent refractive errors and those predicted by preoperative calculations.

Results.—A total of 206 patients met inclusion criteria. The average of the absolute value of the unadjusted second eye error ($|E_{UNADJ}|$) was +0.44 diopters (D) compared with +0.42 D for the fully adjusted second eye error ($|E_{FULL}|$). The optimal amount of adjustment of the second eye IOL power was determined to be 50%; the average of the absolute value of this partially adjusted second eye error ($|E_{PARTIAL,50\%}|$) was +0.36 D; this was statistically different from ($|E_{UNADJ}|$) ($P < 0.0001$) and ($|E_{FULL}|$) ($P = 0.001$). The statistically significant benefit was observed for patients with either myopic or hyperopic errors in the first eye. The percentages of patients achieving postoperative refractions within 0.5 D and 1.0 D of the predicted refraction were 66.5% and 90.3%, respectively, for the unadjusted second eye, 67.0% and 90.8%, respectively, for the hypothetic fully adjusted second eye, and 74.3% and 93.7%, respectively, for the hypothetic partially adjusted (50%) second eye.

Conclusions.—Accounting for 50% of the observed error of predicted refraction of the first eye reduced the error of predicted refraction in the second eye. This novel methodology has the potential to improve the refractive outcomes in the second eye of patients with cataract.

▶ This interesting retrospective study considered an important question for cataract surgeons: Can adjusting for the refractive outcome of a patient's first operative eye increase the accuracy of the outcome for the second eye? Intuitively, one would think the answer to this question is yes, and indeed most surgeons, at least heuristically, adjust their intraocular lens (IOL) power selection for the second eye when the first eye has a greater than expected deviation from the target refraction. However, an earlier study by Jabbour et al[1] showed no benefit to adjusting the second eye for the prediction error of the first eye. The novel approach in this study involves correcting for only part of the first eye prediction error. Specifically, the authors found that the ideal correction amount was 50%, which improved the percent of second eyes within 0.5 D of target refraction from 65% to 74%, as shown in Table 3 in the original article.

A controlled prospective study testing this conclusion would provide stronger evidence and should be undertaken in the future.

M. F. Pyfer, MD

Reference

1. Jabbour J, Irwig L, Macaskill P, Hennessy MP. Intraocular lens power in bilateral cataract surgery: whether adjusting for error of predicted refraction in the first eye improves prediction in the second eye. *J Cataract Refract Surg*. 2006;32:2091-2097.

Risk Factors for Acute Endophthalmitis after Cataract Surgery: A Population-based Study

Hatch WV, Cernat G, Wong D, et al (Ophthalmology and Vision Sciences at the Univ of Toronto, Canada; The Inst for Clinical Evaluative Sciences, Toronto, Canada; St Michael's Hosp, Toronto, Canada)

Ophthalmology 116:425-430, 2009

Objective.—To identify risk factors for suspected acute endophthalmitis after cataract surgery.

Design.—Population-based retrospective cohort.

Participants.—Administrative data from more than 440,000 consecutive cataract surgeries in Ontario, Canada, from April 1, 2002, to March 31, 2006.

Methods.—Consecutive physician billing claims for cataract surgery and specific intraoperative and postoperative procedures related to complications of cataract surgery were identified. Acute endophthalmitis was defined using surrogate markers for intraocular infection, including vitrectomy, vitreous injection, or aspiration procedures not in combination with air/fluid exchange or dislocated lens extraction, performed 1 to 14 days after cataract surgery. Anterior vitrectomy performed on the day of surgery was used as a surrogate marker for capsular rupture.

Main Outcome Measures.—Overall rates of endophthalmitis were calculated and grouped by patient demographics, surgical facility, season, year, and association with capsular rupture.

Results.—There were 617 suspected acute endophthalmitis cases of 442,177 cataract surgeries over the 4 years. The overall unadjusted and adjusted rates of suspected acute endophthalmitis were both 1.4 per 1000 cataract surgeries. Men had higher rates than women (1.70 vs. 1.19/1000 surgeries, $P<0.0001$) with an adjusted odds ratio of 1.40 (95% confidence interval, 1.19–1.64). The oldest age group (≥85 years) had the highest rate (2.18/1000), and the youngest group (20–64) had the second highest rate (1.76/1000). The endophthalmitis rates for these age groups were significantly different from those aged 65 to 84 years. The endophthalmitis rate was approximately 10-fold higher in those with capsular rupture compared with those without (13.11 vs. 1.34/1000, $P<0.0001$), with an adjusted odds ratio of 9.56 (95% confidence interval, 6.43–14.2).

Conclusions.—The overall rates of suspected acute endophthalmitis are low but significantly higher in certain patient groups. Our population-based analysis can be used as a benchmark for quality-improvement initiatives and can assist clinicians in educating their patients regarding the risks associated with cataract surgery. Future work is required to address the higher rate of endophthalmitis in men, those with capsular rupture, and the oldest patients undergoing cataract surgery.

▶ The authors of this article examined a medical billing database to identify cases of suspected acute postoperative endophthalmitis from among over 440 000 cataract surgeries over a 4-year period in Ontario, Canada. They also created a useful summary of the recent large studies on incidence of endophthalmitis. As a rare event, any study of postoperative endophthalmitis requires a large number of surgical cases to reach statistical significance, as is achieved in this article. Contrary to the findings of West et al from 2005 in the United States,[1] this study found no trend toward increased rates of endophthalmitis during the study period (2002-2006). This is reassuring because the conversion to nonsutured temporal corneal incisions by most cataract surgeons from about 1998-2002 was suggested as a cause for the increased incidence of endophthalmitis over time in the article by West et al. After converting to sutureless corneal incisions, most cataract surgeons have not significantly modified their technique since 2002, except for a trend toward smaller incision sizes. The findings in this study imply that our incisions are adequately sealed, and the endophthalmitis rate has stabilized. Older age, likely due to decreasing immune function and other comorbidities, and intraoperative complications, such as vitreous loss, have been well established as risk factors for postoperative endophthalmitis, as is supported by this article. Interestingly, men had a slightly higher risk for endophthalmitis (1.4×) as did younger patients aged 20 to 64 years (about 1.25×). The mechanism for this difference in risk is not clear but should motivate further study. This article should be read along with the article by Freeman et al,[2] which is also reviewed.

M. F. Pyfer, MD

References

1. West ES, Behrens A, McDonnell PJ, Tielsch JM, Schein OD. The incidence of endophthalmitis after cataract surgery among the U.S. Medicare population increased between 1994 and 2001. *Ophthalmology.* 2005;112:1388-1394.
2. Freeman EE, Roy-Gagnon MH, Fortin E, Gauthier D, Popescu M, Boisjoly H. Rate of endophthalmitis after cataract surgery in quebec, Canada, 1996-2005. *Arch Ophthalmol.* 2010;128:230-234.

Rate of Endophthalmitis After Cataract Surgery in Quebec, Canada, 1996-2005

Freeman EE, Roy-Gagnon M-H, Fortin E, et al (Univ of Montreal, Quebec, Canada; et al)

Arch Ophthalmol 128:230-234, 2010

Objective.—To estimate the annual incidence of endophthalmitis after cataract surgery from January 1, 1996, through December 31, 2005, in Quebec, Canada.

Methods.—Deidentified data were obtained from an outpatient physician billing database (Quebec State Control for Health Insurance [RAMQ]) with regard to all cataract surgical procedures performed from January 1, 1996, through December 31, 2005, in Quebec. For this cohort, records of an *International Classification of Diseases, Ninth Revision (ICD-9)* code for endophthalmitis during the same years were requested from 2 sources: the RAMQ outpatient database and an inpatient hospital discharge database (Maintenance and Exploitation of Data for the Study of Hospitalized Patients [MED-ECHO]). Endophthalmitis after cataract surgery was assumed if it occurred within 90 days of the surgery. Risk factors were examined using χ^2 tests and logistic regression.

Results.—After exclusions, 490 690 cataract surgical procedures were performed from January 1, 1996, through December 31, 2005. A total of 754 cases of endophthalmitis occurred within 90 days after surgery for an overall incidence rate of 1.5 per 1000 surgical procedures (95% confidence interval [CI], 1.4-1.7). Factors associated with endophthalmitis included age of 85 years or older (odds ratio [OR], 1.34; 95% CI, 1.06-1.70), male sex (1.44; 1.24-1.66), later year of surgery (0.94; 0.92-0.97), and region of cataract surgery, because regions 6 (2.21; 1.91-2.55) and 9 (4.00; 2.48-6.43) had higher rates compared with all other regions.

Conclusion.—Reasons that explain the apparent decrease in endophthalmitis, especially in 2005, should be explored and further research performed to understand why certain patients and regions have higher risks of endophthalmitis after cataract surgery.

▶ This epidemiologic study of a state health insurance billing database examined the rate of postoperative endophthalmitis after cataract surgery in Quebec, Canada over a 10-year period ending in 2005. The results echo a similar study,[1] finding the overall incidence of endophthalmitis to be about 1.5 cases per 1000, with increased risk for those over age 85 and for males.

The results are shown graphically in Fig 1 in the original article, which the authors interpret to show a decrease in endophthalmitis incidence over the study period, while the number of cataract surgeries per year doubled over the same 10-year period. The authors do not make this point, but for any event with a built-in lag time for occurrence, including the delay in presentation of endophthalmitis after cataract surgery and the inherent delay in submission to a billing database, there is a tail of cases that could result in over-counting the first year, and undercounting the last year, as that tail is cut off by the discrete start and end times of the study. Even a small number of cases could skew the data for this rare event. Therefore, I suggest discarding the first and last year data, which also happen to be the highest and the lowest incidence, respectively. This changes the graph to indicate an almost stable rate of endophthalmitis over the 8 years (1997-2004).

This again is reassuring in light of the study by West et al in the United States,[2] which showed a sustained increase in endophthalmitis from 1998-2001 that the authors suggested was at least partially related to the migration to sutureless corneal incisions during that time.

This article should be read along with the article by Hatch et al, which is also reviewed in this journal.

M. F. Pyfer, MD

References

1. Hatch WV, et al. Risk factors for acute endophthalmitis after cataract surgery: a population-based study. *Ophthalmology*. 2009;116:425-430.
2. West ES, et al. The incidence of endophthalmitis after cataract surgery among the U.S. Medicare population increased between 1994 and 2001. *Ophthalmology*. 2005;112:1388-1394.

Effect of cefuroxime and moxifloxacin on *Staphylococcus epidermidis* adherence to intraocular lenses

Karadağ S, Özkan B, Karabaş VL, et al (Kocaeli Univ, Turkey)
Can J Ophthalmol 44:663-667, 2009

Objective.—To investigate and compare the effect of cefuroxime and moxifloxacin on adhesion of *Staphylococcus epidermidis* to intraocular lenses (IOLs).

Design.—Experimental study.

Methods.—The 3-pieced hydrophobic acrylic lenses were contaminated with *S. epidermidis* (American Type Culture Collection 35983) solutions containing 10^8 colony-forming units. IOLs were inoculated into test tubes containing tryptic soy broth after being held in antibiotic solutions for 15 minutes. Sonication and vortex procedures were performed in order to remove all the remaining bacteria. From each tube 10 μL and 100 μL was taken and inoculated into sheep blood agar. The colonies were counted overnight. The statistical analyses were made using oneway ANOVA, Tukey Honestly Significant Differences test (HSD) and independent t tests, and a p value less than 0.05 was considered statistically significant.

Results.—Overall, the mean numbers of colony-forming units on the lenses that were held in control, cefuroxime, moxifloxacin 0.5 mg/0.1 mL and moxifloxacin 0.1 mg/0.1 mL solutions were 1398 (SE 10.01×10^3), 29.9 (SE 1.16×10^3), 0.23 (SD 0.04×10^3), and 0.41 (SD 0.05×10^3), respectively. The evaluation using one-way ANOVA and Tukey HSD tests revealed significant statistical differences among the groups ($p = 0.000$). The evaluation using independent t tests revealed significant statistical differences between the 2 moxifloxacin groups ($p < 0.05$).

Conclusion.—Our results suggest that moxifloxacin and cefuroxime significantly inhibit bacterial adherence to IOLs. The effect of moxifloxacin on inhibition of bacterial adherence was significantly greater than that of cefuroxime. For this reason moxifloxacin might be considered as a better prophylactic agent.

▶ The use of intracameral antibiotics during cataract surgery to reduce postoperative endophthalmitis is a controversial topic. At least 1 recent article from the Endophthalmitis Study Group of the ESCRS[1] demonstrated a reduction of endophthalmitis when cefuroxime was administered into the anterior chamber during surgery.

This is an interesting laboratory study that demonstrates the effectiveness of treating hydrophobic acrylic intraocular lenses (IOLs) with antibiotics in decreasing adherence of *Staphylococcus epidermidis*. A previous study by the same group compared cefuroxime with vancomycin in a similar experiment, showing cefuroxime to be somewhat more effective than vancomycin. This study compared cefuroxime with 2 concentrations of moxifloxacin against a buffered saline control solution. Bacterial adherence to an acrylic IOL was reduced by a factor of 40 when treated with cefuroxime versus control, but moxifloxacin treatment was significantly more effective, resulting in a factor of 3000 reduction at the lower concentration and 6000 at the higher concentration.

When the 2 studies are considered together, moxifloxacin appears to be the most effective of the commonly used intracameral antibiotics in reducing *S epidermidis* adherence to hydrophobic acrylic IOLs.

M. F. Pyfer, MD

Reference

1. Endophthalmitis Study Group, European Society of Cataract & Refractive Surgeons. Prophylaxis of postoperative endophthalmitis following cataract surgery: results of the ESCRS multicenter study and identification of risk factors. *J Cataract Refract Surg*. 2007;33:978-988.

Association Between Tamsulosin and Serious Ophthalmic Adverse Events in Older Men Following Cataract Surgery

Bell CM, Hatch WV, Fischer HD, et al (Keenan Res Centre in the Li Ka Shing Knowledge Inst of St Michael's Hosp, Toronto, Ontario, Canada; Inst for Clinical Evaluative Sciences, Toronto, Ontario, Canada; Univ of Toronto, Ontario, Canada; et al)

JAMA 301:1991-1996, 2009

Context.—Both benign prostatic hyperplasia (BPH) and cataract formation are common in older men. The α-adrenergic receptor blocker tamsulosin is frequently prescribed to treat BPH, and research suggests this drug may increase the intraoperative difficulty of cataract surgery. No studies have documented whether use of tamsulosin or other α-blocker drug therapies affect the risk of serious postoperative adverse events.

Objective.—To assess the risk of adverse events following cataract surgery in older men prescribed tamsulosin or other α-blocking drugs used to treat BPH.

Design, Setting, and Patients.—Nested case-control analysis of a population based retrospective cohort study using linked health care databases from Ontario, Canada. We included all men aged 66 years or older who had cataract surgery between 2002 and 2007 (N = 96 128).

Main Outcome Measures.—A composite of procedures signifying retinal detachment, lost lens or lens fragment, or endophthalmitis occurring within 14 days after cataract surgery. The risk of these adverse events was compared between men treated with tamsulosin or other α-blockers and men with no exposure to these medications in the year prior to cataract surgery. We separately examined the association of drug exposure that was either recent (within the 14 days before surgery) or previous (15-365 days before surgery).

Results.—Overall, 3550 patients (3.7%) in the cohort had recent exposure to tamsulosin and 7426 patients (7.7%) had recent exposure to other α-blockers. Two hundred eighty-four patients (0.3%) had an adverse event. We randomly matched 280 of the cases to 1102 controls according to their age, surgeon, and year of surgery. Adverse events were significantly more common among patients with recent tamsulosin exposure (7.5% vs 2.7%; adjusted odds ratio [OR], 2.33; 95% confidence interval [CI], 1.22-4.43) but were not associated with recent exposure to other α-blockers (7.5% vs 8.0%; adjusted OR, 0.91; 95% CI, 0.54-1.54) or to previous exposure to either tamsulosin (≤1.8% vs 1%; adjusted OR, 0.94; 95% CI, 0.27-3.34) or other α-blockers (2.9% vs 2.1%; adjusted OR, 1.08; 95% CI, 0.47-2.48). This corresponds to an estimated number needed to harm (NNH) of 255 (95% CI, 99-1666).

Conclusions.—Exposure to tamsulosin within 14 days of cataract surgery was significantly associated with serious postoperative ophthalmic adverse events. There were no significant associations with exposure to other α-blocker medications used to treat BPH.

▶ Cataract surgeons are now quite familiar with the phenomenon of intraoperative floppy iris syndrome (IFIS) and the difficulties it presents during anterior segment ophthalmic surgical procedures. The association of IFIS with previous systemic use of tamsulosin (Flomax) has been well established and published in the general medical, urologic, and ophthalmic literature.

This is a large population-based study of health records in Ontario, Canada, covering 12 million residents. Patients with early postoperative complications after cataract surgery were identified over a 5-year period by selecting codes for any of the 4 procedures (vitrectomy, vitreous aspiration or injection, dislocated lens extraction, or air or fluid exchange) between 1 and 14 days after cataract surgery. These procedures were used as a surrogate marker for postoperative complications of retained lens fragments, endophthalmitis, and retinal detachment because clinical data were not available. All women, plus men under age 65, were excluded, along with those having combined procedures or any other eye surgery in the preceding 5 years. Matched controls were selected from the database, resulting in 280 cases with complications and 1102 controls without complications. By aligning this database with the Ontario drug registry, the authors determined that patients using systemic tamsulosin within 2 weeks before cataract surgery were about 3 times more likely to experience one of the above postoperative complications compared with patients not exposed to tamsulosin. Those taking other alpha-blocking medications, or who had stopped tamsulosin more than 2 weeks before cataract surgery, had no significant increased risk for postoperative complications.

This study neither examined the cause of the complications nor did it establish that stopping tamsulosin decreased complication risk. It is significant in documenting the public health risk for serious adverse events after cataract surgery in patients taking tamsulosin. Some of these could be avoided not just by informing the cataract surgeon about tamsulosin use, as currently recommended in the package literature, but by seeking ophthalmic consultation before starting the medication. This would allow the surgeon a chance to complete cataract extraction if required before tamsulosin exposure, at least for patients who could safely delay starting the medication, and to counsel all patients appropriately.

M. F. Pyfer, MD

Change in Corneal Sensitivity and Corneal Nerve after Cataract Surgery

Kim JH, Chung JL, Kang SY, et al (Yonsei Univ College of Medicine, Seoul, Korea)

Cornea 28:S20-S25, 2009

Purpose.—To compare corneal sensitivity and recovery of corneal innervation between temporal and superior clear corneal incisions in cataract surgery.

Methods.—We compared the change in corneal sensitivity in patients with cataract who had received phacoemulsification using either temporal clear corneal incisions (group 1) or superior clear corneal incisions (group 2). The changes were measured at 1 week, 1 month, and 3 months after surgery using the Cochet–Bonnet esthesiometer. For a different study population, changes of corneal sensitivity in 25 eyes of 20 patients and corneal nerve density with confocal microscopy in 20 eyes of 20 patients who had undergone cataract surgery were also assessed. All parameters were measured preoperatively and at 1 week, 1 month, and 3 months after surgery.

Results.—There was a significant decrease in sensitivity at the incision site in both groups. At 3 months after surgery, corneal sensitivity mostly recovered to preoperative values. Although postoperative change in corneal sensitivity showed similar patterns in both groups, group 1 showed a larger decrease. At temporal clear corneal incision sites, there was significantly decreased sensitivity at 1 week and 1 month postoperatively. However, corneal sensitivity returned to the preoperative levels by 3 months. Confocal microscopy revealed that at 1 week, 1 month, and 3 months after cataract surgery, subbasal nerve density was significantly reduced to 4113 ± 1421, 3555 ± 1448, and 4198 ± 1239 $\mu m/mm^2$, respectively.

Conclusions.—Corneal sensitivity after cataract surgery returned to near preoperative levels by 3 months before complete restoration of normal corneal innervation. Regeneration of subbasal nerve fibers determined by confocal microscopy seems to require more time than the return of corneal sensation after cataract surgery.

▶ Reduction of corneal sensitivity due to the interruption of the sub-basal nerve plexus is felt to be the primary cause of reversible dry eye syndrome following cataract surgery with a corneal incision as well as laser-assisted in situ keratomileusis (LASIK) surgery. A nasal- or temporal-hinged LASIK flap has been suggested to spare more of the nerve plexus that enters primarily at the 3-o'clock and 9-o'clock positions. Extending this analogy, one could conclude that a temporal corneal incision during cataract surgery is more likely to cause dry eye syndrome than an incision in an alternative location.

This study demonstrates that corneal sensitivity measured with a Cochet-Bonnet esthesiometer is reduced primarily adjacent to the incision after cataract surgery for both temporal and superior corneal incisions. The interesting finding is that central corneal sensitivity is not reduced significantly, even at 1 week after cataract surgery, for both temporal and superior incisions. Also, corneal sensitivity recovers to normal at all locations by 3 months post operation. The authors also used confocal microscopy to measure sub-basal nerve density temporally in a subset of patients with temporal corneal incisions, which showed that by 3 months only about half of the reduction in nerve density had recovered, despite complete recovery of corneal sensation.

This study should reassure most cataract surgeons who use a temporal corneal incision that in normal eyes a reduction in corneal sensitivity is found only adjacent to the incision and that this fully recovers by 3 months. Of course, a patient with other risk factors for dry eye syndrome, even a small reduction of sensitivity combined with the perioperative stress to the corneal epithelium from topical medications, requires extra vigilance to avoid healing problems after cataract surgery

M. F. Pyfer, MD

Progression of Age-Related Macular Degeneration After Cataract Surgery

Dong LM, Stark WJ, Jefferys JL, et al (Stony Brook Univ School of Medicine, NY; Johns Hopkins Univ School of Medicine, Baltimore, MD)

Arch Ophthalmol 127:1412-1419, 2009

Objective.—To document age-related macular degeneration (AMD) progression after cataract surgery.

Methods.—Surgeons prospectively enrolled patients with nonneovascular AMD who were awaiting cataract surgery. Fluorescein angiography was performed preoperatively and at the postoperative week 1, month 3, and month 12 visits. Incidence of neovascular AMD development within 12 months after operation was the primary outcome measure.

Results.—A total of 108 subjects were enrolled. Of 86 eyes with preoperatively photographically confirmed nonneovascular AMD, 71 had gradable images by month 12. Neovascular AMD was observed in 9 of 71 eyes (12.7%; 95% confidence interval, 6.0%-22.7%). The progression rate between week 1 and month 12 decreased to 3 of 65 eyes (4.6%; 95% confidence interval, 1.0%-12.9%) after excluding 5 neovascular events identified on the postoperative week 1 visit and 1 case with missing photographs at this visit.

Conclusion.—The low incidence rate of neovascular AMD development between 1 week and 1 year after cataract surgery did not support the hypothesis that cataract surgery increases the risk of AMD progression. Several eyes appeared to have disease progression on postsurgery week 1 fluorescein angiograms, suggesting that many cases of presumed progression to neovascular AMD following cataract surgery may have been present prior to cataract surgery, but not recognized owing to lens opacity.

▶ The issue of whether cataract surgery is a risk factor for progression of age-related macular degeneration (AMD) is important for cataract surgeons and their patients. Cataract surgery involves at least a temporary increase in ocular inflammation and macular light exposure, and both factors have been postulated to play a role in AMD. There is conflicting evidence in the literature to date, with some large observational studies suggesting an association between pseudophakia and advanced AMD (eg, Blue Mountains Eye Study and Beaver Dam Eye Study), while others finding no association (eg, Age-Related Eye Disease Study). Confounding issues are that both cataract and AMD share significant known risk factors, especially age and tobacco use, so an association is not surprising. Also, decreased visual function with a significant cataract is an indication for cataract surgery, but this may also be a symptom of early-undetected AMD.

This article presents a prospective study of 108 patients with non-neovascular (dry) AMD scheduled for cataract surgery, who were evaluated before and for 12 months after surgery with intravenous fluorescein angiography (IVFA) and fundus photography by independent graders. The primary outcome measure was incidence of neovascular (wet) AMD within 12 months after surgery. The key point of this study was that IVFA was also performed at 1 week postoperatively to detect cases with presumed pre-existing wet AMD that were missed due to the lens opacity. With 71 patients eligible at month 12, the authors found that wet AMD was observed in 9 eyes (12.7%), more than the expected incidence of about 5% or less found in other studies. However, *5 of these 9 eyes already had wet AMD at 1 week after cataract surgery*, and 1 had no photographs at week one. Excluding these eyes decreases the incidence of new-onset wet AMD post cataract surgery to 3 of 65 eyes, or 4.6%. Therefore, this study showed no increase in the development of wet AMD after cataract surgery, and, in fact, demonstrated that over half of the new cases of wet AMD in the year following cataract surgery had actually developed undetected wet AMD before surgery, but the presence of the cataract made the diagnosis difficult. Although not intended as a control group, the authors also analyzed the contralateral nonsurgical eye. Of the 33 phakic fellow eyes eligible for study, 1 developed wet AMD in 12 months, for an incidence rate of 3.3%—not significantly different from the 4.6% rate found in the surgical eyes.

Limitations of this study include the lack of a control group and relatively short-term follow-up. Also, ocular coherence tomography that has become almost essential to detect macular thickening associated with early wet AMD was not included. The accompanying editorial by Klein[1] suggests a larger multicenter, prospective, randomized clinical trial regarding AMD after cataract surgery in which the fellow eye serves as a control. This would indeed provide stronger evidence, but until this trial is undertaken, cataract surgeons and retinal specialists can now reassure their patients with dry AMD that at least 1 well-performed study showed no significant increase in progression to wet AMD after cataract surgery.

M. F. Pyfer, MD

Reference

1. Klein BE. Is the risk of incidence or progression of age-related macular degeneration increased after cataract surgery? *Arch Opthalmol.* 2009;127:1528-1529.

Analysis of surface whitening of extracted hydrophobic acrylic intraocular lenses

Matsushima H, Mukai K, Nagata M, et al (Dokkyo Med Univ, Tochigi, Japan)
J Cataract Refract Surg 35:1927-1934, 2009

Purpose.—To identify the cause of light scattering on the surface (ie, whitening) of extracted AcrySof intraocular lenses (IOLs).

Setting.—Department of Ophthalmology, Dokkyo Medical University, Tochigi, Japan.

Methods.—Dislocated IOLs extracted from 3 patients were stored and the IOL surfaces examined under light microscopy. The effect of whitening on visual function was evaluated by measuring light transmission with a spectrophotometer. To determine the cause of opacification, the IOLs were examined for calcium phosphate deposits using an electron probe X-ray microanalyzer. The IOL surface, including the presence of organic deposits and evidence of hydrolysis, was also examined by Fourier-transform infrared spectrophotometry. The IOLs were then dried, immersed again in physiological saline, and serially examined for changes in opacification.

Results.—The optic surfaces of all IOLs had opacification due to whitening. Light transmission in the visible range of 360 to 800 nm was 4% less than that of unused IOLs. The X-ray microanalysis showed no calcium phosphate deposits. Fourier-transform infrared spectrophotometry of the

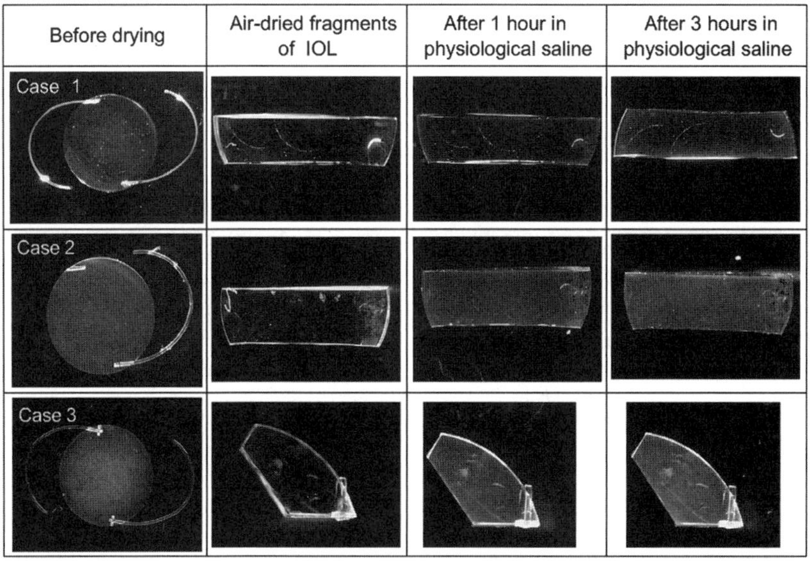

FIGURE 8.—Mechanism of development of whitening (IOL = intraocular lens). (Reprinted from Matsushima H, Mukai K, Nagata M, et al. Analysis of surface whitening of extracted hydrophobic acrylic intraocular lenses. *J Cataract Refract Surg*. 2009;35:1927-1934, with permission from ASCRS and ESCRS.)

IOL optic material showed no evidence of hydrolysis. Opacification disappeared after the IOLs were dried and then reappeared over time when the IOL was immersed again in physiologic saline.

Conclusions.—The findings strongly suggest that whitening of the hydrophobic acrylic IOL was due to trace water molecules that infiltrate the optic. Within the 3-dimensional network of the polymeric lens material, the molecules are too small to form observable voids but can form water aggregates of sufficient size to scatter visible light, causing opacification (ie, whitening) (Fig 8).

▶ Several different causes for partial loss of transparency over time in implanted acrylic intraocular lenses (IOLs) have been described. These include surface deposition of cells or cellular debris, accumulation of calcium or other minerals on the surface or within the substance of the lens, and appearance of presumed water vacuoles (termed glistenings). Optically significant calcification requiring removal of the IOL has affected mainly hydrophilic acrylic material. Most of the time these lens implant opacities are not visually significant. Cells or cellular debris on the anterior or posterior lens surface can usually be cleared with Nd-YAG laser application if they impair vision.

This article describes a new form of partial transparency loss in hydrophobic acrylic IOLs. These lenses were removed years after implantation due to subluxation but preoperatively were observed to have a mild white haze on the surface under diffuse illumination. The authors analyzed these explanted IOLs. They demonstrated that the haze decreased light transmission by an insignificant 4% compared with a new lens of the same material and that calcium or organic material do not account for the surface whitening. Convincing photographs (Fig 8) show that the haze disappears when the lens is dried in air and then reappears when immersed in normal saline. The authors postulate that the mechanism for surface whitening is diffuse infiltration of water molecules into the lens polymer, in contrast to the larger discrete water vacuoles deeper in the material that create the appearance of glistenings described previously.

Although not usually significant clinically, any loss of transparency of implanted IOLs over time should be understood and corrected to achieve the best possible results from increasingly refined advanced design lens implants.

M. F. Pyfer, MD

Anterior capsulotomy with a pulsed-electron avalanche knife

Palanker D, Nomoto H, Huie P, et al (Stanford Univ, CA; et al)

J Cataract Refract Surg 36:127-132, 2010

Purpose.—To evaluate a new pulsed-electron avalanche knife design for creating a continuous curvilinear capsulotomy (CCC) and compare the CCC with a mechanical capsulorhexis.

Setting.—Department of Ophthalmology, Stanford University, Stanford, California, USA.

Methods.—In this study, CCCs were created in freshly enucleated bovine eyes and in rabbit eyes in vivo. The cutting velocity was adjusted by controlling the burst repetition rate, voltage amplitude, and burst duration. Tissue samples were fixed and processed for histology and scanning electron microscopy (SEM) immediately after surgery.

Results.—The study included 50 bovine eyes and 10 rabbit eyes. By adjusting the electrosurgical waveforms, gas-bubble formation was minimized to permit good surgical visualization. The optimum voltage level was determined to be ±410 V with a burst duration of 20 μs. Burst repetition rate, continuously adjustable from 20 to 200 Hz with footpedal control, allowed the surgeon to vary linear cutting velocity up to 2.0 mm/s. Histology and SEM showed that the pulsed-electron avalanche knife produced sharp-edged capsule cutting without radial nicks or tears.

Conclusions.—The probe of the pulsed-electron avalanche knife duplicated the surgical feel of a 25-gauge cystotome and created a histologically smooth capsule cut. It may improve precision and reproducibility of creating a CCC, as well as improve its proper sizing and centration, especially in the face of surgical risk factors, such as weak zonules or poor visibility.

▶ This article describes animal testing of a new pulsed-electron avalanche knife (PEAK) originally designed for vitreoretinal surgery and adapted for creation of the continuous curvilinear capsulotomy (CCC) in cataract surgery. It is of interest mainly because it includes high quality scanning electron micrographs of the capsule edge after both standard mechanical capsulorhexis (Fig 4 in the original article) and CCC with the PEAK device (Fig 5 in the original article). Both show a remarkably smooth edge without radial extensions or adjacent tissue damage.

A properly sized and centered anterior capsulotomy is a key component to consistent results in modern cataract surgery. The continuous curvilinear capsulorhexis maneuver, originally described by Gimbel and Nuehann,[1] was revolutionary due to its high tensile strength and flexibility relative to other capsulotomy techniques allowing development of a new generation of intraocular lenses (IOLs), including the current multifocal and accommodating models that require precise stable positioning for optimal performance. For experienced surgeons, the CCC is a quick and straightforward maneuver in the large majority of cases, so it is hard to justify the use of an additional device at this time. However, future IOL options may require a very small, very large, or noncircular capsulorhexis, which are difficult to create manually. Time will tell whether this technology or others being evaluated, such as the plasma (Fugo) blade or the femtosecond laser, eventually supplant the mechanical CCC.

M. F. Pyfer, MD

Reference

1. Gimbel HV, Neuhann TT. Development, advantages, and methods of the continuous circular capsulorhexis technique. *J Cataract Refract Surg*. 2001;27: 1346-1347.

2 Refractive Surgery

Four-Year Follow-up of Posterior Chamber Phakic Intraocular Lens Implantation for Moderate to High Myopia

Kamiya K, Shimizu K, Igarashi A, et al (Univ of Kitasato School of Medicine, Kanagawa, Japan)

Arch Ophthalmol 127:845-850, 2009

Objective.—To assess the long-term clinical outcomes of implantation of a lens consisting of a biocompatible collagen copolymer (Visian implantable Collamer lens [ICL]; STAAR Surgical, Nidau, Switzerland) for moderate to high myopia.

Methods.—We evaluated 56 eyes of 34 patients with myopic refractive errors of −4.00 to −15.25 diopters (D) who underwent ICL implantation and routine postoperative examinations. Before and 1, 3, and 6 months and 1, 2, and 4 years after surgery, we assessed the safety, efficacy, predictability, stability, and adverse events of the surgery.

Results.—Mean (SD) logMAR uncorrected and best spectacle-corrected visual acuities were −0.03 (0.23) and −0.21 (0.09), respectively, at 4 years after surgery. The mean (SD) safety and efficacy indexes were 1.19 (0.25) and 0.83 (0.29), respectively. At 4 years, 44 (79%) and 52 (93%) of the eyes were within ±0.5 and ±1.0 D, respectively, of the targeted correction. Mean (SD) manifest refraction changes of −0.24 (0.57) D occurred from 1 month to 4 years after surgery. No vision-threatening complications occurred during the observation period.

Conclusion.—Implantation of ICLs is safe and effective and provides predictable and stable refractive results in the treatment of moderate to high myopia during a 4-year observation period, suggesting its viability as a surgical option for the treatment of such eyes.

► As I have said and written many times before, I am not overly concerned about the short-term results of phakic intraocular lenses (IOLs); it is the long-term issues that I worry about. This study reviewed 4-year results of the Visian implantable Collamer lens (ICL) in 56 eyes of 34 patients.

Uncorrected and best-corrected visual acuity and stability of refractive results were all excellent at 4 years. Safety results were also quite good. There were no significant intraocular pressure (IOP) rises. One eye developed an implant-related cataract that required removal. However, endothelial cell loss was not insignificant over 4 years. The mean cell loss of 3.7% is higher than physiological cell loss of approximately 0.6% per year, or 2.4% over 4 years. This level of endothelial cell loss is somewhat lower than most previously reported results for phakic IOLs. The bottom line is that as longer term follow-up studies are reported, the results continue to be good. Now, 4 years is certainly not "long-term," but we are getting there.

C. J. Rapuano, MD

AcrySof Phakic Angle-supported Intraocular Lens for the Correction of Moderate-to-High Myopia: One-Year Results of a Multicenter European Study

Kohnen T, Knorz MC, Cochener B, et al (Johann Wolfgang Goethe-Univ, Frankfurt/Main, Germany; Univ Eye Clinic Mannheim, Germany; CHU Morvan, Brest, France; et al)

Ophthalmology 116:1314-1321, 2009

Purpose.—To investigate the safety and effectiveness of the AcrySof phakic angle-supported intraocular lens (IOL) (Alcon Laboratories, Inc., Fort Worth, TX) for correction of moderate-to-high myopia in adults.

Design.—One-year interim analysis of a phase 3, nonrandomized, open-label, prospective, multicenter European clinical study.

Participants.—A total of 190 subjects (190 eyes) with moderate-to-high myopia. The preoperative mean manifest refraction spherical equivalent (MRSE) was −10.38 diopters (D) ±2.43 standard deviation (SD).

Methods.—Unilateral implantation of the AcrySof phakic angle-supported IOL.

Main Outcome Measures.—Best spectacle-corrected visual acuity (BSCVA), uncorrected distance visual acuity (UCVA), predictability and stability of MRSE, adverse events, and endothelial cell density.

Results.—Of 190 subjects enrolled, 161 completed the 1-year postoperative visit. No subjects lost ≥2 lines BSCVA. A UCVA of 20/20 or better was achieved by 57.8%; 99.4% had 20/40 or better. A BSCVA of 20/32 or better was achieved by 100% of subjects; 85.7% had 20/20 or better. The mean MRSE was −0.23 D (±0.50 D: −2.50 to 0.75 D). Residual refractive error was within ±1.0 D from the target for 95.7% of subjects and within ±0.5 D for 72.7% of subjects. The overall mean percentage change in central endothelial cell density 1 year after surgery was −4.77 ± 8.04% (n = 139). No pupil ovalization, pupillary block, or retinal detachment events were observed.

Conclusions.—The AcrySof phakic angle-supported IOL yielded excellent refractive correction and predictability with acceptable safety in subjects with moderate-to-high myopia. These 1-year interim analysis findings demonstrate preliminary support for the safety and efficacy of this IOL (Tables 2 and 3).

▶ The 3 main options for phakic intraocular lenses are (1) posterior chamber (eg, Visian ICL), (2) iris clip (eg, Verisyse), and (3) angle supported phakic intraocular lens (IOL) such as the one reported in this study. While all of

TABLE 2.—Adverse Event Incidence Rates

Adverse Event	Incidence Rate N = 190 n	%
Increased IOP requiring treatment[a]	6	3.2
Prolonged hospitalization for increased IOP[b, c]	5	2.6
Cataract formation[d]	5	2.6
Corneal haze	1	0.5
Synechia (single-strand)	2	1.1
Secondary surgical intervention		
IOL replacement for power exchange[e]	1	0.5
IOL removal because of upside-down placement	1	0.5
New suturing[e]	1	0.5
Endophthalmitis	0	0
Pupillary block	0	0
Pupil ovalization	0	0
Retinal detachment	0	0

IOL = intraocular lens; IOP = intraocular pressure.
Incidence rates are based on the number of eyes with an event divided by the number of eyes implanted.
[a]≥1 mo after surgery.
[b]On day of surgery because of retained OVD.
[c]Prolonged hospitalization was defined as a hospital stay ≥24 hrs beyond the planned stay.
[d]Secondary to concurrent ophthalmic disease (n = 2), upside-down IOL implantation (n = 2), subject age, and family pathology (n = 1).
[e]Observed in the same subject.

TABLE 3.—Change in Central Endothelial Cell Density from Preoperative Visit to One Year after Surgery

Mean Change in Endothelial Cell Density Category, %	Subjects n (%)	Overall Mean Change, %
Loss ≥10	21 (15.1)	
Loss <10 to ≥5	20 (14.4)	
Loss <5 to gain <5	92 (66.2)	
Gain ≥5 to <10	5 (3.6)	
Gain ≥10	1 (0.7)	
Total	139 (100)	−4.77 ± 8.04

these lenses can have adverse events, such as endophthalmitis and iritis, the posterior chamber phakic IOLs are more associated with cataracts and iris clip phakic IOLs are more associated with increased levels of endothelial cell loss (and are also trickier to insert properly).

This study reported interim 1-year data of a 5-year study on a foldable, angle-supported phakic IOL. Again, as seen with the other phakic IOLs, the visual results are quite good. Overall, the procedure was safe (see Table 2). Elevated intraocular pressure and cataract were the most common issues. My biggest concern is endothelial cell loss. Mean endothelial cell loss at 1 year was 4.8%, but 15% of eyes lost greater than or equal to 10% of cells (see

Table 3). Given that the haptics of this lens are in the angle, long-term endothelial cell loss results will be critical to determine the long-term success and safety of this lens.

C. J. Rapuano, MD

LASIK World Literature Review: Quality of Life and Patient Satisfaction

Solomon KD, Fernández de Castro LE, Sandoval HP, et al (Med Univ of South Carolina, Charleston; et al)
Ophthalmology 116:691-701, 2009

Purpose.—To analyze the patient reported outcome of satisfaction after LASIK surgery.

Design.—Systematic review.

Participants.—Patient data from previously reported studies.

Methods.—A literature search conducted for the years 1988 to 2008 that included pertinent LASIK surgery information from the review of 2915 retrieved citations. All abstracts from these citations were reviewed and 1581 were deemed to be relevant for review. Complete copies of each of these relevant (1581) articles were obtained, and after thorough analysis each was rated based on the strength of the study design and weight of evidence. A level I rating was assigned to properly conducted, well-designed, randomized clinical trials; a level II rating to well-designed cohort and case-control studies; and a level III rating to case series, case reports, and poorly designed prospective and retrospective studies. Level I and II rated, peer-reviewed articles were entered into a database, and level III articles were eliminated. A total of 309 articles were incorporated into this database, representing level I and level II well-controlled studies of primary LASIK surgery.

Main Outcome Measures.—Patients' satisfaction rates and factors associated with dissatisfaction.

Results.—Nineteen of the 309 database articles (6.1%) reported on both patient quality of life and satisfaction and together encompassed a total of 2198 subjects. The procedures from these 19 articles took place between 1995 and 2003. The overall patient satisfaction rate after primary LASIK surgery was 95.4% (2097 of 2198 subjects; range of patient satisfaction for the 19 articles was 87.2%–100%). The patient satisfaction rate after myopic LASIK was 95.3% (1811 of 1901 patients), and after hyperopic LASIK was 96.3% (286 of 297 subjects).

Conclusions.—Based on this review, worldwide, an average 95.4% of patients were satisfied with their outcome after LASIK surgery. With 16.3 million procedures performed worldwide, and more than a decade of clinical studies and technological innovation, LASIK surgery should be considered among the most successful elective procedures. LASIK

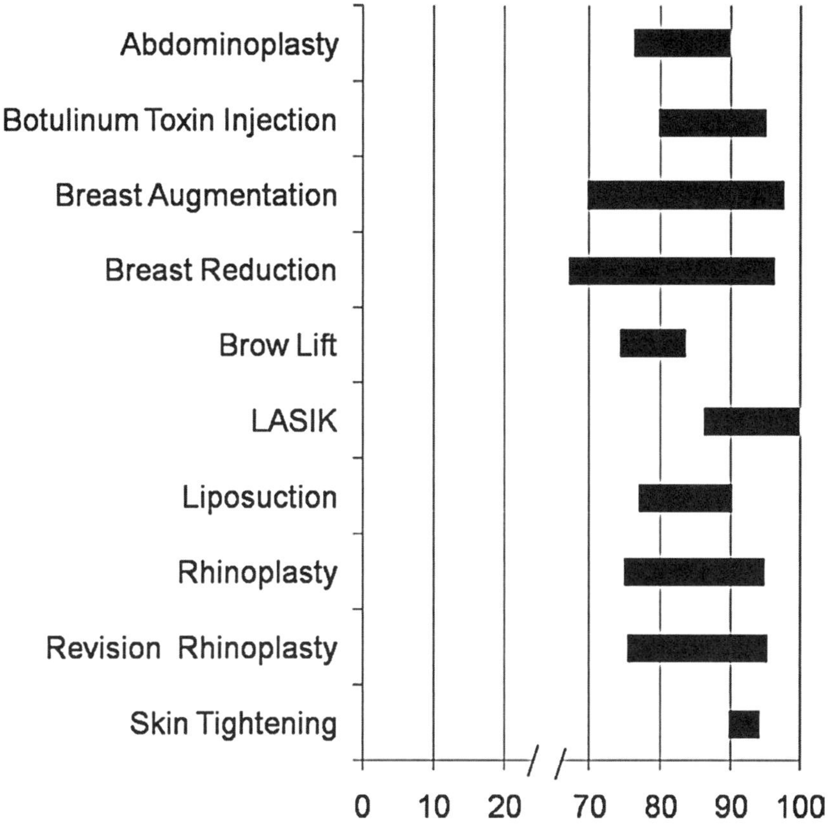

FIGURE 5.—Percentage of patient satisfaction after different elective surgical procedures. (Reprinted from Solomon KD, Fernández de Castro LE, Sandoval HP, et al. LASIK world literature review: quality of life and patient satisfaction. *Ophthalmology*. 2009;116:691-701, with permission from the American Academy of Ophthalmology.)

surgery compares more favorably with other elective surgical procedures in terms of generally higher satisfaction rates (Fig 5).

▶ It goes without saying that no surgical procedure is perfect. It is similarly obvious that cosmetic procedures should come as close to perfect as possible. Patient satisfaction is one way to measure success, especially for cosmetic procedures. There are a number of infamous Web sites describing (often in disturbing detail) poor results after laser-assisted in situ keratomileusis (LASIK). A vocal minority became so loud that the FDA convened a special session in April 2008 to review the results of LASIK.

This systematic review of the world literature confirmed that patient satisfaction and quality of life are excellent in the vast majority of patients after LASIK. Patient satisfaction was consistently very high using both nonvalidated and validated questionnaires, whether it was anonymous or not, and also whether it was performed within 6 months of surgery or later. Satisfaction was also similarly high between 1995 and 2000 versus 2000 and 2003 both in the United States and abroad, including for patients who had myopic or hyperopic LASIK. Very interesting to me was how favorably patient satisfaction after LASIK compared with other elective cosmetic procedures (see Fig 5).

The authors also point out that the most common reasons for patient dissatisfaction after LASIK may be becoming less common. The need for enhancements and night vision symptoms seem to be declining, which is likely related to newer and better technology. Postoperative dry eye is better appreciated than in the past, leading to improved preoperative and postoperative management. These advances should help further increase patient satisfaction in the future.

C. J. Rapuano, MD

Laser in situ keratomileusis versus long-term contact lens wear: Decision analysis

McGee HT, Mathers WD (Private Practice, Pittsburgh, PA; Oregon Health & Science Univ, Portland)

J Cataract Refract Surg 35:1860-1867, 2009

Purpose.—To compare the risk for vision loss from laser in situ keratomileusis (LASIK) versus long-term contact lens wear using decision analysis.

Setting.—Oregon Health & Science University, Portland, Oregon, USA.

Methods.—Based on previously published data, a decision tree was constructed using Markov modeling to calculate the probability of vision loss from LASIK versus contact lenses over time. An outcome variable, visual acuity–adjusted life-year (VALY), was defined to account for timing and severity of vision loss. The VALYs were tallied over a 30-year simulation to determine whether the risk for vision loss with contacts exceeded that with LASIK. Sensitivity analyses were performed to test the effect of changes in key variables including probability of contact lens–related keratitis, probability of ectasia after LASIK, and probability of early post-LASIK vision loss.

Results.—The model's conclusions were highly sensitive to changes in several variables tested, especially risk for post-LASIK ectasia, risk for early vision loss after LASIK, and risk for contact lens–related keratitis (which correlated with type of lenses worn). Rigid gas-permeable lenses were safer than LASIK in every analysis. The safety of LASIK exceeded that for daily-wear soft lenses only when assumptions were most favorable to LASIK, whereas the safety of LASIK always exceeded that for extended-wear lenses except when assumptions were least favorable to LASIK.

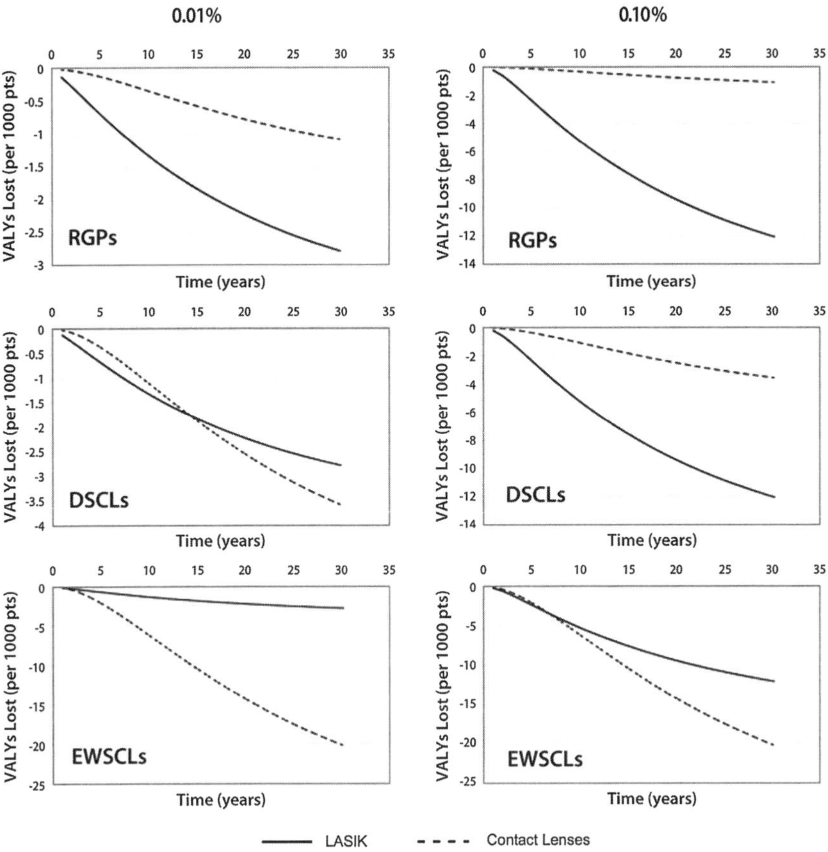

FIGURE 2.—One-way sensitivity analyses on time (years) showing cumulative number of VALYs per 1000 patients (DSCLs = daily-wear soft contact lenses; EWSCLs = extended-wear soft contact lenses; pts = patients; RGPs = rigid gas-permeable contact lenses; VALYs = visual acuity–adjusted life-years). Low risk of ectasia depicted in the left column of graphs (0.01%) and high risk in the right column of graphs (0.1%). (Reprinted from McGee HT, Mathers WD. Laser in situ keratomileusis versus long-term contact lens wear: decision analysis. *J Cataract Refract Surg*. 2009;35:1860-1867, with permission from ASCRS and ESCRS.)

Conclusion.—This decision analysis found that the risk for vision loss associated with LASIK and with long-term contact lens wear might be closer than generally assumed.

▶ About 15 years ago I went to a lecture by a prominent refractive surgeon. He started off the lecture showing a photograph of an eye that had undergone treatment for myopia and now had a severe central corneal ulcer after the treatment and ended up with 20/400 best-corrected vision from severe corneal scarring. After much fanfare, he revealed that the treatment the patient had undergone for myopia was soft contact lenses. The audience was shocked, expecting it to have been laser refractive surgery. While I do not feel that

1 case of a contact lens ulcer should condemn the use of contact lenses, I certainly agree with the point that contact lenses are not without risk. As a tertiary care cornea specialist, I see several new contact lens-related ulcers, severe enough to culture, every week. Most heal well with good best-corrected vision, but some do not.

The authors of this article present a decision tree analysis comparing laser in situ keratomileusis (LASIK) and long-term contact lens use. They attempt to objectively compare the risk of vision loss after LASIK with contact lenses. Our brains do these analyses all the time, every day, for example, comparing the risk of being hit by a truck while jaywalking with crossing at the traffic light. To make a good decision, you need correct information. You may decide to jaywalk if you believe the cars are going 25 miles an hour and the road is dry. If that is true, you will likely make it across the street safely. If, however, in reality the road has an oil spill in the middle and the cars are going 60 miles an hour, you may not fare as well.

In this study, too, the key is the assumptions that are made. When favorable assumptions regarding the safety of LASIK are made, LASIK is safer than the daily-wear soft contact lens use. When less favorable assumptions are made regarding LASIK, daily-wear soft contact lens use is safer than LASIK. Interestingly, using any of the assumptions, rigid gas-permeable contact lens use is always safer than LASIK and extended-wear contact lens use is almost always less safe than LASIK (Fig 2). This study only considers visual loss, not spectacle independence (which includes the ability to change the contact lens power over time), comfort, cost, and a host of other outcomes, but it demonstrates in an objective fashion that daily-wear soft contact lens is not vastly safer than LASIK, which is useful information.

C. J. Rapuano, MD

Ten years after photorefractive keratectomy (PRK) and laser in situ keratomileusis (LASIK) for moderate to high myopia (control-matched study)

Alió JL, Ortiz D, Muftuoglu O, et al (Miguel Hernandez Univ, Alicante, Spain; Ankara Univ School of Medicine, Turkey)

Br J Ophthalmol 93:1313-1318, 2009

Objective.—To compare the long-term outcomes of photorefractive keratectomy (PRK) and laser in situ keratomilesis (LASIK) for myopia between −6 and −10 D.

Methods.—A retrospective, control-matched study including 68 eyes, 34 which underwent PRK and 34 LASIK, with myopia between −6 and −10 D, operated using the VISX 20/20 excimer laser, was performed. Optical zones of 5.5 to 6 mm were used. All PRK-treated eyes were matched with LASIK-treated eyes of the same age, spherical equivalent within ±1.25 D, sphere within ±1.5 D and cylinder within ±2.5 D. All patients were evaluated 3 months, 1 year, 2 years, 5 years and 10 years after surgery. The main

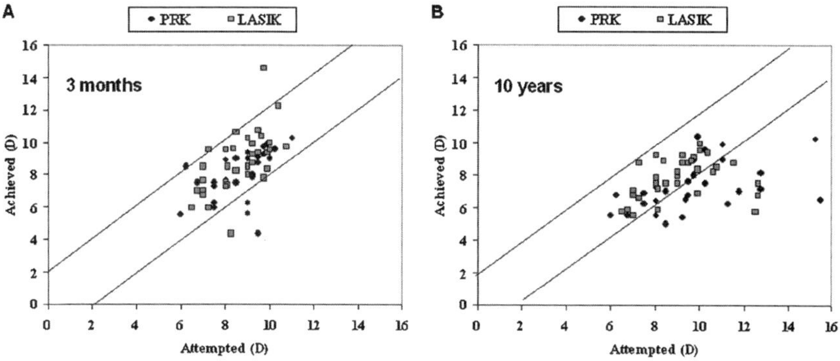

FIGURE 1.—Scattergram of attempted versus achieved correction (A) at 3 months and (B) at 10 years postoperatively for the 68 matched eyes that underwent laser in situ keratomilesis (LASIK) or photorefractive keratectomy (PRK) treatment for myopia between −6 and −10 D. (Reprinted from Alió JL, Ortiz D, Muftuoglu O, et al. Ten years after photorefractive keratectomy (PRK) and laser in situ keratomileusis (LASIK) for moderate to high myopia (control-matched study). *Br J Ophthalmol.* 2009;93:1313-1318, with permission from BMJ Publishing Group Ltd.)

outcomes measures were refractive predictability and stability, safety, efficacy and re-treatment rate.

Results.—At 10 years, 20 (71%) and 23 (88%) were within ±1.00 D after PRK and LASIK respectively. The retreatment rate was 35% and 18% respectively. No eye lost more than two lines of BSCVA in both groups. The efficacy was 0.90 for PRK and 0.95 for LASIK.

Conclusions.—Both PRK and LASIK were safe for moderate myopia. LASIK demonstrated slightly better efficacy, predictability, and less rate of re-treatment after 10 years. The technical improvements should be taken into account when comparing these results with those obtained more recently.

▶ It is difficult to compare the results of laser corneal refractive surgery performed during its infancy (1992-1995—even before Food and Drug Administration's (FDA) approval in the United States) with those performed nowadays. Having said that, studies such as this one are quite valuable to give us long-term safety data. While significant refinements in laser ablations, nomograms, techniques, and adjunctive therapy have occurred in the past 15 years, the photorefractive keratectomy (PRK) and laser in situ keratomileusis (LASIK) procedures are fundamentally unchanged.

Among the 4800 eyes that underwent PRK and LASIK at the authors' center between April 1992 and December 1995, 34 PRK-treated eyes of 33 patients and 34 LASIK-treated eyes of 32 patients who had a spherical equivalent between −6 and −10 D were matched for age and refraction. While that is a small number compared with the number of procedures performed, a 10-year follow-up is rather hard to get.

The refractive results were much better for the LASIK-treated eyes than for the PRK-treated eyes (Fig 1). Additionally, twice as many PRK-treated eyes were retreated compared with LASIK-treated eyes (35% vs 18%). There was important long-term follow-up data. Similar myopic regression rates and stability of refraction were found in the 2 groups. No sight-threatening complications, such as significant corneal haze or any ectasia, were found in either group. Pretty good results for 10 years.

C. J. Rapuano, MD

Seven-year follow-up of LASIK for myopia

Zalentein WN, Tervo TM, Holopainen JM (Univ of Helsinki, Finland)

J Refract Surg 25:312-318, 2009

Purpose.—To assess the long-term refractive results, subjective parameters, and late sequelae of LASIK.

Methods.—A retrospective follow-up study was conducted on 38 eyes of 21 patients (17 with bilateral treatment and 4 with unilateral treatment) who had LASIK surgery between 1999 and 2000. Laser ablations were done with an excimer laser (VISX STAR and STAR S2). Follow-up was 2 months, 2 years, and > 7 years postoperatively. Uncorrected visual acuity (UCVA), best spectacle-corrected visual acuity (BSCVA), manifest refraction, indirect ophthalmoscopy, and wavefront analysis were measured at the last follow-up and a questionnaire was answered.

Results.—Postoperatively, BSCVA ≤ 0.0 (logMAR) was obtained in 91%, 100%, and 89% of eyes at 2 months, 2 years, and at last follow-up, respectively. Postoperative spherical equivalent refraction within ± 0.50 diopters (D) was obtained in 75%, 63%, and 42% of eyes at 2 months, 2 years, and 7 to 8 years, respectively. At 2 months and 2 years, 83% of eyes were within ± 1.00 D, which decreased to 42% at 7 to 8 years. Mean spherical equivalent refraction at 2 months was −0.41 D, at 2 years −0.57 D, and at 7 to 8 years continued to decrease to −1.38 D. Patient satisfaction was high—100% of patients would have LASIK again.

Conclusions.—LASIK outcomes tend to shift toward undercorrection over time. Postoperative ectasia was not noted 7 to 8 years after LASIK. All patients were satisfied with the postoperative results although emmetropia was not reached.

▶ The good news is that 7 years after laser in situ keratomileusis (LASIK), patient satisfaction was high. One hundred percent of patients would have LASIK again. Additionally, no long-term complications, such as ectasia or scarring, were found. The bad news is regression of refractive effect over time. Starting with a spherical equivalent of approximately −7.0 diopters, an undercorrection of −0.4 diopters was found at 2 months, while it was −0.57 diopters at 2 years and −1.38 diopters at 7 years (see Fig 4 in the original article). While this trend was noted in all eyes, it was most pronounced in eyes with preoperative spherical equivalents greater than −6.0 diopters and in patients less than 30 years old (see Fig 5 in the original article).

This study has some issues. First, it only included 38 eyes of 21 patients, while 101 patients had LASIK in 1999 and 2000 at their laser center. Second, less than one-quarter (21) of patients returned for 7-year follow-up. The authors did not compare the preoperative data of patients who returned for long-term follow-up versus those who did not return for long-term follow-up to determine whether this was a representative sample.

I am hopeful that improvement in excimer laser technology from 1999 to 2000 (eg, larger treatment zones, larger blend zones, wavefront treatments, etc) will decrease the amount of refractive shift over time, but only further follow-up studies will tell.

C. J. Rapuano, MD

Ten-year Follow-up of Excimer Laser Surface Ablation for Myopia in Thin Corneas

de Benito-Llopis L, Alió JL, Ortiz D, et al (Vissum Madrid, Spain; Vissum Instituto Oftalmológico de Alicante, Spain; et al)

Am J Ophthalmol 147:768-773, 2009

Purpose.—To evaluate the long-term outcomes of excimer laser surface ablation performed on thin corneas.

Design.—Retrospective study.

Methods.—We included in the study 75 eyes (49 patients) with a preoperative central corneal thickness (CCT) thinner than 500 μm that had undergone surface ablation to correct their myopia and that had at least 10 years of follow-up. We evaluated the stability of visual acuity (VA) and refraction, the predictability, corneal keratometry, safety, efficacy, and postoperative complications at the examinations 3 months and 1, 2, 5, and 10 years after surgery.

Results.—Preoperative CCT was 481.54 ± 15.7 μm (range, 438 to 499 μm). Preoperative spherical equivalent was −6.12 ± 2.67 diopters (D) (range, −2 to −14 D). The best spectacle-corrected VA significantly improved ($P < .01$) during the follow-up. The uncorrected VA showed significant improvement in all visits when compared with the 3-month postoperative visit. Both the sphere and cylinder showed a slight but significant regression ($P < .01$) only in the comparison between 3 months and 10 years after the surgery. Ten years after the surgery, 30 eyes (40%) were within 0.50 D and 43 eyes (57.33%) were within 1.00 D of emmetropia. The safety index improved over the 10 year period and was always higher than 0.9. The efficacy index remained stable around 0.8. The topography did not show signs of corneal ectasia and the keratometry showed no increase in corneal power. Thirty eyes (40%) needed enhancement.

Conclusion.—Surface ablation seems to be safe and effective to correct myopia in corneas thinner than 500 μm, with stable visual and refractive outcomes in a 10-year follow-up.

▶ During the time period studied the authors performed surface ablation on 160 eyes with corneal thicknesses of less than 500 μm. This study included approximately half (75) of the eyes, all examined at 10 years. Presumably those not examined at 10 years had similar demographics and refractive errors, but that information was not provided. Forty percent of the eyes underwent an enhancement during the 10-year follow-up period—a number the authors say is consistent with other studies but I personally feel is rather high.

Even so, this study demonstrates several important findings for patients with thin corneas and their refractive surgeons. Seventy-five eyes were treated with transepithelial photorefractive keratectomy (PRK) using a 6.0-mm optic zone without mitomycin C and followed for 10 years. The refractive and haze results were comparable with eyes with "normal" corneal thicknesses. Most important (at least to me) is the fact that no eyes developed postoperative ectasia. Additionally, no eyes developed late-onset haze after 2 years postoperatively.

The main risk factor for postoperative ectasia after refractive surgery in the literature is abnormal preoperative topography in the involved eye or the fellow eye. The authors state that they know of only 1 case of ectasia after surface ablation in which preoperative topography was normal. That patient's corneal thicknesses were 509/508 μm. Additionally, that patient admitted to rubbing his eyes frequently and had a sibling who underwent corneal transplantation (for an unknown cause, but it could have been keratoconus). Personally, I am extremely wary of performing refractive surgery, especially laser in situ keratomileusis (LASIK), in someone with a close family member with keratoconus.

I am still extremely cautious about performing LASIK in any eye with a corneal thickness less than 500 μm. The results for this study support the use of surface ablation in these eyes. Questions remain. How low can we go in preoperative central corneal thickness and residual stromal bed thickness? Other excellent long-term studies such as this one are needed to begin to answer these questions.

C. J. Rapuano, MD

One-year outcomes of a bilateral randomised prospective clinical trial comparing PRK with mitomycin C and LASIK

Wallau AD, Campos M (Federal Univ of São Paulo, Brazil)

Br J Ophthalmol 93:1634-1638, 2009

Aim.—To compare 1-year follow-up results of photorefractive keratectomy (PRK) with mitomycin C (MMC) and laser in situ keratomileusis (LASIK) for custom correction of myopia.

Methods.—Eighty-eight eyes of 44 patients with moderate myopia were randomised to PRK with 0.002% MMC for 1 min in one eye and LASIK in the fellow eye. The 1-year follow-up was evaluated.

Results.—There were no differences between LASIK and MMC-PRK eyes preoperatively. Forty-two patients completed the 1-year follow-up. MMC-PRK eyes achieved better uncorrected visual acuity ($p = 0.03$) and better best-spectacle-corrected visual acuity ($p < 0.001$) 1 year after surgery. SE did not differ in the two groups during follow-up ($p = 0.12$). Clinically significant haze was not found in surface ablation eyes. LASIK eyes showed a greater higher-order aberration ($p = 0.01$) and lower contrast sensitivity ($p < 0.05$) than MMC-PRK eyes postoperatively. Excellent vision was reported in 64% of LASIK and 74% of MMC-PRK eyes 1 year after surgery. The corneal resistance factor and corneal hysteresis (ORA, Reichert) were higher in LASIK than in MMC-PRK eyes ($p < 0.01$) at the last follow-up.

Conclusions.—Wavefront-guided PRK with 0.002% MMC was more effective than wavefront-guided LASIK for correction of moderate myopia. Further research is necessary to determine the optimal concentration, exposure time and long-term corneal side effect of MMC.

▶ This type of study is exactly what we need more of in ophthalmology. This is a fairly large, bilateral, randomized prospective clinical trial with good follow-up, where one eye is treated in one fashion and the fellow eye in another fashion. The authors looked at custom photorefractive keratectomy (PRK) with mitomycin C (MMC) versus custom laser in situ keratomileusis (LASIK) in moderately myopic eyes (mean SE, approximately −4 D) with 1-year follow-up. For the PRK group, 0.002% MMC (1/10th of the usual concentration) was used for 1 minute. For the LASIK group, a Moria M2 microkeratome was used. Postoperative steroids were used 4 times a day for 2 weeks in both groups.

The results were excellent in both groups. There was no clinically significant corneal haze in the PRK group and no LASIK flap complications. While the 2 groups had similar spherical equivalents at 1 year, the uncorrected visual acuity and best-corrected visual acuity were better in the PRK eyes. Additionally, 52% of the PRK eyes and only 31% of the LASIK eyes achieved 20/15 vision or better at 1 year. Similarly, 74% of PRK eyes and only 64% of LASIK eyes were reported to have excellent vision at 1 year. The PRK group also had better contrast sensitivity ($P < .05$) and fewer higher order aberrations ($P = .01$) than the LASIK group.

Interestingly, the postoperative corneal thickness was statistically thinner in PRK eyes than the LASIK eyes. The corneal resistance factor and corneal hysteresis were also statistically significantly lower in the PRK eyes than the LASIK eyes ($P < .01$). Whether these results were less due to lower biomechanical integrity of the cornea or due to thinner corneal thickness is unknown. Also unknown is whether these results would hold true for a more standard concentration of MMC, lower degrees or higher degrees of myopia, or the use of a femtosecond laser LASIK flap. Perhaps these are some ideas for additional excellent studies.

C. J. Rapuano, MD

Comparison Between Three- and Six-month Postoperative Refractive and Visual Results After Laser Epithelial Keratomileusis With Mitomycin C

de Benito-Llopis L, Teus MA, Hernández-Verdejo JL (Vissum Madrid, Spain)
Am J Ophthalmol 147:71-76, 2009

Purpose.—To compare the residual refraction and visual results between the three- and six-month postoperative visits to detect the optimal moment for enhancement after myopic laser epithelial keratomileusis (LASEK) with mitomycin C (MMC).

Design.—Nonrandomized, interventional, prospective study.

Methods.—One hundred and forty-one consecutive eyes that underwent LASEK with MMC to correct their myopia using the Esiris excimer laser (Schwind Eye Tech Solutions, Kleinostheim, Germany), and that showed three months postoperatively a residual defect or a suboptimal uncorrected visual acuity (UCVA) or best spectacle-corrected visual acuity (BSCVA) were included in the study. We compared the residual spherical refraction and cylinder, the UCVA, and the BSCVA between the three- and six-month postoperative examinations.

Results.—Preoperative spherical refraction was -5.2 ± 2.90 diopters (D). Preoperative cylinder was -1.66 ± 1.20 D. The residual sphere was $+0.43 \pm 0.90$ D three months and $+0.21 \pm 0.90$ D six months after surgery ($P = .0001$). The cylinder was -0.71 ± 0.60 D and -0.67 ± 0.60 D, respectively ($P = .4$). The UCVA was 0.75 ± 0.2 and 0.81 ± 0.2 ($P = .0001$) and the BSCVA was 0.94 ± 0.1 and 1.01 ± 0.1 ($P = .0001$), respectively. Those patients with a myopic defect (sphere or cylinder) three months postoperatively did not show any significant change in UCVA or refractive defect six months after surgery, while those with a hyperopic defect (sphere or cylinder) showed an improvement in UCVA and residual refraction six months postoperatively ($P < .05$).

Conclusions.—Our results suggest that retreatment after myopic LASEK with MMC may be performed three months after surgery when the residual refraction is myopic, but it seems wise to wait at least six months after surgery when the residual refraction is hyperopic.

▶ Refractive stability is generally defined as less than or equal to 0.25 D change in manifest refraction at least 1 month apart, with stable topography. Using the Esiris excimer laser (Schwind Eye Tech Solutions) for laser epithelial keratomileusis (LASEK) with mitomycin C 0.02% for 30 seconds, the authors evaluated refractive stability at 3 and 6 months. Eyes with residual myopia at 3 months were stable at 6 months, while the refractions of eyes with postoperative hyperopia changed between 3 months and 6 months. As the study ended at 6 months, it is unclear whether these eyes were stable after 6 months. While refractive stability should be present before enhancement, eyes after LASEK with mitomycin C with residual myopia are likely to be stable at 3 months, and those with postoperative hyperopia will probably take 6 months or longer to stabilize.

C. J. Rapuano, MD

Comparative Study of Higher-Order Aberrations After Conventional Laser In Situ Keratomileusis and Laser Epithelial Keratomileusis for Myopia Using the Technolas 217z Laser Platform

Kirwan C, O'Keefe M (The Mater Private Hosp, Dublin, Ireland)

Am J Ophthalmol 147:77-83, 2009

Purpose.—To examine changes in higher-order aberrations (HOAs) after PlanoScan laser in situ keratomileusis and (LASIK) and laser epithelial keratomileusis (LASEK).

Design.—Prospective, comparative study.

Methods.—Myopic patients undergoing LASIK (65 eyes of 36 patients) and LASEK (50 eyes of 28 patients) at a private practice were selected randomly. Surgery was performed using the Technolas 217z laser (Bausch & Lomb, Surrey, United Kingdom). Main outcome measures included uncorrected visual acuity (UCVA), manifest refractive spherical equivalent (MRSE), and aberrometry (Zywave; Bausch & Lomb, Rochester, New York, USA) and were recorded before surgery and at three and 12 months after surgery.

Results.—There was no statistical difference between both groups in terms of MRSE ($P = .91$), ablation depth ($P = .47$), scotopic pupil size ($P = .38$), or optical zone ($P = .07$). Before surgery, there was no statistical difference in root mean square (RMS) of total ($P = .70$), third- ($P = .79$), fourth- ($P = .23$), and fifth- ($P = .33$) order aberrations and individual terms. Three months after surgery, RMS of total HOA was raised significantly more ($P = .03$) after LASIK (1.46-factor increase) than LASEK (1.25-factor increase). One year after surgery, a reduction in total HOAs was observed in 13.8% of LASIK- and 48.5% of LASEK-treated eyes compared with preoperative levels.

Conclusions.—Postoperative increases in total HOA and vertical coma were significantly greater in LASIK-than in LASEK-treated eyes. Postoperative reduction in total HOAs was observed in a number of eyes with high

TABLE 6.—Overall Change in Total Higher-Order Aberrations One Year after Surgery Compared with Preoperative Levels in Laser In Situ Keratomileusis and Laser Epithelial Keratomileusis Treatment Groups

Procedure	Change in RMS of Total HOA (before Surgery to 1 Year after Surgery)	No. of Eyes (%)	Magnitude of Change, Mean ± SD (Range)	Preoperative RMS of Total HOA, Mean ± SD (Range)
LASIK	Reduction	9 (13.8)	0.11 ± 0.09 (−0.24 to −0.01)	0.58 ± 0.15 (0.32 to 0.78)
	Increase	54 (83.1)	0.23 ± 0.18 (0.01 to 0.79)	0.37 ± 0.13 (0.14 to 0.71)
	No change	2 (3.1)	0	0.40 ± 0.15 (0.14 to 0.78)
LASEK	Reduction	26 (52)	0.14 ± 0.09 (−0.34 to −0.01)	0.51 ± 0.17 (0.25 to 0.82)
	Increase	24 (48)	0.27 ± 0.27 (0.02 to 1.09)	0.33 ± 0.14 (0.17 to 0.63)

HOA = higher-order aberration; LASEK = laser epithelial keratomileusis; LASIK = laser in situ keratomileusis; RMS = root mean square; SD = standard deviation.

preoperative levels and occurred more frequently in LASEK-treated eyes (Table 6).

▶ The increase in higher-order aberrations after refractive surgery in this study has been reported previously. This study compared conventional laser in situ keratomileusis (LASIK) versus laser epithelial keratomileusis (LASEK). Unlike other studies, however, the authors matched the patients in the 2 groups for total third-, fourth-, and fifth-order aberrations and each individual term. They found a statistically significantly greater increase in higher-order aberrations after LASIK compared with LASEK ($P = .03$). In the LASIK group there was no significant change in higher-order aberrations from 3 months to 12 months postoperatively, while there was a small but significant decrease in higher-order aberrations from 3 months to 6 months postoperatively in the LASEK eyes.

Interestingly, even though a conventional laser treatment was performed in all eyes, many eyes had a reduction in higher-order aberrations 1 year after surgery compared with preoperative levels (See Table 6). This was noted in many more eyes in the LASEK group than in the LASIK group. Also, in both groups, the greater the preoperative higher-order aberrations, the more likely there was to be a reduction in higher-order aberrations at 1 year. This is precisely the group that many surgeons feel are best served by a wavefront-guided laser ablation, and yet they did very well with a conventional laser treatment. As each laser is different, these results using the Bausch & Lomb Technolas 217z excimer laser may not be the same as other lasers.

C. J. Rapuano, MD

Comparison of Night Driving Performance after Wavefront-Guided and Conventional LASIK for Moderate Myopia

Schallhorn SC, Tanzer DJ, Kaupp SE, et al (Naval Med Ctr, San Diego, CA)
Ophthalmology 116:702-709, 2009

Purpose.—To compare preoperative and postoperative changes in simulated night driving performance after wavefront-guided (wLASIK) and conventional LASIK (cLASIK) for the treatment of moderate myopia.

Design.—Retrospective, comparative study.

Participants.—All eyes of subjects with a preoperative manifest spherical equivalent (MSE) between −4.50 and −6.00 who underwent night driving simulator (NDS) testing from 2 clinical trials were entered into the study. This comprised 38 cLASIK patients (62 eyes; mean −5.46 diopters [D] MSE) and 21 wLASIK patients (36 eyes, mean −5.20 D MSE).

Methods.—Patients' records were reviewed from 2 LASIK clinical trials that had similar enrollment criteria. One trial treated patients with conventional LASIK using a bladed microkeratome (cLASIK) and the other treated with a wavefront-guided profile using a femtosecond laser

TABLE 5.—Percentage of Subjects who had a Significant Decrement in Night Driving Simulation Performance after LASIK

Procedure	Without Glare		With Glare	
	Detection*	Identification	Detection	Identification
cLASIK	36%	32%	38%	33%
95% CI	24%–47%	21%–44%	26%–53%	21%–45%
wLASIK	0%	3%	0%	0%
95% CI	—	0%–8%	—	—

CI = confidence interval; cLASIK = conventional LASIK; wLASIK = wavefront-guided LASIK.

TABLE 6.—Percentage of Subjects who had a Significant Improvement in Night Driving Simulation Performance after LASIK

Procedure	Without Glare		With Glare	
	Detection*	Identification	Detection	Identification
cLASIK	3%	2%	3%	7%
95% CI	0%–8%	0%–5%	0%–8%	0%–13%
wLASIK	11%	31%	11%	31%
95% CI	1%–21%	16%–46%	1%–21%	16%–46%

CI = confidence interval; cLASIK = conventional LASIK; wLASIK = wavefront-guided LASIK.

(wLASIK). In both trials, patients with moderate myopia were asked to participate in NDS testing.

Main Outcome Measures.—The detection and identification distances of road hazards were measured with and without a glare source before and 6 months after LASIK. Each eye was tested independently in best-corrected trial frames by a masked operator.

Results.—In every category, there was a mean reduction in the preoperative to postoperative NDS performance after cLASIK (mean change, −21.3 to −27.9 ft, −6.5 to −8.5 m; 95% confidence interval [CI], −12.0 to −41.3 ft, −3.7 to −12.6 m); there was a corresponding mean improvement after wLASIK (mean change +15.0 to +29.1 ft, +4.6 to +8.9 m; 95% CI, +8.3 to +41.5 ft, +2.5 to +12.6 m). Significant differences between cLASIK and wLASIK NDS performance was observed in every category ($P < 0.01$, Tukey's honest significant difference for unequal numbers). A clinical relevant loss of NDS performance (>0.5 seconds) was observed in 32% to 38% of cLASIK eyes for all tasks, whereas only 0% to 3% of eyes had this loss after wLASIK. Between 2% and 7% of cLASIK eyes and 11% and 31% of eyes had a significant postoperative improvement in NDS performance in every task.

Conclusions.—Wavefront-guided LASIK to correct myopia combined with a femtosecond laser flap significantly improved mean night driving visual performance and was significantly better than cLASIK using a mechanical keratome (Tables 5 and 6).

▶ The vast majority of metrics used to evaluate results of refractive surgery (or many eye surgeries for that matter) are static, such as uncorrected vision, best-corrected vision, or contrast sensitivity. This study looked at performance in a night-driving simulator. Night driving is thought to be one of the most visually demanding tasks most of us perform on a routine basis, and difficulty with night driving is also a frequently reported complaint after laser-assisted in situ keratomileusis (LASIK).

A few points: The night driving simulator test was performed monocularly. It is unclear what difference doing it binocularly would have had. The patient population in this study was generally young (mean age: early thirties), and no one was older than 51. Over 80% were male. This demographic is not necessarily a typical refractive surgery population. In addition, all the conventional ablation LASIK eye flaps were created with a Hansatome mechanical microkeratome, while all of the wavefront ablation LASIK eye flaps were created with the IntraLase femtosecond laser. Consequently, it is impossible to separate the effect of ablation technique and flap creation technique.

Even so, the wavefront femtosecond laser flap eyes not only had much better night driving simulator results than the conventional mechanical microkeratome flap eyes, but they had better night driving simulator results postoperatively than with their glasses preoperatively, while the other group had worse results postoperatively than preoperatively (see Tables 5 and 6).

In my experience, without changing my surface ablation or LASIK flap creation techniques, I have noted fewer night vision complaints in eyes after wavefront ablations compared to conventional ablations.

C. J. Rapuano, MD

A Prospective, Contralateral Eye Study Comparing Thin-Flap LASIK (Sub-Bowman Keratomileusis) with Photorefractive Keratectomy

Slade SG, Durrie DS, Binder PS (The Slade & Baker Vision Inst, Houston, TX; Durrie Vision, Overland Park, KS; Binder & Weiss Vision Inst, San Diego, CA)

Ophthalmology 116:1075-1082, 2009

Purpose.—To determine the differences in the visual results, pain response, biomechanical effect, quality of vision, and higher-order aberrations, among other parameters, in eyes undergoing either photorefractive keratectomy (PRK) or thin-flap LASIK/sub-Bowman keratomileusis (SBK; intended flap thickness of ± 100 μm and 8.5-mm diameter) at 1, 3, and 6 months after surgery.

Design.—A contralateral eye pilot study.

Participants.—Fifty patients (100 eyes) were enrolled at 2 sites.

Methods.—The mean preoperative spherical refraction was −3.66 diopters (D) and the mean cylinder was −0.66 D for all eyes. Eyes in the PRK group underwent 8.5-mm ethanol-assisted PRK, whereas in eyes in the SBK group, an 8.5-mm, (intended) 100 μm flap was created with a 60-kHz IntraLase femtosecond laser (Advanced Medical Optics, Santa Ana, CA). All eyes underwent a customized laser ablation using an Alcon LADARVision 4000 CustomCornea excimer laser (Alcon Laboratories, Fort Worth, TX).

Main Outcome Measures.—Preoperative and postoperative tests included best spectacle-corrected visual acuity, uncorrected visual acuity (UCVA), corneal topography, wavefront aberrometry, retinal image quality, and contrast sensitivity. Patients completed subjective questionnaires at each visit.

Results.—One- and 3-month UCVA results showed a statistically significant difference: SBK, 88% 20/20 or better vs. 48% 20/20 or better for PRK. At 6 months, UCVA was 94% 20/20 or better for PRK and 92% for SBK. At 1 and 3 months, the SBK group had lower higher-order aberrations (coma and spherical aberration; $P \leq 0.05$); at 1, 3, and 6 months, there was no statistically significant difference in spherical aberration and vertical and horizontal coma between the 2 groups.

Conclusions.—At the 1-month follow-up, the thin-flap/SBK group demonstrated clinically and statistically significant better visual acuity than the PRK group. By 3 months, the vision in the 2 groups had begun to equalize, although the SBK eyes continued to have better vision.

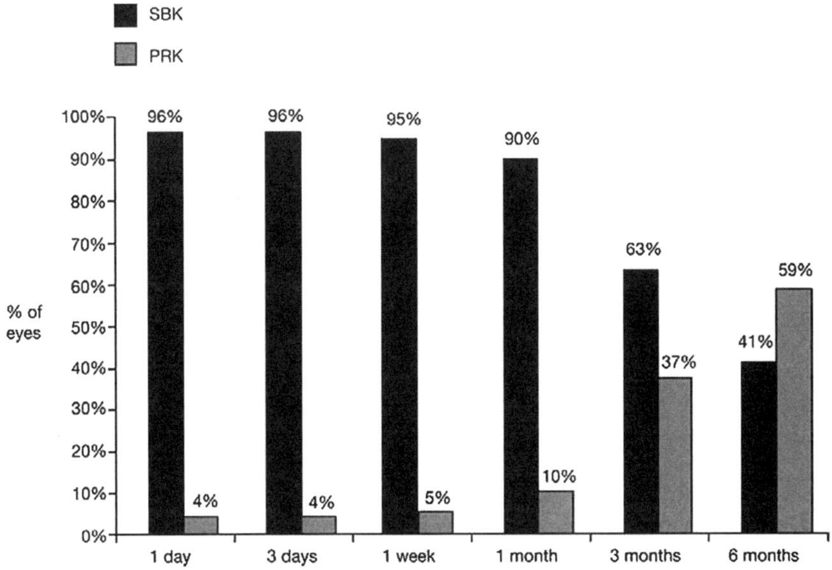

FIGURE 2.—Bar graph showing patient questionnaire results: Which eye has better vision overall? PRK = photorefractive keratectomy; SBK = sub-Bowman keratomileusis. (Reprinted from Slade SG, Durrie DS, Binder PS. A prospective, contralateral eye study comparing thin-flap LASIK (sub-Bowman keratomileusis) with photorefractive keratectomy. *Ophthalmology.* 2009;116:1075-1082, with permission from the American Academy of Ophthalmology.)

TABLE 1.—Uncorrected Visual Acuity Results at 1 Month after Surgery

	20/12.5 or Better (%)	20/16 or Better (%)	20/20 or Better (%)	20/25 or Better (%)	20/40 or Better (%)
SBK	18	46	88	90	100
PRK	2	16	48	48	98

PRK = photorefractive keratectomy; SBK = sub-Bowman keratomileusis.

TABLE 2.—Uncorrected Visual Acuity Results at 6 Months after Surgery

	20/12.5 or Better (%)	20/16 or Better (%)	20/20 or Better (%)	20/25 or Better (%)	20/40 or Better (%)
SBK	24	72	92	98	100
PRK	26	70	94	98	100

PRK = photorefractive keratectomy; SBK = sub-Bowman keratomileusis.

At 6 months, there were no statistical differences between the 2 groups (Fig 2, Tables 1 and 2).

▶ One eye of 50 patients was treated with state-of-the-art thin-flap laser-assisted in situ keratomileusis (LASIK) (8.5 mm diameter, 100 μm thickness) and the fellow eye was treated with state-of-the-art photorefractive keratectomy (PRK) (8.5 mm epithelial defect). This was a well-designed and well-carried-out study. It should be noted that it was supported by Advanced Medical Optics (AMO), the maker of the Intralase femtosecond laser, and 2 of the 3 authors are consultants for AMO.

Not surprisingly, results at 1, 3, and 7 days favor the LASIK group. Somewhat surprising, at least to me, was the fact that LASIK superiority was still present at 1 month (Table 1). However, by 3 and 6 months, the results were fairly equal (Table 2).

Although 50 patients is not a huge number on which to draw major conclusions, there were a few other interesting findings. Although Schirmer test results were very similar in the 2 groups postoperatively, and not very different from baseline, the PRK eyes were generally felt to be drier than the LASIK eyes. Corneal sensitivity was found to be more decreased after LASIK than PRK, even at 6 months. ORA measurements, thought to correlate with the strength of the cornea, were decreased postoperatively in both groups to a similar degree; there did not seem to be an advantage to PRK over LASIK.

Using thin-flap LASIK with a femtosecond laser, the results appear overall better than PRK at least the first month, but do equalize by 3 to 6 months (Fig 2). Whether the advantages of no flap outweigh the delayed recovery is up to the surgeon and the patient.

C. J. Rapuano, MD

Comparison Between Femtosecond Laser-Assisted Sub-Bowman Keratomileusis vs Laser Subepithelial Keratectomy to Correct Myopia

de Benito-Llopis L, Teus MA, Gil-Cazorla R, et al (Vissum Madrid, Spain)

Am J Ophthalmol 148:830-836, 2009

Purpose.—To compare femtosecond laser sub-Bowman keratomileusis (FSBK) vs laser subepithelial keratectomy (LASEK) to correct myopia.

Design.—Retrospective, nonrandomized, interventional, comparative case series.

Methods.—Two thousand one hundred and eight eyes were included in the study. We compared 1,072 eyes treated with FSBK vs 1,036 eyes treated with LASEK with or without mitomycin C (MMC). Visual and refractive results were evaluated 1 day, 1 week, and 1 and 3 months postoperatively.

Results.—Preoperative mean sphere and best spectacle-corrected visual acuity (BSCVA) were −3.93 diopters (D) vs −3.87 D ($P = .5$) and 1.12 vs 1.12 ($P = .8$) in FSBK and LASEK, respectively. Uncorrected visual acuity (UCVA) was 0.92 vs 0.62, 0.98 vs 0.78, 0.96 vs 0.91, and 1.06 vs 1.03 in FSBK and LASEK, respectively, at 1 day, 1 week, and 1 and 3 months after surgery ($P < .01$ for all comparisons). Three months postoperatively, BSCVA was 1.13 and 1.10, respectively ($P = .001$). At that moment, 20 eyes (1.93%) in the LASEK group vs 9 eyes (0.84%) in the FSBK group had lost 2 or more lines of BSCVA. Ten eyes (0.96%) in the LASEK group gained 2 or more lines of BSCVA, whereas 3 eyes (0.28%) in the FSBK group gained 2 lines. Six months postoperatively, only 2 LASEK eyes (0.19%) showed loss of 2 or more lines of BSCVA, compared to 3 FSBK-treated eyes (0.28%).

Conclusion.—Both FSBK and LASEK are safe and effective procedures to correct myopia. Slightly better visual and refractive results were observed in FSBK-treated eyes in a 3-month follow-up.

▶ The strongest part of this study is the large number of eyes (2108). Such large numbers can demonstrate small but important differences that smaller studies would be unable to find. Large numbers can also find statistically significant differences that are not clinically significant. In fact, the second line of the discussion states, "We detected statistically significantly better visual and refractive results after femtosecond laser sub-Bowman keratomileusis (FSBK) 3 months after the surgery, although the differences were very small and probably not clinically relevant."

The weakest part of the study is the short follow-up. When comparing laser in situ keratomileusis (LASIK) with its rapid visual recovery and surface ablation, its more prolonged visual recovery, 6 months to 12 months of follow-up, is important to give a more complete picture, not 3 months as in this study. In fact, in the discussion the authors write of visual acuity, "Maybe a longer follow-up in our study would have allowed these visual differences to decrease," and of the slight overcorrection seen in the laser subepithelial keratectomy (LASEK) eyes, "Perhaps a longer follow-up would make the small differences detected in our study disappear." Large numbers and limited follow-up need to be kept in mind when reviewing the literature.

C. J. Rapuano, MD

Higher-order aberrations after wavefront-optimized photorefractive keratectomy and laser in situ keratomileusis

Randleman JB, Perez-Straziota CE, Hu MH, et al (Emory Univ School of Medicine, Atlanta, GA; Private practices, Atlanta, GA)

J Cataract Refract Surg 35:260-264, 2009

Purpose.—To analyze the changes in higher-order aberrations (HOAs) that occur after wavefrontoptimized photorefractive keratectomy (PRK) and laser in situ keratomileusis (LASIK).

Setting.—Emory Eye Center and Emory Vision, Atlanta, Georgia, USA.

Methods.—This retrospective analysis comprised eyes that had PRK or LASIK from June 2004 through October 2005. Postoperative outcome

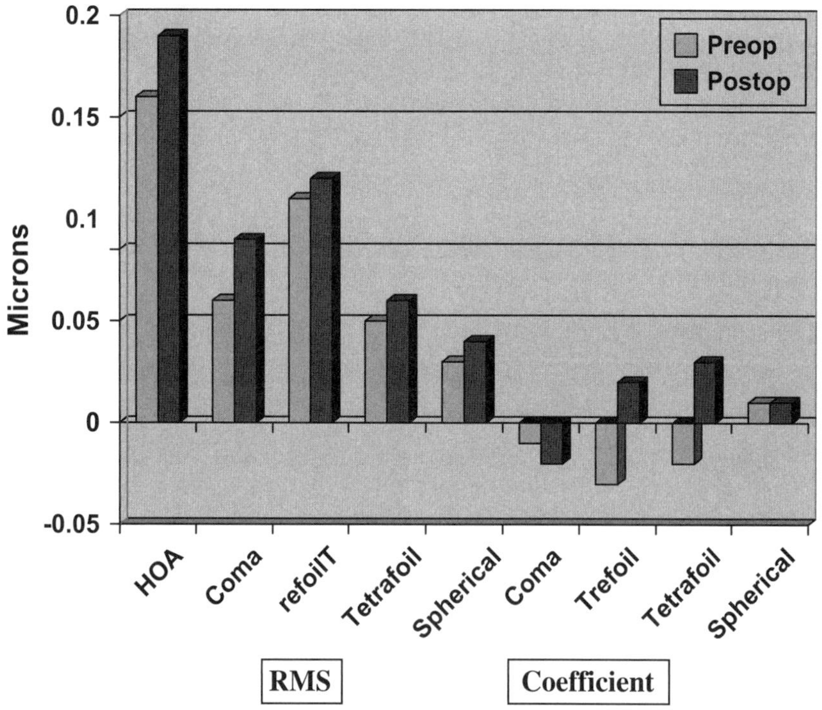

FIGURE 1.—Higher-order aberrations after PRK (RMS = root mean square). (Reprinted from Bradley Randleman J, Perez-Straziota CE, Hu MH, et al. Higher-order aberrations after wavefront-optimized photorefractive keratectomy and laser in situ keratomileusis. *J Cataract Refract Surg*. 2009;35:260-264, with permission from ASCRS and ESCRS.)

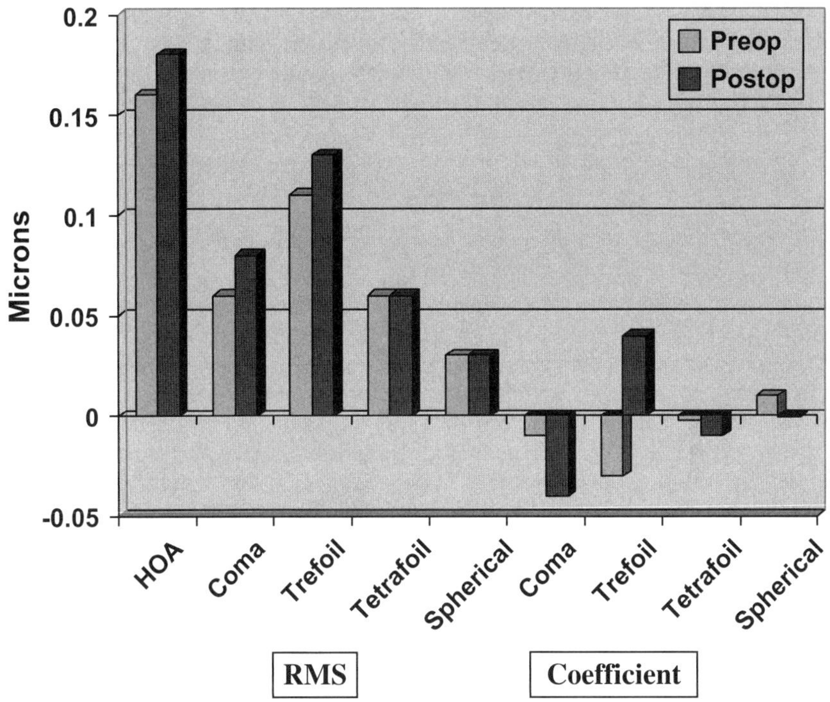

FIGURE 2.—High order aberrations after LASIK (RMS = root mean square). (Reprinted from Randleman JB, Perez-Straziota CE, Hu MH, et al. Higher-order aberrations after wavefront-optimized photorefractive keratectomy and laser in situ keratomileusis. *J Cataract Refract Surg*. 2009;35:260-264, with permission from ASCRS and ESCRS.)

measures included 3-month uncorrected visual acuity (UCVA), best spectacle-corrected visual acuity (BSCVA), manifest refraction spherical equivalent (MRSE), changes in the root mean square (RMS) and grouped coefficient HOAs (microns) measured with a corneal analyzer, and subjective assessment of visual aberrations.

Results.—One hundred consecutive eyes of 54 patients had PRK, and 100 contemporaneous consecutive eyes of 71 patients had LASIK. The PRK and LASIK populations were similar in general demographics, preoperative HOAs, and postoperative UCVA and BSCVA. The mean MRSE was slightly hyperopic after PRK (mean +0.11 diopters [D]) and slightly myopic after LASIK (mean −0.19 D) ($P<.0001$). There were no statistically significant changes in RMS or grouped coefficient HOA values after PRK or LASIK, nor were there significant differences in postoperative RMS or grouped coefficient HOA values between PRK and LASIK. One percent of PRK and LASIK patients reported a subjective increase in postoperative visual aberrations; 5% reported a subjective improvement postoperatively.

Conclusions.—Wavefront-optimized excimer laser surgery did not induce significant HOAs after PRK or LASIK. The 2 techniques were equally efficacious and had equivalent postoperative HOA profiles (Figs 1 and 2).

▶ The WaveLight Allegretto laser used in this study can be used in wavefront-optimized mode or wavefront-guided mode. In the wavefront-optimized mode, the laser treatment is based on the manifest refraction and software adjustments that have been made to retain the cornea's natural asphericity. Wavefront-guided treatments, on the other hand, require a wavefront map of the eye to be treated; the actual laser treatment is based on this. The treatments in this study were all wavefront optimized.

Figs 1 and 2 demonstrate an increase in higher order aberrations after both photorefractive keratectomy (PRK) and laser in situ keratomileusis (LASIK). However, the authors found no statistically significant difference between preoperative and postoperative higher order aberrations for either of these 2 groups. Interestingly, they use a P value of $<.001$ rather than the standard .05 for statistical significance, making it difficult to show a difference, but they do not provide the actual P value. They do provide the P values (all $>.5$) comparing PRK and LASIK, demonstrating no difference in higher-order aberrations in these 2 groups.

It is nice to see that there isn't a large increase in higher-order aberrations using these techniques and this laser, but I am not convinced that there is no increase. The postoperative higher-order aberration data look very similar for PRK and LASIK, suggesting that the LASIK flap does not induce significant higher-order aberrations. The best news is that only about 1% of patients noted worsening in subjective visual aberrations while about 5% of patients noted improvement in subjective visual aberrations after both PRK and LASIK.

C. J. Rapuano, MD

Thresholds for Interface Haze Formation After Thin-Flap Femtosecond Laser In Situ Keratomileusis for Myopia

Rocha KM, Kagan R, Smith SD, et al (Cole Eye Inst, Cleveland, OH)

Am J Ophthalmol 147:966-972, 2009

Purpose.—To evaluate the risk factors for interface haze formation after thin-flap femtosecond laser – laser in situ keratomileusis (LASIK).

Design.—Prospective case series.

Methods.—One hundred and ninety-nine consecutive eyes that underwent femtosecond laser LASIK with a LADAR 4000 excimer laser (Alcon Laboratories, Fort Worth, Texas, USA), were analyzed from January 1 to April 30, 2008. Treated eyes were divided into 2 groups according to desired flap thickness: 90 μm (106 eyes), and 100 to 110 μm (93 eyes). Cycloplegic refraction, spherical equivalent (SE), uncorrected visual acuity, best spectacle-corrected visual acuity (BSCVA), depth

6 months. However, in the 5 myopic and 14 hyperopic eyes followed for 1 year, most eyes had stable manifest refractions from 3 to 12 months (see Fig 5). One hyperopic eye had a +1.50 diopter hyperopic shift from 3 to 12 months. While haze and refractive results were demonstrated to be fairly good in this study, questions still remain. The optimum duration of mitomycin C is still unknown. Long-term stability is also unknown. Hopefully, further studies will help answer these questions.

C. J. Rapuano, MD

Reference

1. Maloney RK, Chan WK, Steinert R, Hersh P, O'Connell M, Summit Therapeutic Refractive Study Group. A multicenter trial of photorefractive keratectomy for residual myopia after previous ocular surgery. *Ophthalmology.* 1995;102: 1042-1052.

Photorefractive keratectomy in eyes with atypical topography

Hardten DR, Gosavi VV (Univ of Minnesota, Minneapolis)

J Cataract Refract Surg 35:1437-1444, 2009

Laser correction of refractive errors is one of the most effective surgical procedures today. Even so, the selection of patients who will have the outcomes they expect remains a major challenge. Corneal ectasia, a frustrating problem that can occur naturally with diseases such as keratoconus, has also been reported after refractive surgery. This review addresses the issues surrounding the use of surface refractive surgery in patients who may have atypical topography, which is a risk factor for ectasia. At present, available tests for predicting future corneal stability can give false positives and false negatives. Although the technology for treating irregular corneal astigmatism has improved, results in eyes with irregular astigmatism are less predictable than in eyes with regular astigmatism, even when wavefront- and topography-driven treatments are used. An increased risk for corneal instability may be associated with laser vision correction (LVC), although instability is generally thought to be less of a risk with surface ablation or photorefractive keratectomy than with laser in situ keratomileusis. Surface LVC has shown good success in improving uncorrected distance visual acuity with a relatively low rate of complications, even in eyes with topographic irregularities.

▶ This article reviews the issue of refractive surgery and ectasia. We know ectasia can occur without refractive surgery—it is called keratoconus. We also know it occurs after refractive surgery, much more commonly after laser in situ keratomileusis (LASIK) than surface ablation; however, the reasons for this are still unclear. Certainly, many more LASIK procedures have been performed than surface ablation procedures. The residual stromal bed is much thinner after LASIK than surface ablation. Common sense would indicate that thinner stromal beds lead to weaker corneas, which increase the risk of ectasia, which is very likely true. The problem is that the correlation of thin corneas and thin residual stromal beds and the development of ectasia is present but weak. Many, many patients with thin corneas and thin residual beds after surface ablation and even LASIK do not develop ectasia. Conversely, some eyes with no known risk factors do develop ectasia after LASIK and even rarely after surface ablation. Irregular corneal topography is also a risk factor for the development of ectasia after refractive surgery.

Another study published this year by de Benito-Llopis et al discusses the safety of surface ablation in eyes with thin corneas. Hardten and Gosavi of this article report very good results for surface ablation in 92 eyes of 59 patients with abnormal preoperative topography; none developed ectasia.

My take-home message from these articles is that surface ablation in eyes with thin corneas or atypical topography can result in good vision. The risk that surface ablation will cause additional irregular topography or frank ectasia is small but not zero. Patients need to understand this situation before surgery.

C. J. Rapuano, MD

Role of depressive symptoms in patient satisfaction with visual quality after laser in situ keratomileusis

Morse JS, Schallhorn SC, Hettinger K, et al (Naval Med Ctr, San Diego, CA)
J Cataract Refract Surg 35:341-346, 2009

Purpose.—To assess the role of depressive symptoms in patient satisfaction with visual quality after laser in situ keratomileusis (LASIK).

Setting.—Navy Refractive Surgery Center, Ophthalmology Department, Naval Medical Center, San Diego, California, USA.

Methods.—This was a prospective study of active-duty military patients having bilateral conventional LASIK to treat low to moderate myopia with or without astigmatism. Patients completed the Armstrong Laboratory Personality Survey Depression scale preoperatively. Patients were also given a 10-point Navy questionnaire that included an assessment of patient satisfaction with visual quality at the 1- and 6-month follow-up examinations. Patients were stratified by their visual quality rating after LASIK as highly satisfied, satisfied, and less satisfied and by their depression scale score into low, medium, and high groups. A proportional odds model was developed to compare the visual quality rating between the 3 depression groups 1 and 6 months post LASIK.

Results.—The study comprised 370 patients. An uncorrected visual acuity of at least 20/20 was achieved in 88.6% of eyes. Patients with higher levels of depressive symptoms had 3.0 times higher odds (95% confidence interval [CI], 1.2 to 7.4) of being less satisfied than those with low levels of depressive symptoms 1 month after LASIK ($P \leq .02$) and 2.5 times higher odds (95% CI, 1.0 to 6.5) of being less satisfied at 6 months ($P \leq .06$).

Conclusion.—Preoperative depressive symptoms were a significant contributor to patient satisfaction with visual quality after LASIK.

▶ This study confirms what most surgeons (not just refractive surgeons) know already, namely that "upbeat, happy" patients are generally more satisfied with their surgical results than "downbeat, unhappy" patients. However, this study was in a very select patient population: active duty military personnel. Only 21% were women, and all military personnel are screened for psychiatric disorders, including depression. This is certainly not a typical refractive surgery population.

How we can use this information in clinical practice is not obvious. It isn't practical to use a 240-item questionnaire such as the Armstrong Laboratory Personality Survey used in this study on patients, but hopefully it will make us a little bit more aware of this issue.

C. J. Rapuano, MD

Prophylaxis of diffuse lamellar keratitis with intraoperative interface steroids in LASIK

Ng EY, Thinagaran S, Kinsella F, et al (Univ College Hosp Galway, Republic of Ireland)

J Refract Surg 25:306-311, 2009

Purpose.—To investigate the safety and efficacy of intraoperative interface steroids for the prophylaxis of diffuse lamellar keratitis (DLK).

Methods.—Two centers analyzed 1210 consecutive procedures in a prospective interventional trial. Center A irrigated the lasered stromal bed with balanced salt solution (BSS), instilled a drop of preserved dexamethasone 0.1% suspension on the stromal bed, and replaced the corneal flap. Center B replaced the flap, inserted a multiple port cannula to irrigate the stromal interface with BSS, then introduced 0.5 mL preservative-free prednisolone sodium phosphate 0.5% solution into the stromal interface with another multiple port cannula. All LASIK procedures after a fixed date received intraoperative interface steroids. Consecutive procedures immediately before this date were used as controls.

Results.—Center A performed 405 intraoperative interface steroids procedures and contributed 405 controls. Center B performed 200 intraoperative interface steroids procedures and contributed 200 controls. Preoperative refraction and postoperative visual acuity were similar in control and intraoperative interface steroids groups. In center A, 5.7% (30% were stage II) and 2% (all only stage I) of controls and intraoperative interface steroid eyes, respectively, developed DLK; intraoperative interface steroids decreased the rate of DLK by 3.0 times (95% confidence interval: 1.3 to 6.8). In center B, 6.5% of controls developed DLK (15% were stage II); with intraoperative interface steroids, only 1 procedure

(0.5%) developed DLK. In both centers, no bilateral DLK or DLK beyond stage I were noted when intraoperative interface steroids were used.

Conclusions.—Intraoperative interface steroids safely reduced the incidence and severity of DLK.

▶ The incidence of diffuse lamellar keratitis (DLK) in the control (noninterface steroids) group was 5.7% and 6.5% at their 2 centers. These numbers seem a bit higher than I would expect, but 70% and 85% were only grade 1, so that is probably reasonable. This study demonstrated a significant drop in the likelihood of DLK when topical steroids were added to the laser-assisted in situ keratomileusis (LASIK) flap interface (see Table 3 in the original article).

Given the relatively low number of eyes with DLK and the fact that they were mostly grade I in the control group, it is not a surprise that the postoperative vision was similar in the control and study groups. There was also no difference in complications between the study and control groups.

Interestingly, at one center they used 1 drop of preserved dexamethasone 0.1% micro suspension, and at the other center they used preservative-free prednisolone phosphate 0.5% solution. All patients received fluorometholone 0.1% 4 times a day for 5 days postoperatively. The prednisolone phosphate group had a lower incidence of DLK than the dexamethasone group, perhaps because it was of a higher concentration, it was preservative-free, it was a solution and not a suspension, or some other reason.

If your DLK rate is low, below 1% to 2%, then it may not be worth adding steroids directly to the flap interface. However, if your DLK rate is much higher than that, it may be worth trying. Whether it should be preservative-free or a solution rather than a suspension is still not known.

C. J. Rapuano, MD

Corneal Endothelial Cell Loss 9 Years After Excimer Laser Keratorefractive Surgery

Patel SV, Bourne WM (Mayo Clinic, Rochester, MN)

Arch Ophthalmol 127:1423-1427, 2009

Objective.—To determine the long-term changes in the corneal endothelium after laser in situ keratomileusis (LASIK) and photorefractive keratectomy (PRK).

Methods.—Twenty-nine eyes (16 patients) received myopic LASIK or PRK, with intended correction to emmetropia. Central endothelial photographs were taken before and 9 years after surgery and were analyzed by the same masked investigator after appropriate calibration for magnification. Comparisons were made by using generalized estimating equation models to account for any correlation between fellow eyes of the same patient. The annual exponential rate of cell loss was compared with cell loss during a 10-year period in 42 normal (unoperated) corneas of 42 subjects.

TABLE 1.—Endothelial Cell Density and Morphology Before and After Keratorefractive Surgery[a]

Group	Endothelial Cell Density Mean (SD), Cells/mm²	MDD	*P* Value	Coefficient of Variation of Cell Area Mean (SD)	MDD	*P* Value	% of Hexagonal Cells Mean (SD)	MDD	*P* Value
All Eyes (n = 29)									
Preoperative	2837 (336)		<.001	0.34 (0.05)	0.03	.24	54 (8)	5.7	.19
At 9 years	2685 (351)			0.33 (0.03)			56 (5)		
LASIK Eyes (n = 20)									
Preoperative	2925 (303)		<.001	0.33 (0.05)	0.04	.98	55 (9)	7.4	.77
At 9 years	2741 (308)			0.33 (0.03)			56 (5)		
PRK Eyes (n = 9)									
Preoperative	2641 (340)	230	.45	0.36 (0.03)		.009	51 (5)		.01
At 9 years	2559 (423)			0.32 (0.04)			58 (5)		

Abbreviations: LASIK, laser in situ keratomileusis; MDD, minimum detectable difference for nonsignificant comparisons ($\alpha = .05$, $\beta = .20$); PRK, photorefractive keratectomy.

[a]Comparisons between preoperative and 9-year measurements were made by using generalized estimating equation models to account for any correlation between fellow eyes of the same patient.

Results.—Endothelial cell density 9 years after LASIK and PRK had decreased by 5.3% from preoperative density ($P < .001$), whereas coefficient of variation of cell area ($P = .24$) and percentage of hexagonal cells ($P = .19$) did not change. The mean annual rate of cell loss after refractive surgery (0.6% [standard deviation, 0.8%]) was not different from that in normal corneas (0.6% [0.5%], $P = .88$; minimum detectable difference = 0.5%; $\alpha = .05$; $\beta = .20$).

Conclusions.—Laser in situ keratomileusis and PRK had no long-term effect on the corneal endothelium. Corneas that have undergone LASIK or PRK can be considered for use as donors for posterior lamellar keratoplasty procedures (Table 1).

▶ Bill Bourne, one of the gurus of corneal endothelial cell studies, is the senior author of this article. The bottom line of this study was that over a 9-year period, photorefractive keratectomy (PRK) and laser in situ keratomileusis (LASIK) did not seem to cause corneal endothelial cell loss greater than the physiologic cell loss expected (0.6% per year); for a visual representation, see Table 1. Unfortunately, the number of eyes was somewhat small (20 LASIK, 9 PRK), so they were unable to comment on the seemingly higher percent of cell loss in the LASIK eyes (6.3%) compared with the PRK eyes (3.1%). They conclude that from a corneal endothelial cell standpoint, post-PRK and post-LASIK eyes may be suitable donors for posterior lamellar keratoplasty, such as Descemet's stripping endothelial keratoplasty. Regarding using such tissue as donor material, I am more concerned by (1) a poor quality cut due to instability of a LASIK flap, and (2) unusual contour of the donor graft due to the refractive surgery, which may cause an unpredictable refractive change. But, if that occurred, perhaps PRK or LASIK could be performed without significant risk to the new donor endothelium.

C. J. Rapuano, MD

Straylight measurements before and after removal of epithelial ingrowth

Lapid-Gortzak R, van der Meulen I, van der Linden JW, et al (Retina Total Eye Care, Driebergen, the Netherlands; et al)

J Cataract Refract Surg 35:1829-1832, 2009

In 3 eyes with epithelial ingrowth after laser in situ keratomileusis, straylight was measured before and after the ingrowth was removed. In 2 eyes of 1 patient, epithelial ingrowth reached the pupillary axis. Straylight decreased (improved) significantly after ingrowth removal: a 3.6-fold decrease in the right eye and a 10-fold decrease in the left eye. The uncorrected distance visual acuity (UDVA) improved from 0.25 (20/80) in both eyes to 1.0 (20/20) and 0.8 (20/25), respectively. In 1 eye of another patient, from which epithelial ingrowth was removed to prevent flap melting and distortion, the pupillary opening was not obscured and no significant change in straylight was found. The UDVA improved from 0.32 (20/60) to 1.0 (20/20) after the ingrowth was removed. An increase in straylight can be a significant complication of epithelial ingrowth. After the interlamellar space is cleared, the improvement in straylight is several factors larger than the gain in UDVA.

▶ We are always looking for better ways to measure visual function. Snellen visual acuity, while important, certainly does not tell the whole story. The straylight meter discussed in this small case report may give us some additional useful information regarding vision. Two eyes with central epithelial ingrowth improved their Snellen visual acuity somewhat, but their straylight measurements greatly improved after the ingrowth was removed. It would be interesting to see if other patients with good Snellen visual acuity but severe complaints of poor visual quality have abnormal straylight measurements. I believe entities, such as epithelial basement membrane dystrophy or superficial punctate keratopathy, are often responsible for such symptoms. If we could obtain objective and accurate measurements of compromised visual function (even in eyes with good Snellen visual acuity measurements), we could begin to develop more effective treatments. Having removed epithelial ingrowth after laser in situ keratomileusis (LASIK) in numerous eyes, the improvement in the subjective quality of vision is frequently much more impressive than improvement in Snellen visual acuity. I wish I had a straylight meter to have evaluated my patients pre- and postoperatively.

C. J. Rapuano, MD

Arcuate Keratotomy for High Postoperative Keratoplasty Astigmatism Performed With the Intralase Femtosecond Laser

Buzzonetti L, Petrocelli G, Laborante A, et al (IRCCS–"Casa Sollievo Della Sofferenza" Hosp, San Giovanni Rotondo (Foggia), Italy)

J Refract Surg 25:709-714, 2009

Purpose.—To evaluate the refractive and keratometric effect of arcuate keratotomy performed using the IntraLase femtosecond laser (Abbott Medical Optics) in patients with high postoperative keratoplasty astigmatism.

Methods.—Nine eyes of nine patients (mean age 45 ± 7.5 years; mean spherical equivalent refraction −2.50 ± 3.60 diopters [D]) who had undergone a penetrating keratoplasty were considered. The subjective refraction was measured, and corneal thickness and keratometric parameters were calculated by the Pentacam (Oculus Optikgeräte). All uncomplicated surgeries were performed with the IntraLase femtosecond laser. Paired 70° arc length incisions were performed at 80% depth of the corneal thickness. The mean optical zone was 5.9 mm. The side cut was 90°. All incisions were performed in the graft itself. Mean change in best spectacle-corrected visual acuity (BSCVA), refractive and keratometric astigmatism, and spherical equivalent refraction was evaluated. Follow-up was 3 months. Refractive and keratometric data were analyzed using vector analysis as described by Alpins. A paired Student *t* test was used to compare preoperative and 3-month postoperative data. A P value <.05 was considered significant.

Results.—Mean preoperative BSCVA was 20/30, increasing to 20/25 postoperatively ($P > .05$). The mean refractive astigmatism decreased by 6.00 D ($P < .05$), whereas the mean keratometric value decreased by 4.60 D ($P < .05$). The mean spherical equivalent refraction did not change significantly. The surgical vectors in the refractive and keratometric analysis were calculated, showing good predictability.

Conclusions.—Arcuate keratotomy performed with the IntraLase femtosecond laser could be an effective, safe, and relatively predictable treatment of high postoperative keratoplasty astigmatism.

▶ Advances in medical, pharmaceutical, and surgical technology have greatly improved corneal transplantation results over the years, with more and more grafts remaining clear. However, astigmatism is still a major issue. Toric soft contact lenses, rigid gas permeable contact lenses, and hybrid contact lenses can be used successfully by many patients, but not by everyone. Refractive surgery using surface ablation and laser in situ keratomileusis (LASIK) can also be performed, but is more effective for myopia (and to a lesser degree, hyperopia) than for astigmatism. Relaxing incisions can be successful but are quite unpredictable. One reason for this unpredictability may be the variety of techniques used to perform relaxing incisions. They can be performed in the graft/host junction or in the graft. They can also be done with a "cut-down" technique or a guarded diamond blade.

This study reports the results of using the IntraLase femtosecond laser to create astigmatic keratotomy (AK) incisions in grafts of 9 patients followed for 3 months. The mean optical zone was 5.9 mm and ranged from 4.8 to 6.8 mm. The depth was 80% of the thinnest corneal point at the optical zone diameter. Mean refractive cylinder decreased from 9.1 D to 3.1 D. Spherical equivalent didn't change significantly. The results appeared better in eyes where the optical zone was > 6.0 mm and AK depth was over 500 μm. More eyes with longer follow-up are needed, but this new technology appears very promising for an extremely frustrating condition for patients and surgeons.

C. J. Rapuano, MD

Phakic Intraocular Lens Implantation for the Correction of Myopia: A Report by the American Academy of Ophthalmology

Huang D, Schallhorn SC, Sugar A, et al

Ophthalmology 116:2244-2258, 2009

Objective.—To review the published literature for evaluation of the safety and outcomes of phakic intraocular lens (pIOL) implantation for the correction of myopia and myopic astigmatism.

Methods.—Literature searches of the PubMed and Cochrane Library databases were conducted on October 7, 2007, and July 14, 2008. The PubMed search was limited to the English language; the Cochrane Library was searched without language limitations. The searches retrieved 261 references. Of these, panel members chose 85 papers that they considered to be of high or medium clinical relevance to this assessment. The panel methodologist rated the articles according to the strength of evidence.

Results.—Two pIOLs have been approved by the US Food and Drug Administration (FDA): one iris-fixated pIOL and one posterior-chamber IOL. In FDA trials of iris-fixated pIOLs, uncorrected visual acuity (UCVA) was ≥20/40 in 84% and ≥20/20 in 31% after 3 years. In FDA trials of posterior-chamber pIOLs, UCVA was ≥20/40 in 81% and ≥20/20 in 41%. Satisfaction with the quality of vision with both types of pIOLs was generally high. Toric anterior- and posterior-chamber pIOLs have shown improved clinical results in European trials compared with spherical pIOLs. Comparative studies showed pIOLs to provide better best spectacle-corrected visual acuity (BSCVA) and refractive predictability and stability compared with LASIK and photorefractive keratectomy and to have a lower risk of retinal detachment compared with refractive lens exchange. Reported complications and long-term safety concerns include endothelial cell loss, cataract formation, secondary glaucoma (pupillary block, pigment dispersion), iris atrophy (pupil ovalization), an traumatic dislocation.

Conclusions.—Phakic IOL implantation is effective in the correction of myopia and myopic astigmatism. In cases of high myopia of −8 diopters or more, pIOLs may provide a better visual outcome than keratorefractive surgeries and better safety than refractive lens exchange. The short-term rates of complications and loss of BSCVA are acceptable. Comprehensive preoperative evaluation and long-term postoperative follow-up examinations are needed to monitor for and prevent serious complications, and to establish long-term safety.

► Last year I wrote a comment on the American Academy of Ophthalmology's (AAO) Ophthalmic Technology Assessment (OTA) on wavefront-guided laser in situ keratomileusis (LASIK) for myopia and astigmatism. This year the AAO published their OTA on phakic intraocular lenses (IOLs) for myopia. The AAO created the OTA Committees many years ago to provide unbiased, evidence-based evaluations of new technology for the AAO membership. Disclosure note: I was the Chair of the Refractive Surgery OTA Committee several years ago.

With incredible help and support from the AAO staff, the OTA Committee obtains all related articles on the subject, selects the appropriate ones, and has a methodologist review them. The group generates the OTA document, which is reviewed by the relevant subspecialty societies, gets revised, and then gets approved by the AAO Board.

This OTA reviewed the literature on 2 types of phakic IOLs that are FDA-approved (iris clip anterior chamber IOL and posterior chamber IOL) and also angle-supported anterior chamber IOLs. I agree with their conclusion that phakic IOLs may be appropriate in eyes that are at higher risk for problems with keratorefractive surgery (eg, > -8 D), although long-term follow-up is needed to establish long-term safety for these lenses.

C. J. Rapuano, MD

3 Glaucoma

Anterior Segment Optical Coherence Tomography as a Screening Tool for the Assessment of the Anterior Segment Angle

Pekmezci M, Porco TC, Lin SC (Univ of California, San Francisco)

Ophthalmic Surg Lasers Imaging 40:389-398, 2009

Background and Objective.—Anterior segment optical coherence tomography (AS-OCT) is an alternative method for the assessment of angle width. The purpose of this study is to assess the accuracy of AS-OCT for detecting occludable angles and compare the results of high- and low-resolution images with gonioscopy.

Patients and Method.—Visante AS-OCT (Carl Zeiss Meditec, Dublin, CA) images of 303 eyes (155 patients) presenting between February 1 and July 15, 2007, were retrospectively analyzed. Angle recess area (ARA) and angle opening distances (AOD) at 250, 500, and 750 μm were measured and correlated with the corresponding gonioscopic measurements.

Results.—AS-OCT parameters showed a nonlinear relationship with gonioscopy, ARA having the highest correlation. Correlations between high- and low-resolution images were modest. Cut-off values were 0.180 mm^2 (70.3% sensitivity, 87.4% specificity) for ARA and 0.264 mm (71.8% sensitivity, 84.8% specificity) for AOD at 500 μm.

Conclusion.—AS-OCT appears to be a promising screening tool for narrow angles.

▶ Gonioscopy is challenging and underused. Fremont and coworkers found that gonioscopy was performed in less than half of all patients within a year of the diagnosis of glaucoma. It is a difficult skill, and is uncomfortable for some patients.

Anterior segment optical coherence tomography (AS-OCT) can be used to assess the angle, although it gives less detail than gonioscopy. It is, however, noncontact. It does not show structure behind the iris as well as the ultrasound biomicroscope (UBM).

AS-OCT was shown in this article to be able to discern occludable angles. In America, screening for narrow angles would not be cost effective, especially with an expensive device. However, in other parts of the world, where angle closure glaucoma is much more common and skilled gonioscopists are more rare, AS-OCT screening might be worthwhile.

The correlation of AS-OCT parameters to clinical evaluation is not exact, but of course, 2 gonioscopists often disagree as well. With gonioscopy or AS-OCT, we are still unsure of the exact parameters that predict acute or chronic angle closure glaucoma.

For further reading on this subject I suggest an article by Fremont et al.[1]

J. S. Myers, MD

Reference

1. Fremont AM, Lee PP, Mangione CM, et al. Patterns of care for open-angle glaucoma in managed care. *Arch Ophthalmol.* 2003;121:777-783.

Atypical retardation pattern in measurements of scanning laser polarimetry and its relating factors

Yanagisawa M, Tomidokoro A, Saito H, et al (Univ of Tokyo, Japan; et al)

Eye 23:1796-1801, 2009

Purpose.—To assess the prevalence of atypical retardation pattern (ARP) in scanning laser polarimetry (SLP) with variable corneal compensation (VCC) and enhanced corneal compensation (ECC), and to evaluate the factors relating to typical scan score (TSS).

Methods.—Measurements of SLP–VCC, SLP–ECC, and the Humphrey field analyzer (HFA) were performed in 105 normal subjects and 82 open-angle glaucoma (OAG) patients. ARP was defined as an SLP image with TSS <80.

Results.—Prevalence of ARP with SLP–VCC was 13.3 and 14.6% in normal and OAG eyes, respectively, and that with SLP–ECC (2.9% and 1.2%) was lower than SLP–VCC ($P < 0.009$). TSS with SLP–VCC was significantly correlated with age (partial correlation coefficient (PCC) = −0.22, $P = 0.003$) and refractive error (PCC = 0.26, $P < 0.001$) after adjusting for each other. TSS with SLP–ECC was significantly correlated with neither age nor refractive error (PCC = −0.02, $P = 0.788$; PCC = 0.10, $P = 0.177$, respectively). In OAG eyes, mean deviation (MD) of HFA was significantly correlated with TSS with SLP–VCC and SLP–ECC (PCC = 0.35, $P = 0.001$; PCC = 0.23, $P = 0.039$, respectively). In SLP-VCC, MD was significantly correlated with retinal nerve fiber layer (RNFL) thickness only after excluding eyes with ARP ($P < 0.001$).

Conclusions.—ARP in SLP–VCC measurements was found in more than 10% of normal or glaucomatous eyes, and TSS was significantly lower in older subjects, more myopic eyes, or eyes with more advanced glaucomatous damage. The presence of ARP disturbs the accuracy of RNFL thickness measurement by SLP–VCC. In SLP–ECC measurements, prevalence of ARP was considerably lower and TSS was not affected by

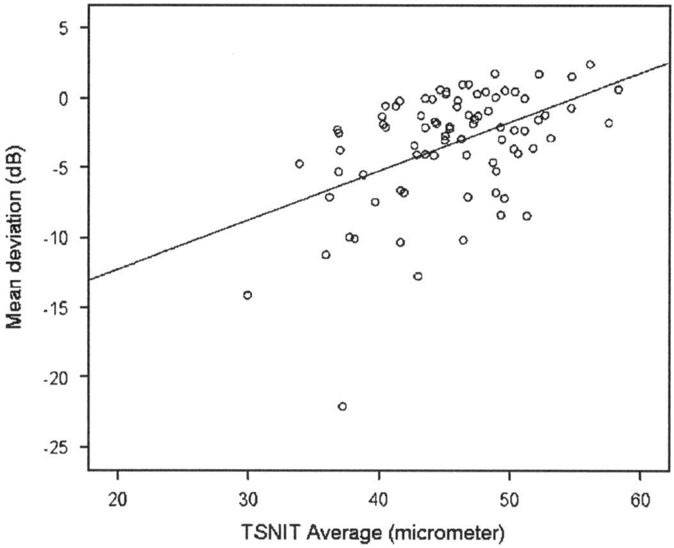

FIGURE 2.—Correlation between RNFL average determined by scanning laser polarimetry with enhanced corneal compensation and mean deviation (MD) of Humphrey perimeter. The correlation was significant in all 82 open-angle glaucoma eyes (Pearson's correlation coefficient, $R = 0.48$, $P < 0.001$). (Reprinted from Yanagisawa M, Tomidokoro A, Saito H, et al. Atypical retardation pattern in measurements of scanning laser polarimetry and its relating factors. *Eye.* 2009;23:1796-1801.)

TABLE 2.—Prevalence of ARP in Measurements of SLP with VCC and that with ECC in 105 Normal and 82 OAG Eyes

	Normal ($N = 105$)			OAG ($N = 82$)			
	N	Prevalence	${}^{a}P$-Value	*N*	Prevalence	${}^{a}P$-Value	${}^{b}P$-Value
VCC	14/105	13.3 (8.1–21.1)%	0.009	12/82	14.6 (8.6–23.9)%	0.002	0.834
ECC	3/105	2.9 (1.0–8.1)%		1/82	1.2 (0.2–6.6)%		0.632

ARP = atypical retardation pattern; ECC = enhanced corneal compensation; Normal = ophthalmologically healthy eyes, OAG = eyes with open-angle glaucoma; SLP = scanning laser polarimetry; VCC = variable corneal compensation.

The numbers of eyes with ARP and the prevalence (95% confidence interval) are shown.

[a]*P*-value between the measurements with SLP–VCC and those with ECC (Fisher's exact test).

[b]*P*-value between the normal and OAG groups (Fisher exact test).

age or refractive error, suggesting the advantages of ECC in clinical practices (Fig 2, Table 2).

▶ The GDx uses scanning laser polarimetry to quantify the thickness of the ganglion cell layer. This technology has been quite helpful in evaluating glaucoma, but over the years the cornea and other sources of polarization artifact have led to errant measurements of the nerve fiber layer. VCC, variable corneal compensation, helped to reduce these errors. This article reports on the latest iteration, enhanced corneal compensation (ECC), in the reduction of atypical retardation patterns (ARPs).

The article shows significant improvement in the performance of the GDx using ECC. These atypical retardation patterns probably account for most of the surprises clinicians see, in which the GDx results do not match the rest of the clinical picture. However, there is still a wide spread between nerve fiber layer measurements and visual field results.

In an era in which Zeiss owns GDx and is a leader in optical coherence technology, the future of the GDx is uncertain. The new generation of spectral domain optical coherence tomography (SD-OCT) instruments shows excellent measurement of the nerve fiber layer without polarization artifacts. The technologies continue to evolve, and SD-OCT is positioned to take a leading role in the future. However, at their best, these technologies supplement rather than replace a good clinical examination, and none have been shown to be better than the expert evaluation of the nerve or disc photos.

J. S. Myers, MD

Clinicians Agreement in Establishing Glaucomatous Progression Using the Heidelberg Retina Tomograph

Vizzeri G, Weinreb RN, Martinez de la Casa JM, et al (Univ of California San Diego, La Jolla; Hosp Clinico San Carlos, Madrid, Spain)

Ophthalmology 116:14-24, 2009

Purpose.—To assess the degree of concordance among clinicians reviewing 3 Heidelberg retina tomograph (HRT) printouts used to detect progression, the Moorfields regression analysis (MRA), the topographic change analysis (TCA), and trend analysis (TA), and to compare with progression identified by stereophotographs.

Design.—Observational cohort study.

Participants.—We longitudinally followed 237 eyes of 168 patients (50 glaucomatous eyes, 187 glaucoma suspects) from the Diagnostic Innovation in Glaucoma Study (mean follow-up, 46.8 ± 14.2 months), with a minimum of 4 HRT images (range, 4–8).

Methods.—Three experienced observers judged the presence of progression using the HRT follow-up printouts available for each HRT method of analysis (MRA, TCA, TA). The overall assessment was based on majority rule, with ≥ 2 graders agreeing on the classification.

Main Outcome Measures.—Observers agreement in assessing HRT progression and agreement for progression or no progression between the HRT methods of analysis and the reference standard represented by masked stereophotograph assessment. The κ test was used to assess the interobserver agreement.

Results.—In general, agreement among clinicians for subjective assessment of progression based on HRT printouts was moderate to good; agreement (κ) ranged from 0.52 to 0.71 for MRA, 0.61 to 0.63 for TCA, and 0.45 to 0.74 for TA. Of the 237 eyes, 16 (6.8%) were found to progress during follow-up based on masked stereophotograph assessment. Agreement for progression/no progression between the HRT

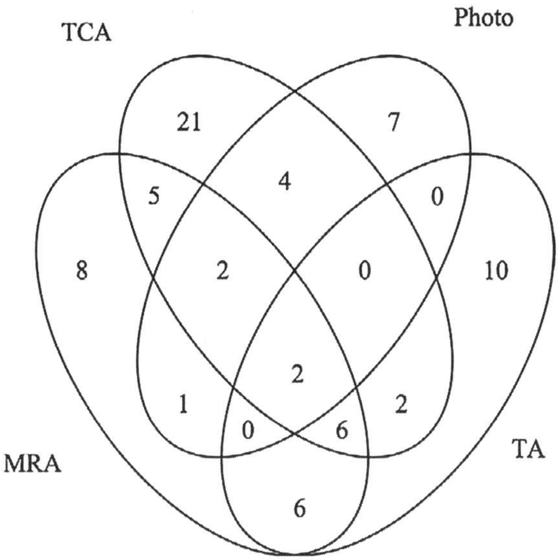

FIGURE 2.—Venn diagram showing the agreement on progression between Moorfields regression analysis (MRA), topographic change analysis (TCA), and trend analysis (TA) and the reference standard. Progression for the MRA, TCA, and TA was defined based on majority rule. The TA is based on the normalized "average" parameter defined as the average of several HRT parameters combined (rim area, rim volume, cup volume, cup shape, mean retinal nerve fiber layer thickness, mean height of contour, mean contour elevation, contour line modulation temporal, mean cup depth, and mean height inside contour line). HRT = Heidelberg retina tomograph. (Reprinted from Vizzeri G, Weinreb RN, Martinez de la Casa JM, et al. Clinicians agreement in establishing glaucomatous progression using the heidelberg retina tomograph. *Ophthalmology.* 2009;116:14-24, with permission from the American Academy of Ophthalmology.)

methods and stereophotography was similar among MRA (84.8%, agreement on 5 progressing eyes and 196 nonprogressing eyes; $\kappa = 0.14$), TCA, (82.3%, agreement on 8 progressing eyes and 187 nonprogressing eyes; $\kappa = 0.2$), and TA (84%, agreement on 2 progressing eyes and 197 nonprogressing eyes; $\kappa = 0.01$).

Conclusions.—Clinicians' agreement in identifying suspected glaucomatous progression using different HRT methods of analysis was moderate to good and was similar among all methods, including MRA, which is not designed to detect progression. Agreement between progression identified by HRT and masked stereophotograph assessment was poor. These results suggest that assessment of the HRT and stereophotography may be identifying different aspects of structural change.

▶ Most articles on imaging for detection of glaucoma or progression focus on algorithms or measures that are not applied clinically. Few studies have looked at the performance of these instruments in the hands of the clinician using the data generated by the machine for clinical use.

TABLE 2.—Kappa Values and Standard Error (SE) for Agreement among Different Observers for the Heidelberg Retina Tomograph Methods of Analysis for Detecting Progression

Agreement between Observers	Kappa	SE
Moorfields regression analysis		
A vs B	0.52	0.08
A vs C	0.61	0.08
B vs C	0.71	0.06
Topographic change analysis		
A vs B	0.61	0.07
A vs C	0.63	0.07
B vs C	0.62	0.06
Trend analysis		
A vs B	0.45	0.09
A vs C	0.74	0.07
B vs C	0.58	0.08

This study considers the issue of detecting progression using the Heidelberg retina tomograph (HRT). Three observers used clinically available HRT parameters to judge progression.

The interobserver agreement was moderate (Table 2). The agreement among any of the parameters and stereo disc photos was limited. In the Venn diagram (Fig 2), none of these 3 HRT parameters in the clinicians' hands identified even half of the 16 eyes found to progress on stereo disc photos.

Among the potential advantages of quantitative imaging is the hope for a more standardized assessment. One of the many valid criticisms of visual fields is that they are not uniformly interpreted and that there is no consensus on how to grade or determine progression. It appears that these same issues are currently present for quantitative optic nerve imaging.

J. S. Myers, MD

Coupling of HRT II and AS-OCT to evaluate corneal endothelial cell loss and *in vivo* visualization of the Ahmed glaucoma valve implant

Mendrinos E, Dosso A, Sommerhalder J, et al (Geneva Univ Hosps, Switzerland)
Eye 23:1836-1844, 2009

Aims.—To report corneal endothelial cell loss and *in vivo* visualization of the Ahmed glaucoma valve implant in eyes with refractory glaucoma.

Methods.—Ten eyes underwent Ahmed valve implant surgery and were followed-up for 12 months. Data collected included intraocular pressure (IOP), number of antiglaucoma medications and surgery-related complications. At 6 and 12 months postoperatively, the intracameral length of the drainage tube (ICL) and the distance between the tube and the cornea (T–C distance), and the iris (T–I distance) were assessed using anterior segment optical coherence tomography (AS-OCT). Heidelberg cornea tomograph II (HRT II) was used to measure the corneal endothelial cell density.

Results.—Mean (±SEM) preoperative IOP was 29.5 ± 4 mm Hg. Mean postoperative IOP was 11.6 ± 2 at 12 months ($P < 0.01$). Over a 6-month period, mean corneal endothelial loss was 7.9% ± 2.5 in the central and 7.5% ± 2.4 in the peripheral cornea ($P < 0.01$). There was no correlation between central or peripheral corneal endothelial cell loss and the T–C, T–I distance or the ICL of the tube.

Conclusions.—Corneal endothelial cell loss occurs following Ahmed valve implant surgery, this appears to be multifactorial. AS-OCT and

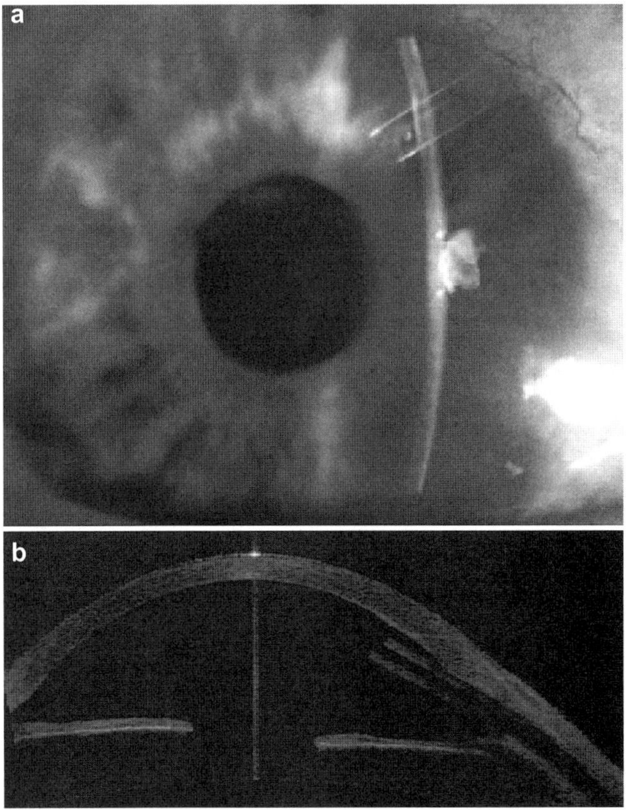

FIGURE 2.—(a) Slit-lamp anterior segment photography showing the drainage tube into the anterior chamber of a patient who underwent Ahmed valve implant surgery. (b) Visante OCT of the anterior segment of the same patient providing details about the anatomic relationship between the drainage tube and the cornea. Note the contact of the tube with the limbus; the distance between the extremity of the tube and the cornea was measured to be 0.6 mm. Corneal endothelial cell density in proximity of the tube measured by *in vivo* confocal microscopy was 590 cells/mm^2. On the basis of the results given by AS-OCT and confocal microscopy, this patient was elicited to be treated by partial tube resection and repositioning. (Reprinted from Mendrinos E, Dosso A, Sommerhalder J, et al. Coupling of HRT II and AS-OCT to evaluate corneal endothelial cell loss and *in vivo* visualization of the Ahmed glaucoma valve implant. *Eye*. 2009;23:1836-1844.)

TABLE 1.—Endothelial Cell Density (cells/mm^2) and the Percentage Change Between 6 and 12 Months After Surgery

Patient No.	CED 6 Months	PED 6 Months	CED 12 Months	PED 12 Months	CED Change	PED Change	Percentage of CED Change	Percentage PED Change
1	2731	2462	2336	2133	−395	−329	−14.5	−13.4
2	2023	1853	1861	1760	−162	−93	−8.0	−5.0
3	1196	590	1170	524	−26	−66	−2.2	−11.2
4	2093	1973	1831	1968	−262	−5	−12.5	−0.3
5	1846	2373	1756	1974	−90	−399	−4.9	−16.8
6	3287	3350	2929	3150	−358	−200	−10.9	−6.0
7	1855	1880	1768	1835	−87	−45	−4.7	−2.4
8	2172	1842	2049	1709	−123	−133	−5.7	−7.2
9	1226	1141	1143	1068	−83	−73	−6.8	−6.4
10	2158	1968	1964	1850	−194	−118	−9.0	−6.0
Mean	2059	1943	1881	1797	−178	−146	−7.9	−7.5
±SEM	197	234	164	215	39	40	2.5	2.4

CED = central endothelial cell density; PED = peripheral endothelial cell density.

HRT II are promising methods for the follow-up of patients with a glaucoma drainage device (Fig 2, Table 1).

▶ Tube shunts are increasingly used and have been of tremendous help in the management of glaucoma. However, it has long been recognized that tubes close to the endothelium can lead to corneal decompensation.

This article shows that corneal endothelial cell counts dropped even when the tube was not close to the endothelium. This is a small, uncontrolled series of eyes. However, it is worth noting that in every case corneal endothelial cell counts dropped at least a few percent between 6 and 12 months postoperatively. This concern should be considered in choosing the best treatment for each patient.

J. S. Myers, MD

Scanning laser polarimetry with variable corneal compensation in migraine patients

Martinez A, Proupim N, Sanchez M (Galician Inst of Ophthalmology, Santiago de Compostela, La Coruña, Spain; Health Centre Conxo, Santiago de Compostela, La Coruña, Spain; Galician Inst of Ophthalmology, Santiago de Compostela, La Coruña, Spain)
Acta Ophthalmol 87:746-753, 2009

Purpose.—This study aimed to compare scanning laser polarimetry measurements of retinal nerve fibre layer (RNFL) thickness in eyes of migraine patients with those in eyes of age-matched, healthy subjects.

Methods.—The study was designed as an observational, prospective, cross-sectional study. It included 57 eyes of 57 patients with migraine with or without aura according to the criteria of the International Headache Society and 44 eyes of 44 age-matched healthy controls. Scanning laser polarimetry images were obtained using a commercial GDx VCC system (Version 5.3.1; Laser Diagnostic Technologies, Inc.). At each sitting, three sets of GDx VCC measurements were acquired for each

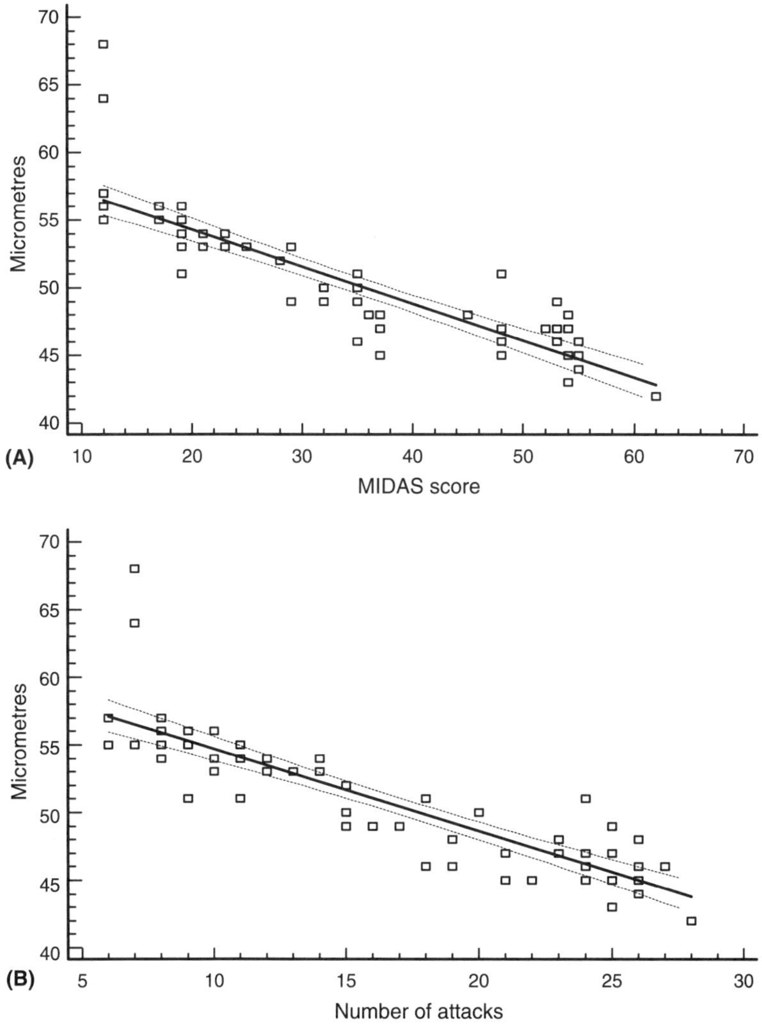

FIGURE 2.—Evaluation of the relationship between retinal nerve fibre layer average parameter (TSNIT.Av) and migraine values. (A) There was a significant relationship between TSNIT.Av and MIDAS score ($r = -0.87$, 95% confidence interval [CI] -0.92 to -0.78; $p < 0.001$). (B) There was a significant relationship between TSNIT.Av and number of attacks ($r = -0.87$, 95% CI -0.92 to -0.78; $p < 0.001$). MIDAS = Migraine Disability Assessment. (Reprinted from Martinez A, Proupim N, Sanchez M, Scanning laser polarimetry with variable corneal compensation in migraine patients. *Acta Ophthalmol.* 2009;87:746-753.)

patient and used in the analysis. Image acquisition was performed in undilated eyes in all subjects.

Results.—The mean ± standard deviation RNFL average thickness parameter in the migraine subjects was significantly lower than in the control group, at 50.4 ± 4.8 μm versus 54.7 ± 3.4 μm, respectively ($p < 0.0001$). However, there were no differences between migraine subjects and controls in mean RNFL thickness in superior and inferior areas. In the migraine group the mean migraine disability assessment (MIDAS) score was 34.3 ± 15.3 and the mean number of attacks per year was 17.1 ± 6.9 (range 6–28). The mean RNFL average thickness parameter was significantly correlated with MIDAS score ($r = -0.86$, $p < 0.0001$) and frequency of attacks ($r = -0.86$, $p < 0.0001$).

Conclusions.—The mean RNFL average thickness parameter was found to be thinner in migraine patients. In addition, we found a strong correlation between migraine severity and RNFL average thickness parameters (Fig 2).

▶ An association between normal-tension glaucoma and migraines has long been recognized. This article shows a clear association between migraine and nerve fiber layer thickness measured by the GDx with variable corneal compensation. Although the loss was diffuse and not clearly aligned along the vertical areas as seen in glaucoma, the findings raise questions regarding the pathophysiology of migraine. We know that glaucoma damage propagates upstream to lead to neuronal loss in the brain. Perhaps cerebral events in migraine lead to downstream damage in the eye. It should be noted that 1 previous study of similar design did not see this relation, although multiple other studies have shown related issues, such as field loss in patients with migraine.

J. S. Myers, MD

Prediction of Functional Loss in Glaucoma From Progressive Optic Disc Damage

Medeiros FA, Alencar LM, Zangwill LM, et al (Univ of California–San Diego, La Jolla)

Arch Ophthalmol 127:1250-1256, 2009

Objective.—To evaluate the ability of progressive optic disc damage detected by assessment of longitudinal stereophotographs to predict future development of functional loss in those with suspected glaucoma.

Methods.—The study included 639 eyes of 407 patients with suspected glaucoma followed up for an average of 8.0 years with annual standard automated perimetry visual field and optic disc stereophotographs. All patients had normal and reliable standard automated perimetry results at baseline. Conversion to glaucoma was defined as development of 3 consecutive abnormal visual fields during follow-up. Presence of progressive optic disc damage was evaluated by grading longitudinally acquired

TABLE 2.—Results of the Univariable and Multivariable Cox Models Evaluating the Relationship Between Predictors and Risk of Development of Visual Field Loss

Predictor	Univariable HR (95% CI)	Univariable *P* Value	Multivariable HR (95% CI)	Multivariable *P* Value
Optic disc progression	25.8 (16.0-41.7)	<.001	16.0 (9.8-25.9)	<.001
Baseline glaucomatous optic disc grading	3.76 (2.04-6.94)	<.001	2.47 (1.35-4.52)	.003
Baseline vertical cup-disc ratio, per 0.1 larger	1.45 (1.22-1.71)	<.001	1.35 (1.15-1.59)	<.001
Baseline IOP, per 1 mm Hg higher	1.06 (1.02-1.11)	.003		
Central corneal thickness, per 40 μm thinner	1.87 (1.28-2.72)	<.001		
Baseline PSD, per 0.1 dB higher	1.25 (1.16-1.35)	<.001		
Age, per decade older	2.24 (1.67-3.01)	<.001		

Abbreviations: CI, confidence interval; HR, hazard ratio; IOP, intraocular pressure; PSD, pattern standard deviation.

simultaneous stereophotographs. Other predictive factors included age, intraocular pressure, central corneal thickness, pattern standard deviation, and baseline stereophotograph grading. Hazard ratios for predicting visual field loss were obtained by extended Cox models, with optic disc progression as a time-dependent covariate. Predictive accuracy was evaluated using a modified R^2 index.

Results.—Progressive optic disc damage had a hazard ratio of 25.8 (95% confidence interval, 16.0-41.7) and was the most important risk factor for development of visual field loss with an R^2 of 79%. The R^2s for other predictive factors ranged from 6% to 26%.

Conclusions.—Presence of progressive optic disc damage on stereophotographs was a highly predictive factor for future development of functional loss in glaucoma. These findings suggest the importance of careful monitoring of the optic disc appearance and a potential role for longitudinal assessment of the optic disc as an end point in clinical trials and as a reference for evaluation of diagnostic tests in glaucoma (Table 2).

▶ This study clearly shows that progressive glaucomatous optic nerve change leads to visual field loss. Although clinicians are all aware of this, rigorous research demonstrating this has been limited.

This study confirmed many known risk factors, such as IOP, corneal thickness, age, and baseline cup-to-disc ratio.

This study is important, as it lays the groundwork for imaging of the nerve, in this case serial stereodisc photographs, as an endpoint in clinical trials of drugs. This endpoint will be critical if non-IOP therapies are to be developed and proven for glaucoma treatment. Since disc change preceded visual field change by many years in this study, the use of disc endpoints will greatly speed validation of any neuroprotective treatments.

J. S. Myers, MD

Glaucoma With Early Visual Field Loss Affecting Both Hemifields and the Risk of Disease Progression

De Moraes CGV, Prata TS, Tello C, et al (Einhorn Clinical Res Ctr, NY; et al)
Arch Ophthalmol 127:1129-1134, 2009

Objective.—To evaluate whether damage to both hemifields in glaucomatous eyes predicts more rapid disease progression than does single-hemifield involvement.

Methods.—We reviewed the medical records of 43 660 consecutive patients. Eyes with glaucomatous optic neuropathy, 10 or more Swedish Interactive Threshold Algorithm standard 24-2 visual fields in at least 5 years, and mean deviation (MD) smaller than −6.0 dB were included. Pointwise linear regression was used to determine progression. Cox proportional hazards analysis was used to calculate risk of progression based on different baseline covariates.

Results.—We enrolled 205 eyes (205 patients; mean [SD] age, 64.2 [11.0] years; follow-up, 6.5 [1.8] years; number of visual fields, 12.3 [2.9]). Patients were divided into 3 groups: initial superior defect (group A; n = 79; MD, −3.4 [1.9] dB), initial inferior defect (group B; n = 61; MD, −3.4 [1.8] dB), and both hemifields affected (group C; n = 65; MD, −4.2 [1.5] dB). Group C progressed faster than did groups A and B ($P < .02$). Multivariate analysis showed significant effect of higher baseline intraocular pressure, thinner central corneal thickness, and initial damage to both hemifields.

Conclusions.—Initial damage to both hemifields increases the risk of glaucoma progression. More aggressive therapy should be considered for these eyes.

► In a landmark article, Grant and Burke reviewed cases of blindness in the glaucoma clinic at the Massachusetts Eye and Ear Infirmary.[1] Their conclusion was that patients who had both hemifields affected on Goldmann visual field testing were much more likely to go blind.

In this article, De Moraes et al use more sophisticated analyses and modern automated static perimetry to show that, indeed, having field defects in both hemifields is a very significant risk factor for progressive loss of visual field (despite treatment) (Table 2). In this data set, having both hemifields involved

TABLE 2.—Distribution of Eyes Based on Rates of Visual Field Progression

Rate of Progression	Eyes, No. (%) Group A (n = 79)	Group B (n = 61)	Group C (n = 65)[a]
Fast (>1.5 dB/y)	5 (6.3)	2 (3.3)	13 (20.0)
Moderate (0.5-1.5 dB/y)	27 (34.2)	17 (27.9)	28 (43.1)
Slow (<0.5 dB/y)	47 (59.5)	42 (68.8)	24 (36.9)

[a]The χ^2 test showed significant differences between groups ($P < .01$).

TABLE 3.—Cox Proportional Hazards Including Each Variable Independently (Univariate Model)

Variable	HR (95% CI)	*P* Value
Age	1.01 (0.99-1.03)	.10
MD	1.05 (0.94-1.17)	.27
No. of points with $P < 1\%$	1.01 (0.97-1.05)	.54
CCT, per 40-μm decrease	1.32 (1.08-1.61)	<.01
Baseline IOP	1.08 (1.03-1.13)	<.01
Exfoliation syndrome	1.11 (0.63-1.96)	.70
Baseline damage to both hemifields	1.58 (1.07-2.32)	.02

Abbreviations: CCT, central corneal thickness; CI, confidence interval; HR, hazard ratio; IOP, intraocular pressure; MD, mean deviation.

was a stronger predictor of visual field deterioration than age, baseline intraocular pressure (IOP), exfoliation syndrome, 40-micron thinner central corneal thickness, or mean deviation on field testing (Table 3).

The presence of field loss in 2 hemifields should be strongly considered in formulating a treatment plan and goal pressure as well as in counseling patients.

J. S. Myers, MD

Reference

1. Grant WM, Burke JF. Why do some people go blind from glaucoma? *Ophthalmology.* 1982;89:991-998.

Visual field index rate and event-based glaucoma progression analysis: comparison in a glaucoma population

Casas-Llera P, Rebolleda G, Muñoz-Negrete FJ, et al (Ramón y Cajal Hosp, Madrid, Spain)

Br J Ophthalmol 93:1576-1579, 2009

Aims.—The aim of the study was to compare event-based glaucoma progression analysis (GPA) I with new GPA II software and pattern deviation-based trend analyses (visual field index [VFI]) to detect progression in a glaucoma population.

Methods.—This was a retrospective study that included 90 eyes of 90 patients with a minimum of five reliable visual field tests and a follow-up period of at least 2 years.

Results.—Event-based GPA II detected progression in 16.7% of eyes in which trend analysis VFI failed. GPA detected progression 6.8 months earlier than VFI. GPA I and II showed excellent agreement ($k = 0.94$). Agreement between VFI and mean deviation (MD) linear analysis and with GPA criteria was $k = 0.52$ and $k = 0.48$, respectively. Mean rates of progression of MD and VFI were −0.41 dB and −1.30% annually, respectively ($rho = 0.824$; $p<0.0001$). Using VFI, mean follow-up time was

TABLE 4.—Kappa Statistics for Pairs of Progression Criteria

	Event-Based GPA I vs GPA II	Event-Based GPA II vs Trend Analysis VFI	Event-Based GPA II vs Trend Analysis MD	Trend-Analysis VFI vs MD
Kappa value	0.94	0.48	0.22	0.52
Standard error	0.03	0.10	0.11	0.11
p Value	0.000	0.000	0.031	0.000

GPA, glaucoma progression analysis; MD, mean deviation; VFI, visual field index.

6.12 and 4.89 years ($p = 0.004$) and the mean number of visual field tests was 7.33 and 6.01 ($p = 0.023$) in eyes with and without progression, respectively.

Conclusions.—Event-based software GPA I and II had excellent agreement. Event analysis showed earlier and greater sensitivity for detecting progression than VFI analysis and both had only moderate agreement. Trend analysis VFI is likely to detect progression in patients with a greater number of visual field tests and a longer followup time. The VFI analysis seems to be more accurate than MD analysis for determining rate of progression (Table 4).

▶ Determining progression in a visual field series is at times an arduous task that may appear arbitrary as well. Multiple trials in glaucoma have each used their own methods for determining progression, and comparison studies have shown that these methods do not yield equivalent results. Given the lack of consensus in the research community and the fact that these research algorithms are completely unwieldy for clinical use, it is no surprise that there is no consensus on grading field progression in clinical practice.

This study compares the newer software provided by Humphrey visual field machines to aid in the evaluation of progression. The Glaucoma Progression Analysis (GPA) compares each point in follow-up fields to the average of that point on 2 baseline fields. Open and closed triangles at each point alert the clinician to repeated changes at given points. This approach helps clinicians to identify progressing points more easily.

The Visual Field Index (VFI) is essentially an enhanced mean deviation (MD) emphasizing the central field. Linear regression of the VFI is used to assess for progressive loss.

This study shows that these different methods do not always agree. In fact, the GPA and the VFI have only moderate correlation.

Event-based change detection methods (eg, the GPA, in which a field is compared with a baseline) are very different than trend-based methods (eg, the VFI, in which a series of fields are analyzed for progressive loss). Each have their strengths and limitations. Event-based methods will generally pick up change sooner but with less confidence and more potential error from fluctuation. Trend-based methods are generally more specific or certain but less sensitive. Octopus field testing has moved to trend-based analysis for clusters of points, such as a nasal step, in an attempt to increase sensitivity while reducing fluctuation from scotomas, which move slightly based on small changes in patient alignment.

Clinicians must use either method with care and judgment given the inherent fluctuations in the fields. The addage, measure twice, cut once, is very applicable in this circumstance. Change should be confirmed by repeated testing or other related measures such as structural change.

J. S. Myers, MD

Visual Field Progression in the Collaborative Initial Glaucoma Treatment Study: The Impact of Treatment and Other Baseline Factors

Musch DC, Gillespie BW, Lichter PR, et al (The Univ of Michigan, Ann Arbor)

Ophthalmology 116:200-207, 2009

Purpose.—To evaluate factors associated with visual field (VF) progression, using all available follow-up through 9 years after treatment initiation, in the Collaborative Initial Glaucoma Treatment Study (CIGTS).

Design.—Longitudinal follow-up of participants enrolled in a randomized clinical trial.

Participants.—Six hundred seven newly diagnosed glaucoma patients.

Methods.—In a randomized clinical trial, 607 subjects with newly diagnosed open-angle glaucoma initially were treated with either medication or trabeculectomy. After treatment initiation and early follow-up, subjects were evaluated clinically at 6-month intervals. Study participants in both arms of the CIGTS were treated aggressively in an effort to reduce intraocular pressure (IOP) to a level at or below a predetermined, eye-specific target pressure. Visual field progression was analyzed using repeated measures models.

Main Outcome Measures.—Visual field progression, measured by Humphrey 24-2 full-threshold testing and assessed by the change in the mean deviation (MD), and an indicator of substantial worsening of the VF (MD decrease of ≥3 dB from baseline), assessed at each follow-up visit.

Results.—Follow-up indicated minimal change from baseline in each initial treatment group's average MD. However, at the 8-year follow-up examination, substantial worsening (≥3 dB) of MD from baseline was found in 21.3% and 25.5% of the initial surgery and initial medicine groups, respectively. The effect of initial treatment on subsequent VF loss was modified by time ($P<0.0001$), baseline MD ($P = 0.03$), and diabetes ($P = 0.01$). Initial surgery led to less VF progression than initial medicine in subjects with advanced VF loss at baseline, whereas subjects with diabetes had more VF loss over time if treated initially with surgery.

Conclusions.—The CIGTS intervention protocol led to a lowering of IOP that persisted over time in both treatment groups. Progression in VF loss was seen in a subset, increasing to more than 20% of the subjects. The findings regarding initial surgery being beneficial for subjects with

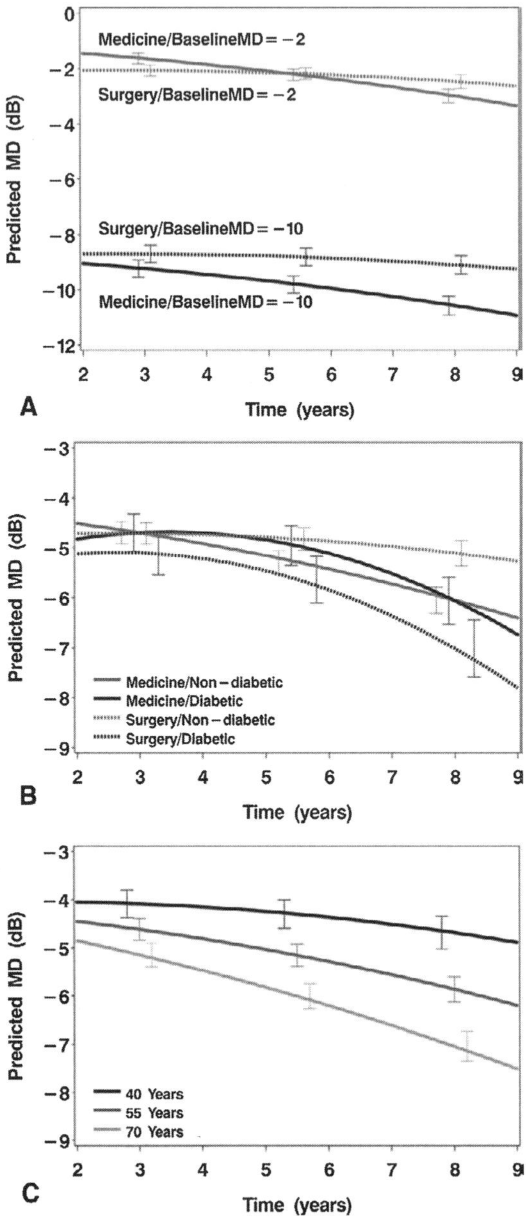

FIGURE 2.—A, Graph showing the model estimates of mean deviation (MD) over follow-up time as a function of initial treatment (medicine or surgery) and baseline MD (−2 or −10 dB). **B**, Graph showing the model estimates of MD over follow-up time as a function of initial treatment (medicine or surgery) and diabetes status (diabetic or nondiabetic). **C**, Graph showing the model estimates of MD over follow-up time as a function of age at enrollment (40, 55, or 70 years). (Reprinted from Musch DC, Gillespie BW, Lichter PR, et al. Visual field progression in the collaborative initial glaucoma treatment study: the impact of treatment and other baseline factors. *Ophthalmology.* 2009;116:200-207, with permission from the American Academy of Ophthalmology.)

more advanced VF loss at presentation, but detrimental for patients with diabetes, are noteworthy and warrant independent confirmation.

▶ The Collaborative Initial Glaucoma Treatment Study compared initial medical treatment versus initial trabeculectomy for primary open-angle glaucoma. Previous reports have shown that with aggressive pressure reduction of 30% to 40%, both groups did well at 5 years with little overall progression.

This report looks at long-term outcomes and investigates visual field loss as a function of treatment group and other characteristics. Key findings are that the surgery group had lower visual field loss rates at 7 years and above for patients with more significant field loss at baseline. Older patients were seen to lose field more quickly (Fig 2).

These findings suggest that there may be a role for trabeculectomy earlier in the treatment algorithm for patients with advanced field loss (eg, a mean deviation of—10 dB). Clinicians should share these results with affected patients, and especially in cases where there are concerns regarding adherence, consider surgical alternatives.

J. S. Myers, MD

Natural History of Open-Angle Glaucoma

Heijl A, for the Early Manifest Glaucoma Trial Group (Lund Univ Malmö, Sweden; et al)

Ophthalmology 116:2271-2276, 2009

Objective.—This article, based on the Early Manifest Glaucoma Trial (EMGT), provides prospective natural history data on progression of glaucomatous field defects in 3 of the most common glaucoma types.

Design.—Cohort of EMGT patients randomized to the untreated control group and followed up to the time of progression, when treatment could be initiated.

Participants.—We evaluated 118 control patients: 46 with high-tension glaucoma (HTG), 57 with normal-tension glaucoma (NTG), and 15 with pseudoexfoliation glaucoma (PEXG).

Methods.—Visual fields were tested every 3 months with the Humphrey 30-2 Full Threshold test program.

Main Outcome Measures.—Linear regression analyses of the perimetric mean deviation (MD) values were performed, and the rate of progression was defined as the regression coefficient in decibels per year. Percentages of progressed eyes and time to progression were determined using EMGT event-based predetermined progression criteria derived from Glaucoma Change Probability Maps.

Results.—The median and interquartile rates of visual function loss were −0.40 (1.05) dB/year overall and −0.46 (1.61) in HTG, −0.22 (0.65) in NTG, and −1.13 (6.13) in PEXG. Thus, interpatient variability was large. Mean rates were considerably higher than medians:

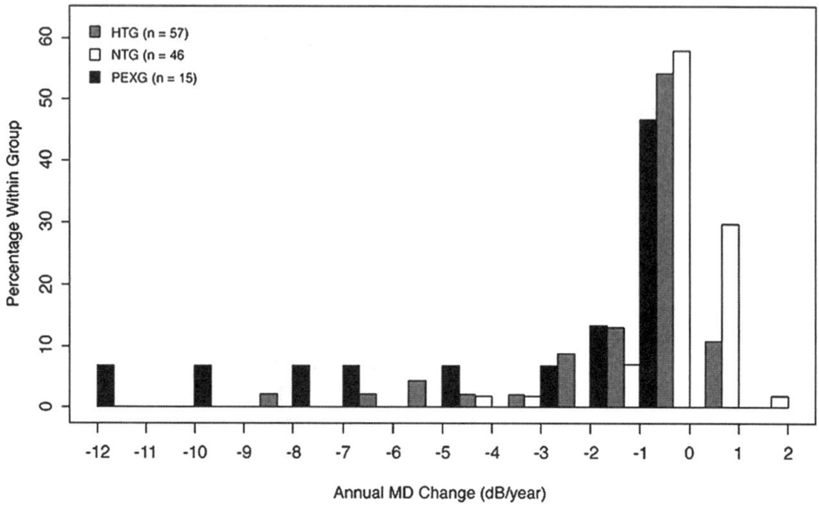

FIGURE 1.—Rates of visual field progression in patients with HTG, NTG, and PEXG. Rate of progression is expressed as annual change of the perimetric MD values. The x axis is divided in intervals of 1 dB, and the y axis displays the percentage of patients within each of the 3 diagnostic categories. Thus, 2% (1 patient) of the 46 patients with NTG showed an improvement of >1 dB/year. HTG = high-tension glaucoma; MD = mean deviation; NTG = normal-tension glaucoma; PEXG = pseudoexfoliation glaucoma. (Reprinted from Heijl A, for the Early Manifest Glaucoma Trial Group. Natural history of open-angle glaucoma. *Ophthalmology.* 2009;116:2271-2276, with permission from the American Academy of Ophthalmology.)

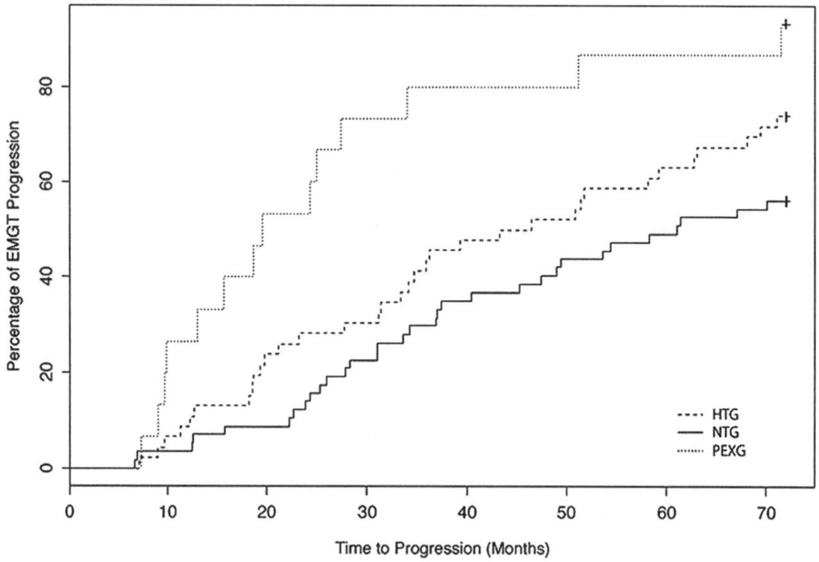

FIGURE 2.—Time to progression in patients with HTG, NTG, and PEXG. The latter progressed faster than the other 2 groups. EMGT = Early Manifest Glaucoma Trial; HTG = high-tension glaucoma; NTG = normal- tension glaucoma; PEXG = pseudoexfoliation glaucoma. (Reprinted from Heijl A, for the Early Manifest Glaucoma Trial Group. Natural history of open-angle glaucoma. *Ophthalmology.* 2009;116:2271-2276, with permission from the American Academy of Ophthalmology.)

−1.08 dB/year overall, −1.31 in HTG, −0.36 in NTG, and −3.13 in PEXG. Differences in median visual function progression rates among groups were statistically significant (NTG vs. HTG, $P = 0.003$; PEXG vs. non-PEXG, $P < 0.001$). Progression was considerably and significantly faster in older than in younger patients ($P = 0.002$). By 6 years, 68% of patients had progressed overall, 74% of those with HTG, 56% of those with NTG, and 93% of those with PEXG ($P = 0.012$). Median time to progression also differed considerably among groups: 19.5 months in PEXG, 44.8 months in HTG, and particularly 61.1 months in NTG ($P < 0.0001$).

Conclusions.—In this 6-year follow-up study, the median untreated rate of progression corresponded to advancing from normal visual function to blindness in approximately 70 years, whereas on the basis of the mean rate, visual function would show the same deterioration in approximately 25 years. Large differences existed among patients and different glaucoma types, with PEXG progressing considerably faster than HTG, and NTG progressing at the lowest rate (Figs 1 and 2).

▶ The Early Manifest Glaucoma Trial (EMGT) compared observation with treatment using betaxolol and laser trabeculoplasty. This trial showed significant benefit to treatment, but as patients were not treated to a target pressure and the average pressure reduction was 20%, the progression rate was high in the treated group.

In the trial reported here, the outcomes of the untreated subjects, 118 control patients, are reported in greater detail. The authors have performed an analysis of the rate of progression without treatment. The sample size is limited, especially as subtypes of glaucoma are evaluated, but the quality of the data in this carefully designed and monitored National Eye Institute-sponsored study is excellent.

The authors found that in this sample, the patients with exfoliative glaucoma got worse most quickly, followed by the patients with high-tension open-angle glaucoma, followed by the patients with normal-tension glaucoma.

The results for the overall group show a mild average rate of progression of the mean deviation (MD) on Humphrey Visual Field (HVF) testing. The mean rate is much higher than the median, indicating that there is a smaller proportion of patients getting worse at a much faster rate. This corresponds to clinical experience, in which many patients are very stable, and a few seem to do very badly. This is why extrapolations based on average rates are not helpful in glaucoma. To illustrate this, consider 2 groups, one in which everyone gets worse than 1-dB per year on MD, and the other in which 90% are stable, but 10% get worse at 10 dB per year. Both have the same average MD, but in the first group, no one goes blind in 10 years. In the second group, 10% of patients are blind in 3 years. Fig 1 shows that indeed most patients in each glaucoma subtype were fairly stable, but that more than 25% of exfoliative and perhaps 15% of high-tension glaucoma subjects were what might be considered fast progressors, with average rates of progression of 2 dB per year or more. Because patients with definite progression were treated (and thus removed from the untreated sample group) and patients with initial intraocular pressure

(IOP) of > 30 mm Hg were excluded from the study, this study may underestimate average progression. In Fig 2 we see that untreated, the march to progression is deliberate.

Glaucoma is a leading cause of blindness worldwide. This study helps us to understand the rate of vision loss in glaucoma and how variable its course can be. Clinical observation of treated and untreated patients remains critical to determine the risk to each patient. Patients who demonstrate rapid progression are at very high risk of symptomatic vision loss and should be treated aggressively.

J. S. Myers, MD

Driving Cessation and Driving Limitation in Glaucoma: The Salisbury Eye Evaluation Project

Ramulu PY, West SK, Munoz B, et al (Johns Hopkins Univ, Baltimore, MD)

Ophthalmology 116:1846-1853, 2009

Objective.—To determine if glaucoma is associated with driving limitation or cessation.

Design.—Cross-sectional analysis within a longitudinal, population-based cohort study.

Participants and Controls.—One thousand one hundred thirty-five ever-drivers between 73 and 93, including 70 subjects with unilateral and 68 subjects with bilateral glaucoma.

Methods.—All subjects reported their driving habits during each of 4 study rounds. During the fourth and final study round, subjects were assessed systematically for the presence of glaucoma.

Main Outcome Measures.—Self-reported driving cessation or driving limitation, including cessation of night driving, driving fewer than 3000 miles annually, or cessation of driving in unfamiliar areas.

Results.—Fifteen percent of subjects without glaucoma no longer were driving at the end of the cohort study, compared with 21% of unilateral glaucoma subjects ($P = 0.2$) and 41% of bilateral glaucoma subjects ($P < 0.001$). Multivariate regression analysis showed that bilateral (odds ratio [OR], 2.6; $P = 0.002$), but not unilateral (OR, 1.5; $P = 0.3$), glaucoma subjects were more likely no longer to be driving when compared with subjects without glaucoma. The odds that bilateral glaucoma subjects no longer were driving doubled for every 5 dB of visual field (VF) worsening in the better eye ($P < 0.001$). Driving cessation within the previous 2 years was analyzed using separate multiple regression models, and both bilateral (OR, 3.6; $P = 0.004$) and unilateral (OR, 2.4; $P = 0.06$) glaucoma subjects were more likely to stop driving over this period than subjects without glaucoma. Driving cessation associated with bilateral glaucoma was present in 0.82% of the population, or 1 in every 122 individuals. Greater numbers of driving limitations were not more likely among subjects with glaucoma than subjects without glaucoma. However, bilateral glaucoma subjects did attribute more driving limitations to difficulties with their vision than subjects without glaucoma (OR, 2.2; $P = 0.02$).

Conclusions.—Bilateral, and possibly unilateral, glaucoma is associated with significantly higher rates of driving cessation among the elderly. The substantial difference in driving patterns seen with different degrees of better-eye VF damage suggests that minimizing VF loss in the better-seeing eye is associated with better functional outcomes.

▶ Driving remains a critical aspect of independence for many people in our society. This study reports on the odds that people in the Salisbury Eye Evaluation Survey stopped driving. People with glaucoma were more likely to stop driving, especially if the glaucoma was bilateral. This is not surprising, although 40% cessation in bilateral glaucoma over 10 years is higher than what might have been predicted.

An interesting finding was that for every 5 dB of increased visual field loss on perimetry, the odds of driving cessation doubled. Often we discuss the risk of glaucoma in terms of the odds of blindness. This study clearly shows that profound impacts to a patient's quality of life occur long before blindness. Functional vision loss, whether visual acuity, contrast sensitivity, or field loss, contributes greatly to activities of daily living.

The requirements for driving vary by state in the United States, as do requirements for reporting drivers who do not meet standards. Many states require at least 20/40 vision for night driving (some allow up to 20/70 during the day) and at least 120 degrees of visual field in the horizontal midline, excluding normal blindspots. These are guidelines for legality, not necessarily safety, and other factors, such as reaction time and concentration, may be just as important.

J. S. Myers, MD

Doctor–Patient Communication in Glaucoma Care: Analysis of Videotaped Encounters in Community-Based Office Practice

Friedman DS, Hahn SR, Quigley HA, et al (Wilmer Eye Inst, Baltimore, MD; Albert Einstein College of Medicine, The Bronx, NY; et al)
Ophthalmology 116:2277-2285, 2009

Purpose.—To assess doctor–patient communication in patients with glaucoma.

Design.—Observational cohort study.

Participants.—Twenty-three ophthalmologists and 50 patients with glaucoma.

Methods.—Doctor–patient encounters were audio- and videotaped and analyzed using validated sociolinguistic approaches. After the visit, the doctor and the patient completed questionnaires, and patients were interviewed using a semistructured, patient-centered protocol.

Main Outcome Measures.—Summary statistics about doctor–patient encounters, assessment of alignment of attitudes between patients and doctors, and patient admission to missing doses.

Results.—Physicians spent an average of 8.0 (standard deviation [SD], 3.1; median, 7.8) minutes in the room with the patient and an average of 5.8 (SD, 2.4; median, 7.5) minutes talking with the patient, delivering 70% of all spoken words and asking two thirds of all questions. Glaucoma-related discussion occupied 50% of talk time and was focused primarily on examinations and treatment (25%). One third of discussions addressed ocular issues other than glaucoma. Virtually all physician questions (94%) were closed ended. Most patient questions were about intraocular pressure (20% of visits), details of the medication regimen (20%), disease status (14%), and testing (12%). Although physicians and patients were aligned in believing that the physician should control the visit agenda, physicians tended to support greater physician control of decision making than did patients. Physicians failed to identify most patients who admitted to missing doses, a surrogate for nonadherence, stating that 10 of 13 in this category were taking drops "all" or "most" of the time. Physician interviews detected 3 of the 11 patients whose postvisit questionnaire indicated missing a dose in the last week compared with 11 of the 11 detected by the postvisit research interview. Patients who stated they had missed doses recently reported being less satisfied with the doctor–patient encounter than those who did not.

Conclusions.—Doctor–patient dialogue was universally physician centered; physicians spoke 70% of the words and asked closed-ended questions that restricted the patient's contribution to "yes/no" or brief responses. A minority of physicians ever asked patients if they had questions. In contrast with the patient-centered research interview, doctors'

TABLE 6.—Example of Doctor-Patient Discussion of Glaucoma: A 61-Year-Old Male Patient with the Ophthalmologist

Doctor	Right now your vision is improved to about 20/40 in that eye. Now the pressure was, at that point last week, 38, which have (sic) been reduced actually from 54, so your medication now you're taking the Lumigan and the Timoptic, right?
Patient	Yeah.
Doctor	And your pressures today are still a little high, 23. We really want you a little lower than that, and we need, when we look at your optic nerve and what have you, we need pressures closer to 15. Okay? In that vicinity. But we're getting there.

TABLE 7.—Doctor–Patient Communication in Assessing Barriers to Adherence

A 76-year-old female patient with the ophthalmologist	
Doctor	Terrific. Okay. Any side effects? Any problems from it?
Patient	No, none at all that I noticed. Nothing.
A 58-year-old male patient with the ophthalmologist	
Doctor	Yeah. So, umm, okay. No side effects? No problems with it?
Patient	No, no.
Doctor	Doesn't bother your eyes?
Patient	A little burning for a couple of minutes, but—
Doctor	But it's tolerable?
Patient	Sure. Not a—not any big deal.
Doctor	Okay. It's—it's tolerable.
Patient	Sure [laughs].
Doctor	It's better—better to use drops that have a little stingy burn than to go blind.
Patient	Yeah, yeah.

physician-centered communication failed to identify most patients who had missed doses (Tables 6 and 7).

▶ This article reports on direct observations of physicians caring for patients with glaucoma. The investigators found that the communication was physician dominated. In follow-up extended interviews with researchers, the patients offered important insights, such as non-adherence, that physicians missed. The investigators suggest that more open-ended questions and a more patient centered discussion could improve communication and care.

As shown in the tables, the conversations were not ideal. In an era in which the volume of care per physician is increasing and is expected to increase much further in the coming decade, it is easy to sympathize with the harried physician. Given that our time with each patient is likely to be further reduced in the future, it is clear that we must make the most of every moment. The suggestions in this article point to a way in which clinicians can be more effective in the time they have by focusing on open-ended questions and by making sure that the patient has a chance to speak and the physician to listen.

J. S. Myers, MD

Silent Cerebral Infarct and Visual Field Progression in Newly Diagnosed Normal-Tension Glaucoma: A Cohort Study

Leung DYL, Tham CCY, Li FCH, et al (The Chinese Univ of Hong Kong)

Ophthalmology 116:1250-1256, 2009

Purpose.—To investigate whether the presence of silent cerebral infarct (SCI) is related to field progression in patients with newly diagnosed normal-tension glaucoma (NTG).

Design.—Prospective cohort study.

Participants.—A total of 286 eyes from 286 NTG patients: 64 with SCI (SCI+) and 222 without SCI (SCI−).

Methods.—Patients were assigned to the SCI+ or SCI− group depending on the presence of SCI as detected by cranial computed tomography scan at baseline. Patients were followed-up at 4-month intervals for 36 months for visual field progression as per Anderson's criteria.

Main Outcome Measures.—The primary outcome was the association between SCI and field progression. Secondary outcomes include the prevalence of SCI in NTG patients and other risk factors associated with progression.

Results.—There were no significant differences in the baseline intraocular pressures (IOPs), fluctuation amplitude of pretreatment IOP, baseline visual acuity, vertical cup-to-disc ratio, vertical disc diameter, presenting field indices, and central corneal thickness (CCT) between the 2 groups. Patients with SCI were significantly older compared with SCI− patients (72.4 ± 10.7 vs. 63.2 ± 14.2 years; P<0.001). Univariate analyses revealed age, fluctuation amplitude of pretreatment IOP, thinner CCT, presence of disc hemorrhage, systemic hypertension, arrhythmia, and SCI were significant for field progression. Silent cerebral infarct was present in 29.6% of field-progressed subjects versus 15.3% of field-stable

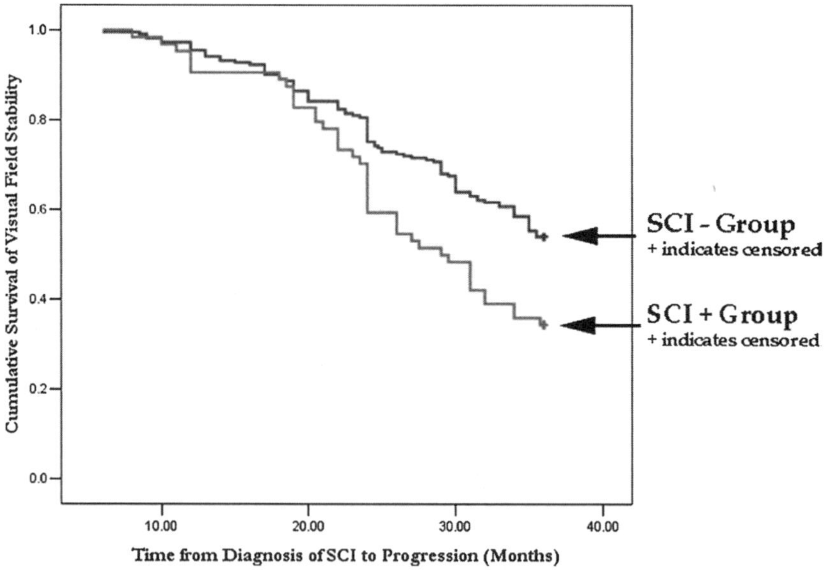

FIGURE 1.—Kaplan-Meier survival analysis for visual field stability in patients with silent cerebral infarct (SCI+) and without silent cerebral infarct (SCI−). A test of equality of survival distributions with Mantel-Cox log rank (P = 0.003), Breslow statistics (P = 0.004), and Tarone-Ware (P = 0.003) statistics showed a significant difference in survival between the 2 groups. (Reprinted from Leung DYL, Tham CCY, Li FCH, et al. Silent cerebral infarct and visual field progression in newly diagnosed normal-tension glaucoma: a cohort study. *Ophthalmology.* 2009;116:1250-1256, with permission from the American Academy of Ophthalmology.)

subjects ($P = 0.004$). Kaplan-Meier survival analysis revealed that 65.6% of SCI+ versus 45.9% of SCI– patients had progressed ($P = 0.003$). Cox proportional hazards regression analysis showed disc hemorrhage (hazard ratio [HR], 2.28; 95% confidence interval [CI], 1.54–3.37; $P<0.001$), SCI (HR, 1.61; 95% CI, 1.09–2.36; $P = 0.016$), systemic hypertension (HR, 1.48; 95% CI, 1.04–2.10; $P = 0.029$), and CCT (per 30 μm of thinning; HR, 1.35; 95% CI, 1.16–1.75; $P<0.001$) were associated with field progression. Other variables significant in the univariate analysis were not significant in the regression model. The most common location of SCI was at the basal ganglia.

Conclusions.—Presence of SCI may be an independent risk factor for visual field progression in patients with NTG.

▶ This article reports on a study of subjects with normal-tension glaucoma who were, prospectively, followed for progressive visual field loss. The study is closely modeled after the Collaborative Normal-Tension Glaucoma Study. In this study, however, the 2 comparison groups are those with a silent cerebral infarct on imaging and those without a silent cerebral infarct on imaging.

The results show that in this group of patients, subjects with a previous silent cerebral infarct were more likely to have progressive glaucomatous field loss (Fig 1).

This study again shows a potential link between vascular pathology and glaucoma. However, there are 2 serious concerns regarding this study.

(1) These patients were untreated. It is completely unknown whether these findings would be true in treated patients. Thus, the clinical utility of this study is limited at best.

(2) The recruitment of subjects with known normal-tension glaucoma into a protocol in which 286 patients were purposely not treated is concerning. The authors state that this study was reviewed by ethics committees, "followed the principles in the Declaration of Helsinki and International Conference on Harmonization–Good Clinical Practice (ICH–GCP) guidelines, and informed consent was obtained from all patients." However, the findings of the Collaborative Normal-Tension Glaucoma Treatment Study suggest that in American patients (these patients were Asian) the risk of progression is 3-fold higher when untreated. Were the subjects informed of this?

Ideally, in studies in which patients are put at greater risk of adverse outcomes, the patients are fully aware and the scientific question has direct clinical relevance to the treatment of the disease.

J. S. Myers, MD

Open-Angle Glaucoma and the Risk of Stroke Development: A 5-Year Population-Based Follow-Up Study

Ho J-D, Hu C-C, Lin H-C (Taipei Med Univ Hosp, Taiwan; Shin Kong Wu-Ho Su Memorial Hosp, Taipei, Taiwan; Taipei Med Univ, Taiwan)

Stroke 40:2685-2690, 2009

Background and Purpose.—Although open-angle glaucoma (OAG) is associated with some of the risk factors of stroke development, there is still no published study addressing whether OAG increases the risk of stroke development. We investigated the risk of stroke development after a diagnosis of OAG.

Methods.—Data were retrospectively collected from the Taiwan National Health Insurance Research Database, which is comprised of 1 073 891 random subjects from among Taiwan's 23 million residents. The study cohort comprised all patients with a diagnosis of OAG (International Classification of Diseases, 9th Revision, Clinical Modification code 365.1 to 365.11) in 2001 (n = 4032). The comparison cohort was comprised of randomly selected patients (5 for every patient with OAG, n = 20 160) matched with the study group in terms of age, gender, geographic location, and comorbid medical disorders. Patients were tracked from their index visits for 5 years. Cox proportional hazard regression was used to compute the 5-year stroke-free survival rate after adjusting for possible confounding factors.

Results.—Stroke developed in 14.9% of patients with OAG and 9.5% of patients in the comparison cohort during the 5-year follow-up period. Patients with OAG had significantly lower 5-year stroke-free survival rates than patients in the comparison cohort. After adjusting for patients' demographic characteristics and selected comorbidities, patients with OAG were found to have a 1.52-fold (95% CI, 1.40 to 1.72) higher risk of having a stroke than the matched comparison cohort.

Conclusions.—Patients with OAG demonstrated a significantly increased risk of stroke development during the 5-year follow-up period.

▶ This retrospective analysis of a database of Taiwanese shows increased rates of stroke in persons with primary open-angle glaucoma (POAG) compared with those without glaucoma. The risk was about 50% greater in glaucoma subjects, and this increased risk was seen even after adjustment for hypertension and diabetes (Table 3). A retrospective database study such as this is subject to many potential biases, but the authors discuss this and it is unlikely these results are purely chance or artifact.

It is unclear why this association exists. The Blue Mountains Eye Study and the Barbados Eye Study both showed increased cardiovascular mortality in glaucoma patients, although only for timolol-treated patients in the latter. In this study, the patients using topical beta-blockers were not seen to have a different stroke risk than those using other medications.

Beyond eye medications, the pathophysiologic connection is not obvious. Many studies have shown that abnormal blood pressure increases the risk of

TABLE 3.—Adjusted HR for Stroke During the 5-Year Follow-Up Period for Patients With OAG as Compared With Patients in the Comparison Cohort, Stratified by Hypertension and Diabetes

	Stroke			
Variables	Patients With Hypertension Adjusted HR* (95% CI)	Patients Without Hypertension Adjusted HR* (95% CI)	Patients Without Diabetes Adjusted HR† (95% CI)	Patients Without Diabetes Adjusted HR† (95% CI)
Cohort				
OAG	1.23‡ (1.02–1.52)	2.05§ (1.73–2.42)	1.20‡ (1.01–1.43)	1.60§ (1.42–1.81)
Comparison	1.00	1.00	1.00	1.00

*Adjusted for gender, age, diabetes, hyperlipidemia, CHD, and geographic region.
†Adjusted for gender, age, hypertension, hyperlipidemia, CHD, and geographic region.
‡$P<0.05$.
§$P<0.001$.

glaucoma, and this could be a common link. However, the association here was even stronger in patients without hypertension.

Underlying vascular abnormalities may be a common pathophysiologic mechanism. Retinal arteriolar narrowing has long been recognized in glaucoma, and this has been associated with vascular abnormalities elsewhere in the body, some of which are also associated with stroke. Another study saw increased rates of glaucoma progression in subjects with silent cerebral infarcts.[1]

This article does not clearly show what, if any, clinical actions should be taken based on these findings. The risk is not high enough to warrant stroke prophylaxis in those with glaucoma. However, in patients with glaucoma, perhaps this suggests that borderline risks for stroke, such as borderline hypertension or diabetes, should be monitored more closely or treated earlier.

J. S. Myers, MD

Reference

1. Leung DY, Tham CC, Li FC, Kwong YY, Chi SC, Lam DS. Silent cerebral infarct and visual field progression in newly diagnosed normal-tension glaucoma: a cohort study. *Ophthalmology*. 2009;116:1250-1256.

Relationship of Incident Glaucoma versus Physical Activity and Fitness in Male Runners

Williams PT (Donner Laboratory, Berkeley, CA)
Med Sci Sports Exerc 41:1566-1572, 2009

Purpose.—To assess the dose–response relationship of vigorous physical activity (running distance, $km \cdot d^{-1}$) or cardiorespiratory fitness (meters-per-second pace during a 10-km footrace) to the risk for incident glaucoma.

Design.—Prospective epidemiologic cohort study.

Methods.—Participant-reported, physician-diagnosed incident glaucoma was compared with distance run per week and 10-km footrace performance in a cohort of 29,854 male runners without diabetes followed prospectively for 7.7 yr. The survival analyses were adjusted for age, hypertension, current and past cigarette use, and intakes of meat, fish, fruit, and alcohol.

Results.—Two hundred incident glaucoma cases were reported during follow-up. The risk for reported glaucoma decreased 37% per meter per second increment in a 10-km race performance ($P = 0.005$). Relative to the least fit men (i.e., slowest, $\leq 3.5\ m \cdot s^{-1}$), the risk for incident-reported glaucoma declined 29% in those who ran 3.6–4.0 $m \cdot s^{-1}$ ($P = 0.06$), 54% for those who ran 4.1–4.5 $m \cdot s^{-1}$ ($P = 0.001$), 51% for those who ran 4.6–5.0 $m \cdot s^{-1}$ ($P = 0.04$), and glaucoma was nonexistent among the 781 men who exceeded 5.0 $m \cdot s^{-1}$ ($P = 0.03$). The risk for incident, reported glaucoma decreased 5% per kilometer per day run at baseline ($P = 0.04$), which remained significant when adjusted for the 10-km race performance (5% reduction per kilometer per day, $P = 0.04$), and both body mass index and race performance ($P = 0.04$). Baseline hypertension was unrelated to the incident glaucoma.

Conclusions.—These data provide preliminary evidence that vigorous physical activity may reduce glaucoma risk, which, in the absence of medical record validation, could represent ocular hypertension in addition to frank glaucoma. Additional follow-up with validation is needed to identify the type of glaucoma affected.

▶ This prospective study of 29 000 male runners tracked incident self-reported glaucoma diagnosis, which occurred in 200 men. In short, runners who ran more and ran quicker were less likely to develop glaucoma.

Patients with glaucoma and at-risk family members are constantly asking whether diet or lifestyle modifications will improve their risks. Other studies have suggested that eye pressure is lower in many with regular exercise. Although there are many potential confounding factors in a nonrandomized study on a self-reported diagnosis, this study suggests that vigorous physical exercise may play a role in reducing the risk.

J. S. Myers, MD

Viscocanalostomy versus trabeculectomy for primary open angle glaucoma: 4-year prospective randomized clinical trial

Gilmour DF, Manners TD, Devonport H, et al (St James's Univ Hosp, Leeds, UK; York District Hosp, UK; Bradford Infirmary, UK; et al)

Eye 23:1802-1807, 2009

Aims.—The purpose of this randomized clinical trial was to compare the effectiveness and safety of viscocanalostomy (visco) with trabeculectomy (trab) in the management of primary open angle glaucoma (POAG).

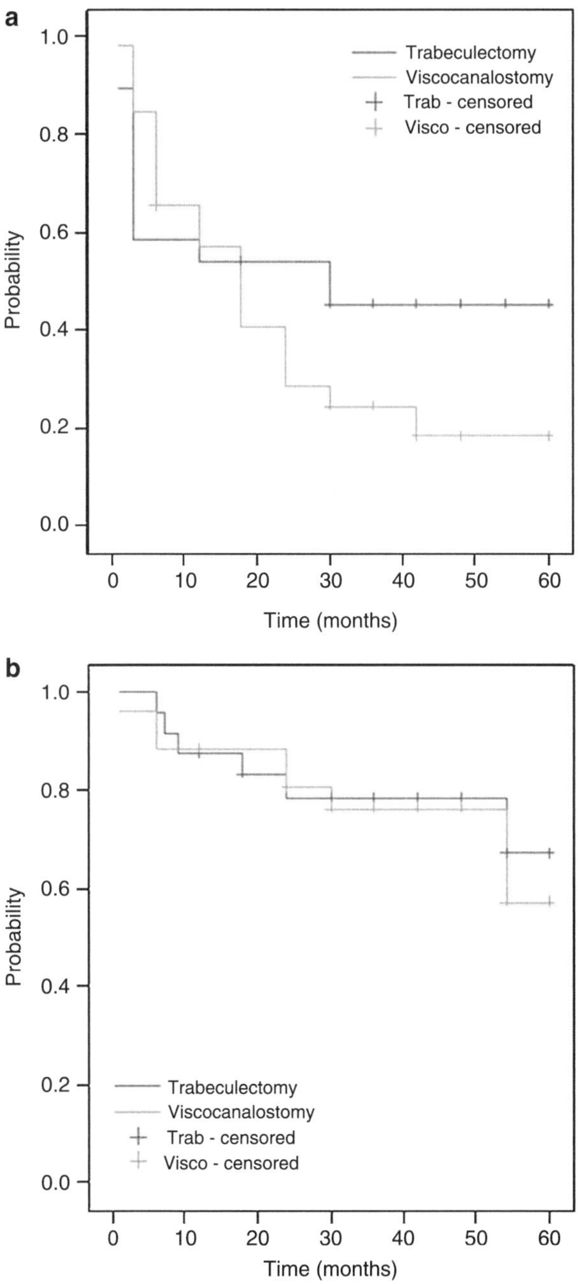

FIGURE 2.—(a) Cumulative probability of complete success (IOP below 18 mm Hg without medication) in eyes having trabeculectomy and viscocanalostomy ($P = 0.3063$). (b) Cumulative probability of qualified success (IOP below 18 mm Hg with or without medication) in eyes having trabeculectomy and viscocanalostomy ($P = 0.7459$). (Reprinted from Gilmour DF, Manners TD, Devonport H, et al. Viscocanalostomy versus trabeculectomy for primary open angle glaucoma: 4-year prospective randomized clinical trial. *Eye*. 2009;23:1802-1807.)

Methods.—Patients were randomized to have a viscocanalostomy (25 eyes) or a trabeculectomy (25 eyes) performed by one surgeon (TDM) and followed up prospectively. Patients were examined preoperatively, at day 1, day 3 if required, day 6, week 2 and thereafter as near as possible to 1, 3, 6, 12, 18, 24, 30, 36, 48, 54, and 60 months. We recorded intraocular pressure (IOP), presence or absence of any complications, presence and description of any bleb, visual acuity with glasses, and full examinations as routine to monitor any progression of the glaucoma. Bleb interventions including needling and antimetabolites were allowed and recorded in both groups. YAG laser goniopuncture was allowed in the viscocanalostomy group.

Results.—Mean follow-up was 40 months (SD 15), with a range from 6 to 60 months. Forty-two percent ($n = 10$) of the patients in the trabeculectomy group had a successful outcome (IOP < 18 mm Hg with no treatment) at last follow-up visit, compared to 21% ($n = 5$) in the viscocanalostomy group. IOP was lower in the trab group with differences in IOP being statistically significant at month 12 ($P = <0.001$), 24 ($P = 0.001$), 30 ($P = 0.030$), 36 ($P = <0.001$), and 48 ($P = 0.018$). The trabeculectomy group required less postoperative topical IOP-lowering medication ($P = 0.011$).

Conclusion.—In this study, we found trabeculectomy to be more effective at lowering IOP than viscocanalostomy in POAG patients (Fig 2).

▶ This study compares trabeculectomy with viscocanalostomy. It reports more long term follow-up than some of the previous single-year studies. In this study, a qualified success consisting of IOP < 18 mm Hg with medications showed a similar survival curve for both groups (Fig 2). However, success without medications favored the trabeculectomy group.

Viscocanalostomy was advanced as a method to lower IOP with fewer postoperative complications and simpler postoperative management. In this study, there was more hypotony in early postoperative period in the trabeculectomy group, but the groups were otherwise similar in complications. The trabeculectomy group had a better overall result for pressure control.

Often, new surgeries are reported with great enthusiasm and then fade quietly away. Fewer clinicians are using viscocanalostomy now, including some of its original strongest proponents. It appears that the technique, which is technically more demanding than trabeculectomy and still results in a filtering bleb in many cases, has not yet delivered the ideal balance of efficacy and safety.

J. S. Myers, MD

Two-Year Survival of Ahmed Valve Implantation in the First 2 Years of Life with and without Intraoperative Mitomycin-C

Al-Mobarak F, Khan AO (The King Khaled Eye Specialist Hosp, Riyadh, Saudi Arabia)

Ophthalmology 116:1862-1865, 2009

Purpose.—To evaluate the effect of intraoperative mitomycin-C (MMC) on polypropylene Ahmed glaucoma valve (AGV) survival 2 years after implantation during the first 2 years of life.

Design.—Retrospective institutional comparative series (1995–2005).

Participants.—Thirty-one eyes of 27 patients (23 unilateral, 4 bilateral; 16 boys, 11 girls) undergoing AGV implantation at a mean age of 11.1 months (standard deviation [SD], 5.46), all of which had 2 years of regular postoperative follow-up. MMC was applied intraoperatively in those cases in the area of AGV implantation in 16 (52%) and was not applied in 15 (48%). In some eyes, MMC was applied intraoperatively in cases done by the surgeons who routinely used MMC for all AGV implantation in young children.

Methods.—Failure was defined as intraocular pressure (IOP) > 22 mmHg with or without glaucoma medications, the need for an additional procedure for IOP control, or the occurrence of significant complications (e.g., endophthalmitis, retinal detachment, persistent hypotony [IOP < 5 mmHg]). Survival was the absence of failure.

Main Outcome Measures.—Failure or significant complications as defined.

Results.—Mean survival for the non-MMC eyes (22.15 months; standard error [SE], 1.93) was significantly longer than survival for the MMC eyes (16.25 months; SE, 2.17) by the log-rank test ($P = 0.025$). The difference in cumulative survival at 2 years was also significantly different by log-rank test ($P = 0.001$): 80.0% (SE 10.3) and 31.3% (SE 11.6), respectively.

Conclusions.—Rather than improved survival, intraoperative use of MMC was associated with shorter survival 2 years after AGV implantation during the first 2 years of life. We speculate that MMC-induced tissue death can stimulate a reactive fibrosis around the AGV in very young eyes (Fig 1).

▶ Juvenile glaucoma is an extremely challenging disease to manage. Although many children do well with primary goniotomy or trabeculotomy, those eyes with more complicated glaucomas often do quite poorly.

In this article, mitomycin was not effective in prolonging Ahmed tube shunt success, and in fact it was associated with a shorter duration of success. Given the many risks associated with mitomycin use, without clear indication of its effectiveness in this surgery mitomycin use is not warranted.

It should be noted that this is a retrospective study, and thus may be biased. If clinicians only used mitomycin in eyes that were judged to be at higher risk of failure, then failure may be related more to the baseline characteristics of the

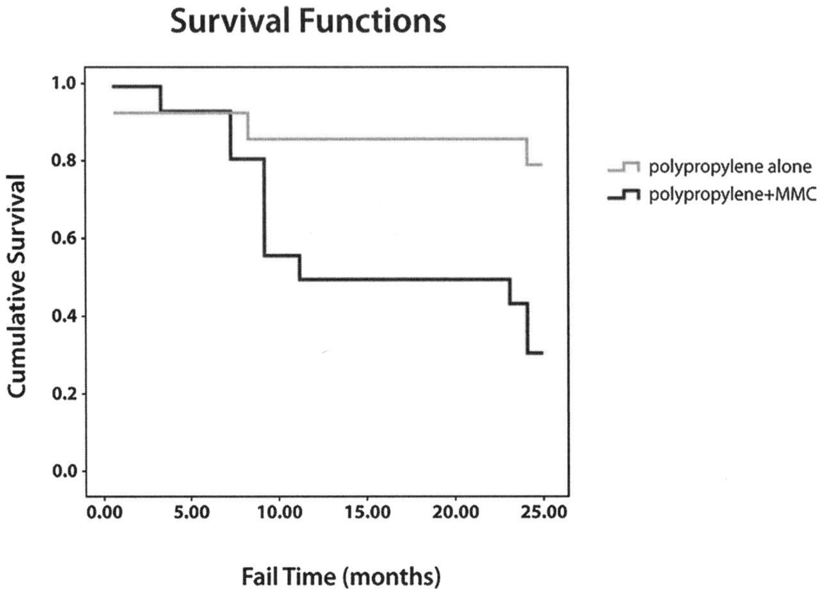

FIGURE 1.—Survival curves for polypropylene Ahmed glaucoma valve implantation with intraoperative mitomycin-C (polypropylene + MMC) and without intraoperative mitomycin-C (polypropylene alone) application show a greater survival at 24 months for the latter group. (Reprinted from Al-Mobarak F, Khan AO. Two-year survival of Ahmed valve implantation in the first 2 years of life with and without intraoperative mitomycin-C. *Ophthalmology.* 2009;116:1862-1865, with permission from the American Academy of Ophthalmology.)

eyes and not to the mitomycin use. However, the authors did not have this impression after careful review of the data and the practicing patterns of the clinicians in the trial.

J. S. Myers, MD

Three-Year Follow-up of the Tube Versus Trabeculectomy Study

Gedde SJ, Schiffman JC, Feuer WJ, et al (Univ of Miami, FL; et al)
Am J Ophthalmol 148:670-684, 2009

Purpose.—To report 3-year results of the Tube Versus Trabeculectomy (TVT) Study.

Design.—Multicenter randomized clinical trial.

Methods.—Setting: Seventeen clinical centers.

Study Population.—Patients 18 to 85 years of age who had previous trabeculectomy, cataract extraction with intraocular lens implantation, or both and uncontrolled glaucoma with intraocular pressure (IOP) $\geq$ 18 mm Hg and $\leq$40 mm Hg on maximum tolerated medical therapy.

Interventions.—A 350-mm^2 Baerveldt glaucoma implant or trabeculectomy with mitomycin C (MMC 0.4 mg/ml for 4 minutes).

Main Outcome Measures.—IOP, visual acuity, use of supplemental medical therapy, surgical complications, and failure (IOP > 21 mm Hg or not reduced by 20%, IOP ≤ 5 mm Hg, reoperation for glaucoma, or loss of light perception vision).

Results.—A total of 212 eyes of 212 patients were enrolled, including 107 in the tube group and 105 in the trabeculectomy group. At 3 years, IOP (mean ± standard deviation [SD]) was 13.0 ± 4.9 mm Hg in the tube group and 13.3 ± 6.8 mm Hg in the trabeculectomy group (P =.78). The number of glaucoma medications (mean ± SD) was 1.3 ± 1.3 in the tube group and 1.0 ± 1.5 in the trabeculectomy group (P =.30). The cumulative probability of failure during the first 3 years of follow-up was 15.1% in the tube group and 30.7% in the trabeculectomy group (P =.010; hazards ratio, 2.2; 95% confidence interval, 1.2 to 4.1). Postoperative complications developed in 42 patients (39%) in the tube group and 63 patients (60%) in the trabeculectomy group (P =.004). Surgical complications were associated with reoperation and/or loss of ≥2 Snellen lines in 24 patients (22%) in the tube group and 28 patients (27%) in the trabeculectomy group (P =.58).

Conclusions.—Tube shunt surgery had a higher success rate compared to trabeculectomy with MMC during the first 3 years of follow-up in the TVT Study. Both procedures were associated with similar IOP reduction and use of supplemental medical therapy at 3 years. While the incidence of postoperative complications was higher following

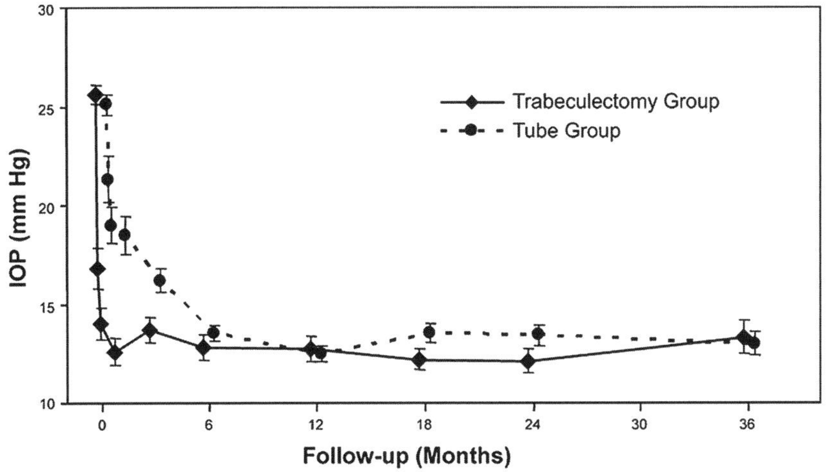

FIGURE 2.—Distribution of intraocular pressure (IOP) at baseline and follow-up in the TVT Study. Data are presented as mean ± standard error of the mean and are censored after a reoperation for glaucoma. (Reprinted from Gedde SJ, Schiffman JC, Feuer WJ, et al. Three-year follow-up of the tube versus trabeculectomy study. *Am J Ophthalmol.* 2009;148:670-684, with permission from Elsevier.)

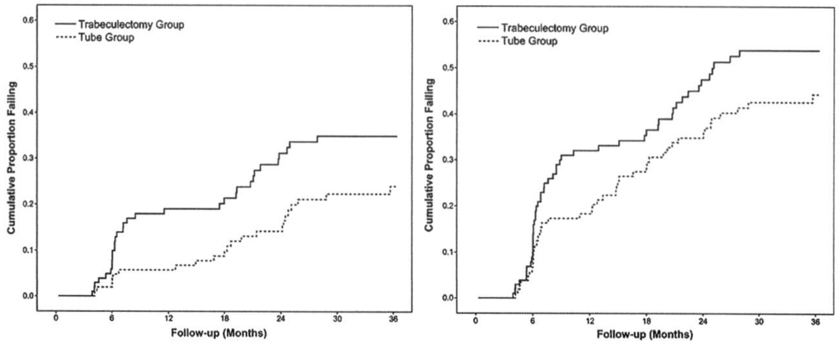

FIGURE 4.—Kaplan-Meier plots of the cumulative probability of failure in the TVT Study defining inadequate intraocular (IOP) reduction as IOP > 17 mm Hg or not reduced by 20% below baseline (Left) or IOP > 14 mm Hg (Right). Inadequate IOP reduction criteria must be present on two consecutive visits after 3 months to qualify as failure. Patients with persistent hypotony, reoperation for glaucoma, and loss of light perception vision are classified as failures. (Reprinted from Gedde SJ, Schiffman JC, Feuer WJ, et al. Three-year follow-up of the tube versus trabeculectomy study. *Am J Ophthalmol.* 2009;148:670-684, with permission from Elsevier.)

TABLE 4.—Reasons for Treatment Failure During Three Years of Follow-up in the Tube Versus Trabeculectomy Study[a]

	Tube Group, n (%) (n = 15)	Trabeculectomy Group, n (%) (n = 28)
Inadequate IOP reduction[b]	7 (47)	10 (36)[d]
Reoperation for glaucoma	6 (40)	9 (32)
Persistent hypotony[c]	2 (13)	8 (29)
Loss of light perception	0	1 (4)

IOP = intraocular pressure.
[a]P = .71 for the difference in distribution of reasons for failure between treatment groups (exact permutation χ^2 test).
[b]IOP >21 mm Hg or not reduced by 20% below baseline on two consecutive follow-up visits after 3 months.
[c]IOP ≤5 mm Hg on two consecutive follow-up visits after 3 months.
[d]Three patients underwent reoperation for glaucoma subsequent to failure because of inadequate IOP reduction.

trabeculectomy with MMC relative to tube shunt surgery, most complications were transient and self-limited.

▶ This major study compares tube shunts (Baerveldts) to trabeculectomy with mitomycin in eyes that underwent surgery previously. This trial considers an earlier role for tube shunt surgery, as opposed to its historic role as a treatment following failure of 1 or more trabeculectomies.

In this trial, the trabeculectomy group had nonsignificant lower pressures, with significantly less medication over the first year, but the results were equivalent by year 3 in terms of average pressure and number of medications (Fig 2).

The failure rate of the trabeculectomy group was higher as time went on than that of the tube shunt group (Fig 4). About a third of trabeculectomy failures were for hypotony (Table 4).

The complications were impressive (Table 7). The rates of occurrence of shallow chambers and wound leaks in the trabeculectomy group were higher

TABLE 7.—Postoperative Complications During Three Years of Follow-up in the Tube Versus Trabeculectomy Study[a]

	Tube Group, n (%) (n = 107)	Trabeculectomy Group, n (%) (n = 105)
Early postoperative complications[b]		
Choroidal effusion	15 (14)	14 (13)
Shallow or flat anterior chamber	11 (10)	10 (10)
Wound leak	1 (1)	12 (11)
Hyphema	2 (2)	8 (8)
Aqueous misdirection	3 (3)	1 (1)
Suprachoroidal hemorrhage	2 (2)	3 (3)
Vitreous hemorrhage	1 (1)	1 (1)
Decompression retinopathy	0	1 (1)
Cystoid macular edema	0	1 (1)
Late postoperative complications[c]		
Persistent corneal edema	10 (9)	6 (6)
Dysesthesia	1 (1)	8 (8)
Encapsulated bleb	2 (2)	6 (6)
Choroidal effusion	2 (2)	4 (4)
Cystoid macular edema	5 (5)	1 (1)
Hypotony maculopathy	1 (1)	4 (4)
Persistent diplopia	5 (5)	0
Bleb leak	0	5 (5)
Tube erosion	5 (5)	—
Endophthalmitis/blebitis	1 (1)	3 (3)
Chronic or recurrent iritis	2 (2)	1 (1)
Tube obstruction	3 (3)	—
Retinal detachment	1 (1)	1 (1)
Corneal ulcer	0	1 (1)
Shallow or flat anterior chamber	1 (1)	0
Total number of patients with postoperative complications[d,e]	42 (39)	63 (60)

[a]Data censored after a reoperation for glaucoma.
[b]Onset ≤1 month.
[c]Onset >1 month.
[d]Some patients had more than one complication.
[e]$P = .004$ for the difference in total number of patients with postoperative complications between treatment groups (χ^2 test).

than some might expect. Corneal edema and eye movement abnormalities (9% each of tube eyes) were also quite common in the tube group.

How should this trial influence practice patterns? That is not clear. Some glaucoma specialists have seen this as a reason to use tube shunts earlier. Other specialists have not been convinced, noting several reservations. First, as noted, the complication rate was higher in this series, and the trabeculectomies were not a standardized approach. Declaring 2 visits with an intraocular pressure (IOP) of 5 mm Hg or less as a failure of trabeculectomy (even in the presence of normal vision) may also have skewed the results. Many clinicians would rather cope with bleb dysesthesia than with eye movement abnormalities. Patients who fail a trabeculectomy can be treated with tube shunts, but the reverse is not usually the case. In young patients, maintaining options for the future may be an important consideration.

Thus, there is no clear consensus. However, even before this trial was completed many in the glaucoma community were using tube shunts at earlier stages in the treatment paradigm, and this study validates that good results can be achieved with excellent pressures for patients receiving tube shunts.

J. S. Myers, MD

Comparison of long-term surgical success of Ahmed Valve implant versus trabeculectomy in open-angle glaucoma

Tran DH, Souza C, Ang MJ, et al (Univ of California Los Angeles)

Br J Ophthalmol 93:1504-1509, 2009

Aim.—To compare the long-term intraocular pressure (IOP) outcomes of Ahmed Glaucoma Valve (AGV) implantation to trabeculectomy with mitomycin C (MMC) in open-angle glaucoma (OAG).

Methods.—78 OAG patients who underwent AGV implantation were matched with respect to age, preoperative surgery, preoperative IOP and preoperative medicines to 88 OAG patients who underwent trabeculectomy with MMC with a minimum of 3 years' follow-up. The cumulative probability of success between the two groups with different criteria was analysed: (1) an IOP≤21 mm Hg and a reduction of IOP≥15% from baseline; and (2) an IOP≤18 mm Hg and a reduction of IOP≥20% from baseline. No loss of light perception, no additional glaucoma surgery and no hypotony were also required.

Results.—The 5-year cumulative probability of success was not statistically significant between eyes that had an AGV or trabeculectomy with MMC when success was defined as criteria A ($p = 0.094$). However, when success was defined according to criteria B, eyes undergoing trabeculectomy with MMC had a higher rate of success ($p = 0.024$).

Conclusions.—Trabeculectomy with MMC has a significantly higher 5-year cumulative probability of success compared with AGV implants when greater reduction IOP is necessary (Figs 1 and 2).

▶ Recent studies have focused attention on the choice between tube shunts and trabeculectomy in the surgical management of glaucoma. This retrospective study of Ahmed tube shunt versus trabeculectomy with mitomycin found that trabeculectomy was much more likely to reduce intraocular pressure (IOP) and require fewer postoperative medications.

The first criteria, intraocular pressure less than or equal to 21 mm Hg and a 15% reduction from baseline, deserves discussion. Although some might consider this as the minimal standard of efficacy for a drug, this is insufficient to justify classification as a surgical success for the vast majority of patients undergoing glaucoma surgery. Research in the last 10 years demonstrates that patient with disc damage or field loss do better with IOPs in the mid to low teens. For ocular hypertension or very early glaucoma, this may be sufficient, but for most patients who come to surgery, a lower goal is required. The authors provide several other more stringent criteria for analysis, and in these trabeculectomy was more effective. Most surgical studies now focus on goals of IOP of 18 mm Hg or less and a 20% or greater reduction in pressure.

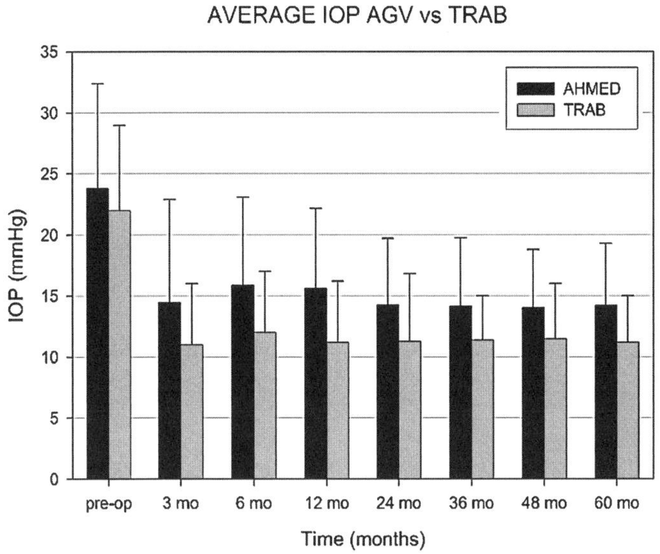

FIGURE 1.—Mean (SD) intraocular pressure (IOP, mm Hg) preoperative and during follow-up. AGV, Ahmed Glaucoma Valve; TRAB, trabeculectomy. (Reprinted from Tran DH, Souza C, Ang MJ, et al. Comparison of long-term surgical success of Ahmed valve implant versus trabeculectomy in open-angle glaucoma. *Br J Ophthalmol.* 2009;93:1504-1509, with permission from the BMJ Publishing Group Ltd.)

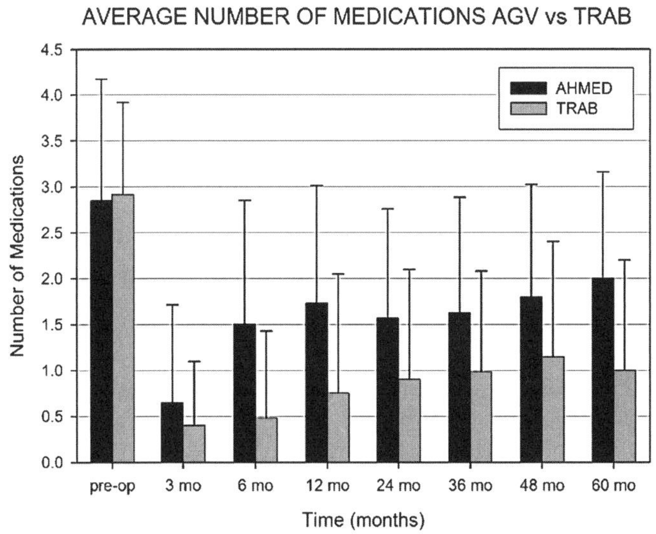

FIGURE 2.—Mean (SD) number of medications preoperative and during follow-up. AGV, Ahmed Glaucoma Valve; TRAB, trabeculectomy. (Reprinted from Tran DH, Souza C, Ang MJ, et al. Comparison of long-term surgical success of Ahmed valve implant versus trabeculectomy in open-angle glaucoma. *Br J Ophthalmol.* 2009;93:1504-1509, with permission from the BMJ Publishing Group Ltd.)

This is a retrospective study, and among its limitations is that despite the authors' attempts, these 2 groups may not have been well matched, and this might favor the trabeculectomy group. Thus, this study is one more to consider but is not a definitive answer. Often, individual patient characteristics, such as conjunctival scarring, may dominate the consideration of tube versus trabeculectomy.

J. S. Myers, MD

Visual Acuity and Intraocular Pressure after Descemet's Stripping Endothelial Keratoplasty in Eyes with and without Preexisting Glaucoma

Vajaranant TS, Price MO, Price FW, et al (Univ of Illinois at Chicago; Cornea Res Foundation of America, Indianapolis, IN; Price Vision Group, Indianapolis, IN; et al)

Ophthalmology 116:1644-1650, 2009

Purpose.—(1) To characterize the pattern of intraocular pressure (IOP) changes after Descemet's stripping endothelial keratoplasty (DSEK) in patients without preexisting glaucoma and in those with preexisting glaucoma, with and without prior glaucoma surgery. (2) To compare vision and IOP outcomes among the 3 groups.

Design.—A retrospective chart review.

Participants.—A total of 805 DSEK cases performed in 641 patients by a single surgeon from December 2003 to August 2007 were available in the database. Only the first-treated eye of each patient with at least 1-year follow-up was included. Four hundred cases qualified: 315 eyes had no glaucoma (C); 64 eyes had glaucoma with no previous glaucoma surgery (G); and 21 eyes had prior glaucoma surgery (GS). Eyes with preexisting retinal problems were included in the analysis.

Methods.—Data analysis included calculation of incidence of postoperative IOP elevation. The study criteria for postoperative IOP elevation were IOP ≥24 mmHg or IOP increase ≥10 mmHg from baseline. Kruskal-Wallis test was used to compare visual acuity (VA) and IOP among the 3 groups preoperatively and at 1-, 3-, 6-, and 12-month postoperative visits.

Main Outcome Measures.—Visual acuity (Snellen) and IOP (millimeters of mercury).

Results.—The incidence of postoperative IOP elevation by the study criteria was 35%, 45%, and 43% for groups C, G, and GS, respectively. Elevated IOP was medically managed by initiating or increasing glaucoma medications or reducing steroids in 27%, 44%, and 38% of the patients in groups C, G, and GS, respectively. A subsequent glaucoma procedure was performed in 0.3%, 5%, and 19% of patients in groups C, G, and GS, respectively. Only the control group had statistically significant IOP elevation at 12 months (median increase of 2 mmHg) when compared with baseline ($P < 0.0001$). All 3 groups had statistically significant improvement in vision at 12 months when compared with baseline

(12-month median VA = 20/40 for C and G; and 20/50 for GS, $P < 0.0001$).

Conclusions.—All groups had a substantial incidence of IOP elevation after DSEK. Close monitoring of IOP is warranted. In this cohort, preexisting glaucoma did not seem to have a negative effect on VA after DSEK.

▶ This study reports a large cohort of patients undergoing Descemet's stripping endothelial keratoplasty (DSEK) and examines the incidence of intraocular pressure (IOP) elevation following DSEK in eyes with and without glaucoma. The eyes with glaucoma had only a slightly higher incidence of IOP elevation but required surgery to address this much more frequently. The eyes without glaucoma required surgery for IOP elevations in 0.3% of cases; for medically controlled glaucoma, surgery was required in 5%, and for eyes with previous glaucoma surgery, additional surgery was required in 19%.

Causes of IOP elevation after DSEK include angle closure, often related to air bubble and pupil block issues, inflammation including graft rejection, and steroid induced glaucoma. The delayed time course of peak IOP at 3 months suggests that the steroid mechanism is most likely.

Eyes with glaucoma are more complicated and difficult in many ways. Glaucoma treatment increases the rate of cataract development and the surgical risks are higher. Glaucoma and its treatment, including surgery, also increase the risk of endothelial decompensation, and it also appears that the complications following DSEK are higher as well. Surgeons should consider these issues carefully in their therapeutic decisions and discussions with patients.

J. S. Myers, MD

Changes in Corneal Endothelial Cells after Ahmed Glaucoma Valve Implantation: 2-Year Follow-up

Lee E-K, Yun Y-J, Lee J-E, et al (Chungnam Natl Univ, Daejeon, Korea; et al)
Am J Ophthalmol 148:361-367, 2009

Purpose.—To evaluate changes in corneal endothelial cells after Ahmed glaucoma valve (AGV) implantation for the treatment of refractory glaucoma.

Design.—Observational case series.

Methods.—We prospectively evaluated the change in density and shape of the corneal endothelium in 41 patients (41 eyes) who had undergone AGV implantation for the treatment of refractory glaucoma. Corneal specular microscopy was performed on the superior, supratemporal, supranasal, and central areas with a noncontact specular microscope before surgery and 1, 6, 12, 18, and 24 months after surgery. The changes at each time point were compared with those at baseline and with those of the control group, which consisted of 20 contralateral glaucomatous eyes receiving antiglaucoma medications.

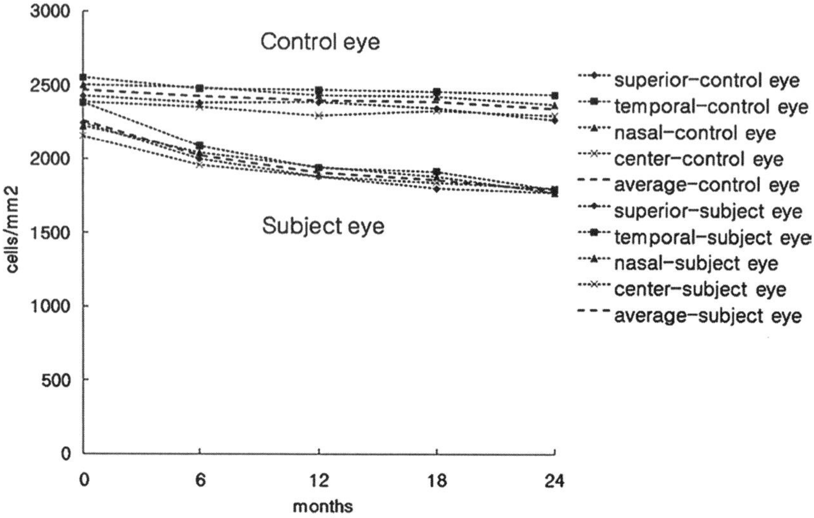

FIGURE 1.—Graph showing the change in endothelial cell count after Ahmed glaucoma valve (AGV) implantation. There was a statistically significant decrease in mean percentage decrease in corneal endothelial cell count in operated eyes in all measurement areas compared with control eyes during the follow-up ($P < .05$, Mann–Whitney U test). (Reprinted from Lee E-K, Yun Y-J, Lee J-E, et al. Changes in corneal endothelial cells after ahmed glaucoma valve implantation: 2-year follow-up. *Am J Ophthalmol.* 2009;148:361-367, with permission from Elsevier.)

Results.—The mean follow-up was 19.1 months. The average percentage decrease in corneal endothelial cell count was 5.8% at 1 month, 11.5% at 6 months, 15.3% at 12 months, 16.6% at 18 months, and 18.6% at 24 months after surgery. The changes were statistically significant compared with those at baseline and those of the control eye at all time points during the study period ($P < .05$). The supratemporal area, the closest site to the tube, showed the greatest decrease in endothelial cell density, by 22.6%, whereas the central cornea showed the smallest decrease, by 15.4%, at 24 months after surgery.

Conclusions.—There was statistically significant corneal endothelial cell loss in the operated eye after AGV implant surgery. The corneal endothelial cell loss increased with time: 15.3% at 12 months and 18.6% at 24 months after surgery, on average, in all measured areas (Fig 1).

► This study shows progressive endothelial cell loss after Ahmed tube shunt implantation. Control eyes (fellow eyes with glaucoma) did much better.

High eye pressure, eye medications, and time, all may take their toll on the cornea. This study suggests that the tube shunt may be more deleterious than time and glaucoma, although the tube eyes likely had worse glaucoma than the control eyes.

It is not clear what the mechanism of damage is. The damage was progressive, suggesting it is not just perioperative trauma. Eyes with tube corneal touch were excluded, although occult episodes of mechanical trauma as may be seen with vigorous eye rubbing are possible. Reflux of shunt capsule fluid into the anterior chamber has been suggested as a possible cause. The tubes' insertion site also has been suggested as a possible source of irritation to the peripheral cornea, and cell loss was greatest in the quadrant of the tube. Some clinicians favor posterior chamber tubes in pseudophakia for these reasons, although it has not been shown to be safer for the endothelium.

Clinicians should be aware that tube shunts may cause significant corneal changes, and this should be considered when choosing among therapeutic options.

J. S. Myers, MD

Measurement of Goldmann Applanation Tonometer Calibration Error

Choudhari NS, George R, Baskaran M, et al (Med Res Foundation, Sankara Nethralaya, Chennai, India)

Ophthalmology 116:3-8, 2009

Objective.—To determine the frequency and possible origins of calibration errors of the Goldmann applanation tonometer and to investigate intraobserver and interobserver agreement in the measurement of such calibration errors.

Design.—Evaluation of diagnostic test or technology.

Participants.—One hundred thirty-two slit-lamp–mounted Haag-Streit Goldmann tonometers (Model AT 900 C/M; Haag-Streit, Bern, Switzerland).

Methods.—Calibration error testing was performed using the standard calibration error check weight bar. A single observer tested 25 instruments on 2 consecutive days. Two observers independently measured calibration errors of another 40 instruments. A single observer performed prospective testing of the remaining Haag-Streit Goldmann tonometers, 6 months after their annual calibration by the bioengineering department of the hospital. Four months later, the same observer retested the instruments that were found to be faulty earlier.

Main Outcome Measure.—Goldmann applanation tonometer calibration error.

Results.—Only 4% of Goldmann tonometers were found to be within the manufacturer's recommended calibration error tolerance (±0.5 mmHg) at 20 mmHg. Twenty-eight percent of instruments had calibration errors of more than ±2 mmHg at the 20-mmHg testing level. An additional 12.12% had calibration errors of more than ±2 mmHg at the 0- or 60-mmHg testing levels, or both. Four months after the initial testing and repair of the 53 faulty instruments, 20.75% again were found to have calibration errors of more than ±2 mmHg at any one or more testing level(s). Intraclass correlation coefficients for intraobserver agreement at 20 mmHg were 0.57 (95% confidence interval [CI], 0.25–0.78) for positive error, 0.82 (95% CI, 0.65–0.92) for negative error, and for interobserver agreement at 20 mmHg, 0.83 (95% CI, 0.70–0.90) for positive error and 0.83 (95% CI, 0.70–0.90) for negative error.

Conclusions.—The authors found good agreement in measurement of Goldmann applanation tonometer calibration error. A significant number of instruments had clinically unacceptable calibration errors. A more frequent calibration error testing and automation of calibration error check is desirable.

▶ Residents studying for the boards of OKAP examinations often review the calibration of Goldmann applanation tonometers. The process is actually quite simple: a metal bar inserted in a small hole in the tonometer provides weighted resistance to allow calibration at 0, 20, and 60 mm Hg. When set correctly, at each point the tonometer head will just tip forward.

However, it is unclear how often clinicians actually calibrate their instruments. In our center, where we do clinical studies, the protocols demand calibration every 30 days. In this study of clinical Goldmann tonometers, 28% were found to be off by more than 2 mm Hg at 20 mm Hg.

Failure to achieve target intraocular pressure (IOP) is a leading reason for patients to undergo incisional glaucoma surgery. Imagine how concerning it would be to a patient to know that this measurement could be off by 2 mm Hg or more because it had not been calibrated recently.

In the study, older instruments were much more likely to be out of calibration. Based on their experience of retesting instruments after re-calibration, the authors suggest checking calibration every 4 months.

J. S. Myers, MD

Interventions Improve Poor Adherence with Once Daily Glaucoma Medications in Electronically Monitored Patients

Okeke CO, Quigley HA, Jampel HD, et al (Univ of Pennsylvania School of Medicine, Philadelphia; Johns Hopkins Univ School of Medicine, Baltimore, MD; et al)

Ophthalmology 116:2286-2293, 2009

Purpose.—To investigate the impact of an intervention program to improve adherence with topical, once daily therapy for glaucoma.

Design.—Randomized controlled clinical trial.

Participants.—Sixty-six patients with glaucoma being treated with a prostaglandin analog in 1 or both eyes at the Scheie Eye Institute or Wilmer Eye Institute between November 2006 and June 2007.

Methods.—In an observational study, participants who took 75% or fewer doses (as measured using the travoprost Dosing Aid [DA]) during an initial 3-month period were randomized into 2 groups. The intervention group watched an educational video, reviewed current barriers to drop-taking and possible solutions with a study coordinator, received regular phone call reminders, and had audible and visible reminders

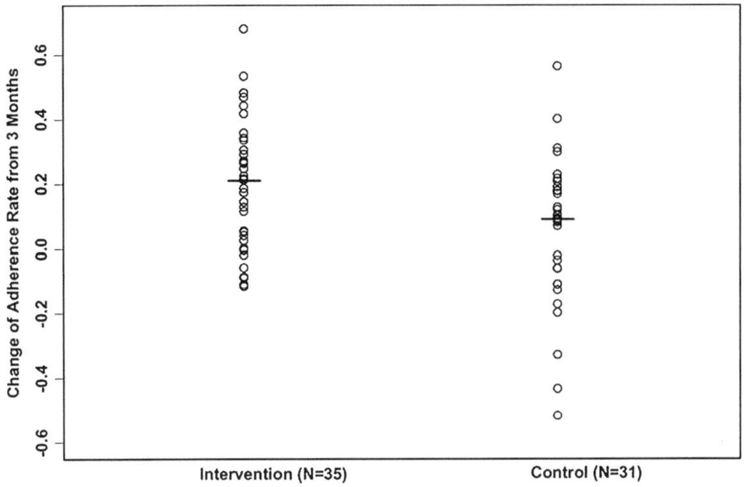

FIGURE 1.—Scatterplot demonstrating distribution of change of adherence rate from 3 months in the nonadherent control group and intervention group. *Circles* indicate adherence rate change for each individual patient; *lines* indicate the median change of adherence rate in each group. (Reprinted from Okeke CO, Quigley HA, Jampel HD, et al. Interventions improve poor adherence with once daily glaucoma medications in electronically monitored patients. *Ophthalmology.* 2009;116:2286-2293, with permission from the American Academy of Ophthalmology.)

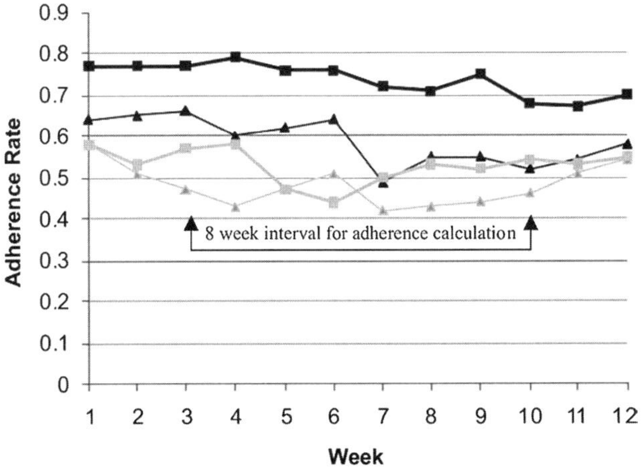

FIGURE 2.—Line graph demonstrating comparison of adherence rate by group at 0 to 3 months (phase 1 before intervention) and 3 to 6 months (phase 2 after the intervention). From bottom to top: *Gray thin line* with *triangles* indicates the mean adherence rate for the nonadherent control group over 12 weeks during phase 1 from 0 to 3 months. *Gray heavy line* with *squares* indicates the mean adherence rate for the nonadherent control group over 12 weeks during phase 2 from 3 to 6 months. *Black thin line* with *triangles* indicates the mean adherence rate for the intervention group over 12 weeks during phase 1 from 0 to 3 months. *Black heavy line* with *squares* indicates the mean adherence rate for the intervention group over 12 weeks during phase 2 from 3 to 6 months. (Reprinted from Okeke CO, Quigley HA, Jampel HD, et al. Interventions improve poor adherence with once daily glaucoma medications in electronically monitored patients. *Ophthalmology.* 2009;116:2286-2293, with permission from the American Academy of Ophthalmology.)

activated on their DA devices. The control group was told to take drops as prescribed and received no additional intervention.

Main Outcome Measures.—Change in drop use adherence as determined by the DA device.

Results.—In the 3-month observation period before randomization, intervention group patients had used a mean of 54 ± 17% of scheduled doses, and this increased to 73 ± 22% during the following 3-month period (P<0.001, n = 35). The control mean adherence rate of 46 ± 23% at baseline was statistically unchanged during the follow-up observation period (51 ± 30%, P = 0.16, n = 31). In a multivariate analysis, intervention, baseline compliance rate of <50%, and white ethnicity were predictors of improved adherence during the 3 months of intervention. The intraocular pressure (IOP) of the intervention and control groups did not change between months 3 and 6 after intervention (P = 0.96, 0.34, respectively), and there was no correlation of IOP change with adherence rate change between both groups (Pearson correlation r = 0.06, P = 0.51).

Conclusions.—A multifaceted intervention significantly increased adherence with glaucoma medications. Those with improved adherence were in the intervention group, had very low adherence rates at baseline, and were white. IOP did not correlate with adherence. Further research is needed to determine which components of this intervention were most effective (Figs 1 and 2).

▶ Adherence to medical therapy and follow-up is a critical component of the successful care of glaucoma. This study reports on an attempt to improve poor adherence to medical therapy by an intervention consisting of a video on adherence, phone call reminders, alarms on a dosing aid, and a meeting with a study coordinator to discuss strategies to improve adherence.

These interventions improved adherence from a dismal 54% ± 17% of scheduled doses, to a mediocre 73% ± 22% during the following 3-month period (P < .001, n = 35).

The authors note that further research is needed to know which aspects of the interventions were most effective. In some studies, researchers have thought that the interest and involvement of others, such as study coordinators, may be important in driving adherence. If this is the case, automated systems, such as prerecorded phone messages, may prove ineffective.

Even when patients know they are being monitored, adherence is poor. Clinicians are poor in judging who is adherent.

Glaucoma is a potentially blinding disease. In those at highest risk of vision loss, such as those with advanced field loss, progressive field loss, or younger age, clinicians should consider and discuss interventions that do not depend on adherence at the earliest signs of nonadherence.

J. S. Myers, MD

Antiglaucoma medications during pregnancy and the risk of low birth weight: a population-based study

Ho J-D, Hu C-C, Lin H-C (Taipei Med Univ Hosp, Taiwan; Shin Kong Wu-HoSu Memorial Hosp, Taipei, Taiwan; Taipei Med Univ, Taiwan; et al)

Br J Ophthalmol 93:1283-1286, 2009

Objective.—To study the relationship between using antiglaucoma medications during pregnancy and the risk of having low-birth-weight (LBW) infants.

Methods.—The study group comprised 244 pregnant women who had been prescribed topical medication to control glaucoma during pregnancy. The comparison group comprised 1952 pregnant women matched for age, year of delivery, maternal hypertension and gestational diabetes. Multivariate logistic regressions were conducted to calculate the adjusted odds ratio of having LBW infants.

Results.—The majority of pregnant women (77.5%) were prescribed beta-blockers to control glaucoma. After adjusting for characteristics of the infant (gender, parity and gestational age), mother (age, the highest educational level, marital status, hypertension and gestational diabetes), father (the highest educational level), parental age difference and family monthly income, there was no significant difference in the risk of LBW infants between mothers prescribed beta-blockers and mothers in the comparison cohort (adjusted odds ratio (OR) 1.48, 95% CI 0.86 to 2.56). However, there was a significantly higher risk of LBW infants for mothers prescribed topical antiglaucoma medications other than beta-blockers (adjusted OR 2.15, 95% CI 1.05 to 5.00).

Conclusions.—Topical beta-blockers can be the first-line drugs when considering medical treatment of glaucoma in a pregnant woman (Table 3).

▶ There has long been appropriate concern regarding the risks of topical glaucoma medications to the fetus in pregnant women. This article presents some reassurance that β-blockers do not pose obvious harm. The finding that other agents may be associated with low birth weight is of great concern, but must be corroborated by other articles. In this cohort, there were only 55 subjects on medications other than β-blockers.

These are not easy studies to complete. Glaucoma is thankfully uncommon in pregnancy. We should continue to seek the safest treatments for all our patients, and counsel the patients who are of childbearing age regarding the medications before the decision is made to conceive. Most glaucoma medications are category C, meaning that animal studies have shown risks to the fetus, but human studies are lacking. An exception is brimonidine, which is category B, showing no harm to the fetus in animal studies, but lacking human studies.

Minimizing medications, choosing the safest medications and punctal occlusion all make good sense. The concern over β-blocker concentration in breast milk and delivery approaches must be kept in mind. Laser and surgical options are sometimes worth discussing, but antimetabolites are contraindicated in pregnancy.

J. S. Myers, MD

TABLE 3.—Crude and Adjusted Odds Ratios of Having Low Birth Weight Infants for Women who Used Topical Antiglaucoma Medication During Pregnancy and Women with no History of Chronic Disease, 2001~2003 (n = 2196)

Variable	Mothers with no History of Chronic Disease n = 1952		Mothers who Used Topical Antiglaucoma Medication (All Categories) During Pregnancy n = 244		Mothers who Used Topical Beta-Blockers During Pregnancy n = 189		Mothers who Used other Topical Antiglaucoma Medication (All Categories Except Beta-Blocker Category) During Pregnancy n = 55	
	No	%	No	%	No	%	No	%
Low birth weight								
Yes	120	6.2	26	10.7	17	9.0	9	16.4
No	1832	93.8	218	89.3	172	91.0	46	83.6
Crude OR (95% CI)	1.00		1.67* (1.05 to 2.64)		1.51 (0.89 to 2.57)		2.23* (1.02 to 5.03)	
Adjusted OR† (95% CI)	1.00		1.63* (1.01 to 2.62)		1.48 (0.86 to 2.56)		2.15* (1.05 to 5.00)	

CI, confidence interval; OR, odds ratio.

*$p<0.05$.

†Adjusted for infant's gender, parity, gestational age; maternal age, highest maternal educational level, maternal marital status, maternal hypertension, gestational diabetes; highest paternal educational level; parental age difference and family monthly income.

4 Cornea

Acanthamoeba Keratitis: Diagnosis and Treatment Update 2009

Dart JKG, Saw VPJ, Kilvington S (Moorfields Eye Hosp NHS Foundation Trust, London, UK; Univ of Leicester, UK)
Am J Ophthalmol 148:487-499, 2009

Purpose.—To describe the current management of Acanthamoeba keratitis (AK).

Design.—A perspective based on the literature and author experience.

Results.—Early diagnosis and appropriate therapy are key to a good prognosis. A provisional diagnosis of AK can be made using the clinical features and confocal microscopy, although a definitive diagnosis requires culture, histology, or identification of *Acanthamoeba* deoxyribonucleic acid by polymerase chain reaction. Routine use of tissue diagnosis is recommended, particularly for patients unresponsive to treatment for AK. Topical biguanides are the only effective therapy for the resistant encysted form of the organism in vitro, if not always in vivo. None of the other drugs that have been used meet the requirements of consistent cysticidal activity and may have no therapeutic role. The use of topical steroids is controversial, but probably beneficial, for the management of severe corneal inflammatory complications that have not responded to topical biguanides alone. The scleritis associated with AK is rarely associated with extracorneal invasion and usually responds to systemic anti-inflammatory treatment combined with topical biguanides. Therapeutic keratoplasty retains a role for therapy of some severe complications of AK but not for initial treatment. With modern management, 90% of patients can expect to retain visual acuity of 6/12 or better and fewer than 2% become blind, although treatment may take 6 months or more.

Conclusions.—Better understanding of the pathogenesis of the extracorneal complications, the availability of polymerase chain reaction for tissue diagnosis, and effective licensed topical anti-amoebics would substantially benefit patients with AK.

▶ This is an excellent review and opinion piece from Moorfields Eye Hospital on the current science and recommended management of *Acanthamoeba* keratitis (AK). The conclusion sums up the frustration of this infection, calling for better understanding of the pathogenesis, more accurate and available diagnosis with polymerase chain reaction (PCR), and effective, licensed treatments. A few points that are worth highlighting are: First, there is a significant difference in national incidence between contact lens wearers in the United Kingdom

(17.53 to 19.50 per million) and the United States (1.65 to 2.01 per million). This not only makes me happy to live on this side of the pond but also demonstrates that the practitioners/scientists in the United Kingdom can offer a lot to our knowledge base on AK. There is also a seasonal rise of infection in summer/early autumn, a finding that we recently confirmed in our patients in Philadelphia. The cause of this is unknown, perhaps resulting from more *Acanthamoeba* in the environment and, perhaps because of more water-based recreation. Second, the authors discuss the difficulty of confirming the diagnosis, calling for a tissue diagnosis based on culture, histology, or PCR. They express concern about the lack of well-designed, masked studies to confirm the findings on confocal, which is becoming the preferred diagnostic technique in some centers. The authors doubt the effectiveness of voriconazole as a cysticidal agent. This is in contrast to another report this year demonstrating the usefulness of voriconazole topically and orally in 2 recalcitrant patients.[1] I have used voriconazole in several patients, especially in those for whom things are not going well. It is unclear to me if it has been of significant value, but the patient for whom you are trying everything given the severity of infection, I think it has a role. The question of whether early surgical intervention, followed by biguanide therapy, is preferred to long-term medical management has been raised in recent literature.[2] The authors remain conservative in their approach to penetrating keratoplasty, recommending it for visual restoration and not for active disease (unless associated with perforation). We continue to struggle with this dilemma with our patients. We not only see the devastating effects of continued inflammation during long treatments but also have cared for the horrific cases of recurrent infections in postgraft cases.

K. M. Hammersmith, MD

References

1. Bang S, Edell E, Eghrari AO, Gottsch JD. Treatment with voriconazole in 3 eyes with resistant Acanthamoeba keratitis. *Am J Ophthalmol.* 2010;149:66-69.
2. Tu EY, Joslin CE, Sugar J, Shoff ME, Booton GC. Prognostic factors affecting visual outcome in Acanthamoeba keratitis. *Ophthalmology.* 2008;115:1998-2003.

Boston Keratoprosthesis Outcomes and Complications

Chew HF, Ayres BD, Hammersmith KM, et al (Thomas Jefferson Univ, Philadelphia, PA; et al)
Cornea 28:989-996, 2009

Purpose.—To evaluate the outcomes of the Boston Keratoprosthesis (KPro) at our institution.

Methods.—A computerized database retrospectively identified all patients who received a Boston KPro from August 2005 to October 2007.

Results.—There were 37 patients, 24 (65%) were male. Mean age was 66.3 years (median 69 years, range: 24–93 years; SD = 18.1 years). Mean follow-up was 16 months (range: 6–28 months; SD = 6.0 months). There were 36 type 1 (97%) and 1 type 2 (3%) KPros. The primary indication was failed penetrating keratoplasty in 29 patients (78%)—22 (59%) from multiple failures. Preoperative comorbidities included glaucoma [27 patients (73%)] and limbal stem cell deficiency [13 patients (35%)]. No intraoperative complications occurred. Postoperative complications included retroprosthetic membrane [24 patients (65%)], increased intraocular pressure [14 patients (38%)], glaucoma progression [5 patients (13.5%)], and endophthalmitis [4 patients (11%)—3 who discontinued prophylactic antibiotics secondary to compliance]. Thirty-six KPros (97%) were retained—1 type 2 KPro (3%) in a patient with ocular cicatricial pemphigoid extruded and was replaced. Mean best-corrected visual acuities were counting fingers preoperatively (range: light perception to 20/100) and 20/90 at last follow-up (range: light perception to 20/25). At last follow-up, 31 patients (84%) improved 2 lines or greater—3 patients (8%) had worse vision.

Conclusions.—Retention rates were excellent, and best-corrected visual acuities improved in the vast majority of patients. Complications can occur and require frequent follow-up to monitor and treat glaucoma progression, endophthalmitis, and inflammation. Patient compliance is of paramount importance. Despite the potential complications, the Boston KPro provides visual improvement in patients with an otherwise poor prognosis.

▶ This article presents our data on the clinical course of 35 patients with the Boston Keratoprosthesis (KPro) over a 26-month period. One of the most concerning complications of this procedure is endophthalmitis, which was seen in 11% of the patients. The clinical course of these patients was further expanded upon in a second article.[1] Three of these patients had gram-positive organisms (*Staphylococcus epidermidis* and *Staphylococcus aureus*), and 3 of the 4 had stopped vancomycin. I am always worried about the compliance with vancomycin and the ability of patients to obtain it. Thus, I usually have them get the first script preoperatively, so that this is not an issue right after surgery. Our rate of endophthalmitis is concerning but is similar to that presented in another case series about Kpro this year.[2] This article from the University of California, Davis presents a study on 30 eyes with the Boston Kpro over a 4-year period. The rate of endophthalmitis was 10%, even though all patients were maintained on topical vancomycin. This article also presents a significant amount of corneal melts, causing loss of retention of the keratoprosthesis. This differs from our article; however, I recently had a patient who 5 years after Kpro developed a late melt, which has been amenable to glue thus far. Certainly, the patients with severe ocular surface disease are at higher risk for these complications. Both articles on Kpro discuss the difficulty in managing and following glaucoma in these patients. There have been some presentations in the past year about an implantable sensor to monitor and follow intraocular pressure. As glaucoma progression was the most likely cause of lost best-corrected visual acuity, we look forward to measures such as this that will aid in glaucoma management.

K. M. Hammersmith, MD

References

1. Fintelman RE, Maguire JI, Ho AC, Chew HF, Ayres BD. Characteristics of endophthalmitis in patients with the Boston Keratoprosthesis. *Cornea.* 2009;28: 877-878.
2. Bradley JC, Hernandex EG, Schwab IR, Mannis MJ. Boston type 1 keratoprosthesis: the University of California Davis experience. *Cornea.* 2009;28:321-327.

Busin Guide vs Forceps for the Insertion of the Donor Lenticule in Descemet Stripping Automated Endothelial Keratoplasty

Bahar I, Kaiserman I, Sansanayudh W, et al (Univ of Toronto, Ontario, Canada)
Am J Ophthalmol 147:220-226, 2009

Purpose.—To compare two insertion methods in Descemet stripping automated endothelial keratoplasty (DSAEK): Busin guide-assisted vs Forceps-assisted insertion of the corneal lenticule graft.

Design.—Prospective, consecutive, comparative, nonrandomized study.

Methods.—Setting: Cornea clinic at the Toronto Western Hospital.

Study Population.—Sixty-three eyes of 63 consecutive patients were included. All patients underwent DSAEK for Fuchs endothelial dystrophy, pseudophakic bullous keratopathy, aphakic bullous keratopathy, failed graft, or iridocorneo endothelial syndrome. Twenty-six consecutive donor discs were inserted with the Busin guide and 37 consecutive eyes underwent forceps assisted insertion of the donor.

Main Outcome Measures.—Uncorrected visual acuity (UCVA), best spectacle-corrected visual acuity (BSCVA), manifest refraction, corneal endothelial cell loss, and postoperative complications.

Results.—Busin guide-assisted DSAEK group had significantly worse UCVA and lower donor endothelial cell counts preoperatively. No significant differences were noted in the intraoperative or postoperative complications. Six months following surgery, BCVA was not significantly different between groups: 20/37 in the Busin guide-assisted DASEK group vs 20/42 in the Forceps-assisted group ($P=.39$). Mean spherical equivalent was −0.02 diopters (D) and 0.82 D ($P=.06$), and mean refractive cylinder was 2.2 D and 1.31 D ($P=.0006$), respectively. Endothelial cell loss was significantly lower in the Busin guide-assisted DASEK group: 25% loss vs 34.3% loss in the Forceps-assisted DSAEK group. ($P=.04$).

Conclusions.—Although visual outcomes were not different between the groups studied, Busin guide-assisted DSAEK resulted in lower percentage of endothelial cell loss compared with forceps insertion, six months following surgery (Tables 3 and 4).

▶ This comparative prospective study of 63 patients undergoing Descemet stripping automated endothelial keratoplasty (DSAEK) provides positive data in support of the use of the Busin guide. The authors find more dislocations and higher rates of primary graft failure in cases that used the forceps technique.

TABLE 3.—Comparison of Six Months Postoperative Results of Busin Guide-Assisted vs Forceps-Assisted Descemet Stripping Automated Endothelial Keratoplasty

	Busin Guide-Assisted DSAEK (n = 16)	Forceps-Assisted DSAEK (n = 25)	*P* (*t* test)
Endothelial cell counts (cells/mm^2)	2035 ± 297	1879 ± 585	.21
Percent of endothelial cell loss	25.0 ± 13.1%	34.3 ± 19.2%	.04
Best-corrected VA (logMAR, in patients without retinal pathology)	0.27 ± 0.14 (20/37)	0.32 ± 0.27 (20/42)	.39
Uncorrected VA (logMAR, in patients without retinal pathology)	0.54 ± 0.13 (20/71)	0.63 ± 0.45 (20/84)	.33
Manifest spherical equivalent (D)	−0.02 ± 1.35	0.82 ± 1.47	.06
Manifest cylinder (D)	2.2 ± 1.0	1.31 ± 0.94	.0006

D = diopter; DSAEK = Descemet stripping automated endothelial keratoplasty; logMAR = logarithm of minimal angle of resolution; VA = visual acuity.

TABLE 4.—Intraoperative and Postoperative Complications in Busin Guide-Assisted vs Forceps-Assisted Descemet Stripping Automated Endothelial Keratoplasty

	Busin Guide-Assisted DSAEK (n = 26)	Forceps-Assisted DSAEK (n = 37)	*P* (χ^2 test)
Disc dislocation	2 (7.7%)	7 (18.9%)	.37
Induced glaucoma	3 (11.5%)	3 (8.1%)	.98
Acute rejection	1 (3.8%)	1 (2.7%)	.62
Primary failure	0 (0%)	1 (2.7%)	.85
Late graft failure	0 (0%)	0 (0%)	—
Interface opacity	0 (0%)	1 (2.7%)	.85
CME	0 (0%)	1 (2.7%)	.85

CME = cystoid macular edema; DSAEK = Descemet stripping automated endothelial keratoplasty.

My personal experience is that both techniques have advantages and disadvantages; however, I prefer the Busin guide. While it is somewhat more cumbersome outside of the eye (with the placement of the anterior chamber maintainer and awkwardness of the guide), it is less so inside the eye as it opens well and requires less manipulation to unfold the graft. This article was criticized by Terry and associates, who are big proponents of the forceps technique. They discussed the different techniques of folding (under vs over). The authors responded to these criticisms satisfactorily and supported their conclusions that, in their hands, the Busin was a superior technique. While I think Dr Terry has been an immense contributor and innovator to partial-thickness corneal transplantation, it does offend me a little that he lectures and writes about the superiority of his technique. Unfortunately, many have been unable to reproduce his technique and outstanding results. I think what is important in DSAEK surgery is that each surgeon finds a technique that works for him/her. The available data can help guide us to what steps may be preferable, but each surgeon needs to find his/her own preferred/successful way to perform this surgery.

K. M. Hammersmith, MD

Corticosteroid-induced intraocular pressure elevation in keratoconus is common following uncomplicated penetrating keratoplasty

Fan JC, Chow K, Patel DV, et al (Univ of Auckland, New Zealand)

Eye 23:2056-2062, 2009

Aims.—To determine the incidence of postkeratoplasty intraocular pressure (IOP) elevation in the eyes of subjects with keratoconus and establish the relationship between IOP and corticosteroid administrations in this population.

Methods.—Following strict inclusion/exclusion criteria, a retrospective analysis was performed on a consecutive series of penetrating keratoplasties performed for keratoconus observing a standardised surgical and postoperative regimen in Auckland, New Zealand. Patient demographics, ocular, medical, and family history, and pre- and postoperative data were recorded until 12 months postkeratoplasty.

Results.—In all, 57 eyes of 48 patients were included—31% New Zealand Europeans, 42% Pacific people, 15% Maori, and 12% other. Eighteen eyes (32%) of 17 patients (35%) exhibited elevated IOP and 12 (21%) eyes exhibited moderate-to-severe elevation of IOP. IOP elevation occurred 3–6 months postkeratoplasty in 78% of eyes. Elevated IOP was significantly less common in Maori and Pacific peoples ($P = 0.02$). All eyes except one required reduction/cessation of corticosteroids to normalise IOP.

Conclusions.—The incidence of presumed steroid-related postkeratoplasty IOP elevation, in 35% of subjects with keratoconus, is markedly higher in this New Zealand study than previously reported in the US and UK studies. Further clinical and genetic analysis of associations between keratoconus and steroid-induced IOP elevation and glaucoma might improve our current understanding of this condition (Table 1).

▶ This article analyzes the incidence of steroid-related postkeratoplasty intraocular pressure (IOP) elevation in 57 eyes of patients with keratoconus. The

TABLE 1.—Postkeratoplasty Pressure Elevation Over 12-Month Follow-up in Keratoconus

	Number of Eyes					
	1 Week	1 Month	3 Months	6 Months	9 Months	12 Months
Mild (22–26 mmHg)	0	0	3	1	1	1
Moderate (27–31 mmHg)	0	1	3	2	0	1
Severe (>31 mmHg)	0	0	3	2	0	0

authors found that over 30% of these patients developed IOP elevation by 12 months. It is interesting that their patients were on a lot of steroids following surgery. They reported that patients took prednisolone acetate 1% every 2 hours for a week and 4 times a day for 6 months. They defined increased IOP as anything greater than 22 mm Hg, thus subdividing the IOP elevation into mild, moderate, and severe. Most patients had a pressure spike from 3 to 6 months following surgery. With these factors, one may conclude that the authors would overestimate IOP elevation following surgery. However, we also looked at this question in an article this year.[1] We found an impressively high rate of IOP elevation in similar patients. Our definition included not only those with an IOP greater than 22 mm Hg but also those with an elevation greater than 5 or 10 mm Hg over their baseline. Our study also included extended follow-up and found that almost a quarter of the patients who have elevated pressure do not develop that until after a year postoperatively. Both of these studies demonstrate the importance of careful follow-up of patients' IOP following keratoplasty.

K. M. Hammersmith, MD

Reference

1. Erdurmus M, Cohen EJ, Yildiz EH, et al. Steroid-induced intraocular pressure elevation or glaucoma after penetrating keratoplasty in patients with keratoconus or Fuchs dystrophy. *Cornea*. 2009;28:759-764.

Descemet's Membrane Endothelial Keratoplasty: Prospective Multicenter Study of Visual and Refractive Outcomes and Endothelial Survival

Price MO, Giebel AW, Fairchild KM, et al (Cornea Res Foundation of America, Indianapolis, IN; Pacific Cataract and Laser Inst, Chehalis, WA; et al)
Ophthalmology 116:2361-2368, 2009

Purpose.—To describe Descemet's membrane endothelial keratoplasty (DMEK) techniques, perioperative challenges, management, and visual and refractive outcomes.

Design.—Prospective, multicenter, consecutive case series.

Participants.—Sixty eyes of 56 patients with Fuchs' endothelial dystrophy, pseudophakic bullous keratopathy, or failed previous graft.

Intervention.—Descemet's membrane (DM) and endothelium were stripped from donor corneas submerged in corneal storage solution in a corneal viewing chamber. Donor DM diameters were 8.5 or 9.0 mm. The central 7 mm of DM was stripped from the recipient cornea. After staining with trypan blue to improve visualization, donor DM was inserted through a 2.8-mm incision. Descemet's membrane endothelial keratoplasty was performed alone (n = 48) or was combined with phacoemulsification and lens implantation (n = 11), pars plana vitrectomy (n = 2), or both.

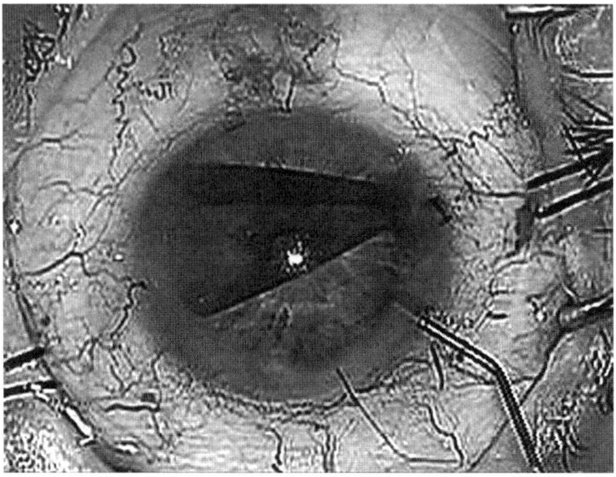

FIGURE 3.—Intraoperative photograph showing the trypan blue-stained donor Descemet's membrane and endothelium being uncurled inside the recipient eye using short bursts of balanced salt solution injected through a cannula. (Reprinted from Price MO, Giebel AW, Fairchild KM, et al. Descemet's membrane endothelial keratoplasty. prospective multicenter study of visual and refractive outcomes and endothelial survival. *Ophthalmology.* 2009;116:2361-2368, with permission from the American Academy of Ophthalmology.)

Main Outcome Measures.—Best spectacle-corrected visual acuity (BSCVA), manifest refraction, and endothelial cell density.

Results.—Median BSCVA was 20/30 at 1 month (range, 20/20–20/60), improving from 20/50 (range, 20/25–hand movements) before DMEK, excluding 4 eyes (7%) with preexisting ocular pathologic features that limited visual potential. At 3 months, 26% had 20/20 vision, 63% saw 20/25 or better, and 94% saw 20/40 or better. Refractive cylinder remained unchanged at 0.9 diopters (D; $P = 0.93$), and a hyperopic shift of 0.49 ± 0.63 D ($P = 0.0091$) was noted in DMEK single procedures. Endothelial cell loss was 30% ± 20% at 3 months and 32% ± 20% in 38 eyes that reached the 6-month examination. Median pachymetry decreased from 660 μm before surgery to 530 μm. Descemet's membrane stripped successfully from 60 of 72 donor corneas; 6 were converted successfully to Descemet's stripping automated endothelial keratoplasty (DSAEK) and 6 (8%) were discarded. Only 1 graft detached completely, but air was reinjected in 38 eyes (63%), mainly for partial detachments. Five DMEK corneas (8%) failed to clear and were replaced successfully with DMEK or DSAEK. All remained clear at last follow-up.

Conclusions.—Compared with DSAEK, DMEK provided a significantly higher rate of 20/20 and 20/25 vision, with comparable endothelial cell loss. Descemet's membrane endothelial keratoplasty restored physiologic pachymetry, but donor preparation and attachment currently are more challenging than with DSAEK.

▶ This is the latest iteration in treatment for endothelial dysfunction, truly transplanting only Descemet's membrane without any posterior stroma. When I saw videos of this presented by Dr Price and others a year ago, it seemed so technically frustrating that I was hoping it would fizzle as a concept. This article illustrates the difficult nature of the procedure with significant numbers of torn grafts and many repeat procedures. However, it also highlights the potential benefits. Perhaps, the most compelling is the financial benefit as the expensive equipment used for Descemet's stripping automated endothelial keratoplasty (DSAEK) is not necessary. Thus, this procedure may be more useful in remote areas. Also, the patients have excellent vision, as there is less interface issue (Fig 3). At this point, however, the technique does not seem ready to be embraced by the larger cornea community. It does seem likely that it will be embraced after refinements.

K. M. Hammersmith, MD

Economic Appraisal of the Boston Ocular Surface Prosthesis

Shepard DS, Razavi M, Stason WB, et al (Brandeis Univ, Waltham, MA; et al)
Am J Ophthalmol 148:860-868, 2009

Purpose.—To perform an economic appraisal of the Boston Ocular Surface Prosthesis in patients with corneal ectasia, irregular astigmatism, or ocular surface disease.

Design.—Cost, incremental cost-effectiveness, and benefit-cost analyses in a prospective observational study.

Methods.—The effects of this scleral lens on visual functioning were measured in 69 patients who received the prosthesis in 2006 and were reassessed 6 months after fitting the prosthesis. Benefits, based on improvements in visual functioning, were converted to quality-adjusted life years (QALYs), and economic values were derived using results from published studies. Costs were estimated from the provider organization's 2006 operating financial statement with additions for donated resources and future scale-up.

Results.—Mean scores on a 100-point visual functioning questionnaire (VFQ-25) improved from 57.0 to 77.8 ($P < .0001$). On average, each fitted patient cost $11 841 ($6001 for clinical services and $5840 to produce the prosthesis). Patients' quality of life improved by 0.10 QALYs per year. Assuming that benefits persist for an average of 5 years, the lifetime gain was 0.48 QALYs; the average cost-effectiveness of the prosthesis was $24 900 per QALY (95% confidence interval $19 100 to $29 600), and the average benefit-cost ratio was 4.0 to 1. In patients with the lowest baseline scores (average VFQ score 38.6), results were even more favorable: cost-effectiveness $17 100 per QALY and benefit-cost ratio 5.6 to 1.

Conclusions.—The Boston Ocular Surface Prosthesis is cost-effective and cost beneficial in patients with severely compromised visual function attributable to ectasia, irregular astigmatism, or ocular surface disease.

▶ While I find these studies on quality-adjusted life years (QALYs) a little too mathematical for my taste, it has been my experience that the Boston Ocular

Surface Prosthesis is a real life changer. It is the most beneficial, in my opinion, for the patient with severe ocular surface disease. The Boston Foundation for Sight has been wonderful to all the patients that I have sent there. The success for an individual patient obviously depends on the level of prefitting functioning and motivation. This foundation is starting to branch out and provide care in more areas of the country, which will bring this super subspecialty care to many more patients.

K. M. Hammersmith, MD

Five-year follow-up on the effect of oral acyclovir after penetrating keratoplasty for herpetic keratitis

Jansen AF, Rijneveld WJ, Remeijer L, et al (Rotterdam Eye Hosp, The Netherlands)

Cornea 28:843-845, 2009

Purpose.—To investigate the long-term effect of oral acyclovir administered during the first 6 months after penetrating keratoplasty (PK) for herpetic eye disease (HED).

Methods.—A 5-year follow-up was undertaken for a patient population from a placebo-controlled, randomized trial on acyclovir prophylaxis after keratoplasty. In this former study the effectiveness of oral acyclovir prophylaxis was significant during the first 2 years after keratoplasty. Prospective data such as graft survival, graft clarity, vascularization, infective events, and rejection episodes were obtained from the national keratoplasty follow-up registry. Additional clinical data were derived from the medical charts.

Results.—For 47 of the original 63 enrolled patients, the 5-year follow-up was completed. Comparing the acyclovir group with the placebo group, we found that with regard to the cumulative clinically evident recurrences, there was a statistically significant lower monthly event rate in the acyclovir group ($P = 0.037$). There were no statistically significant differences in visual acuity or in the use of oral aciclovir between the two treatment groups. The incidences of graft failure, vascularization, and medication or surgery for glaucoma were too low to analyze differences between the two groups.

Conclusion.—The results of our study suggest that oral acyclovir prescribed during the first 6 months after PK for HED protects against clinically evident HED recurrences during the first 5 years following PK.

▶ This article discusses the 5-year follow-up of oral acyclovir after penetrating keratoplasty (PK) for herpes simplex virus (HSV). A previous study from this group compared the 2-year course of patients who had oral acyclovir for 6 months following PK with those who had placebo. This study looks at those patients 3 years later. The authors report that oral acyclovir prescribed during the first 6 months after PK protects against clinically evident HSV during the first 5 years. The outcome parameters in both groups were fairly equivalent.

Twelve of the 47 patients had acyclovir added in their postoperative management. While it may not be surprising that the patients who did receive acyclovir did a little better, it is very shocking that the patients are not routinely kept on acyclovir or some antiviral for an extended period of time following PK. Another recent study showed that long-term oral acyclovir was associated with fewer rejection episodes, HSV recurrences, and longer graft survival.[1] Our group has shown that long-term acyclovir (past 12 months) continues to reduce recurrences in patients with HSV (not just those after PK).[2] It makes intuitive sense that continued antiviral therapy would continue to reduce HSV. We continue to use and recommend long-term oral acyclovir for these patients.

K. M. Hammersmith, MD

References

1. Garcia DD, Farjo J, Musch DC, et al. Effect of prophylactic oral acyclovir after penetrating keratoplasty for herpes simplex keratitis. *Cornea.* 2007;26:930-934.
2. Uchoa UB, Rezende RA, Carrasco MA, Rapuano CJ, Laibson PR, Cohen EJ. Long-term acyclovir use to prevent recurrent ocular herpes simplex virus infection. *Arch Ophthalmol.* 2003;121:1702-1704.

Intraoperative and Postoperative Effects of Corneal Collagen Cross-Linking on Progressive Keratoconus

Vinciguerra P, Albè E, Trazza S, et al (Istituto Clinico Humanitas, Milano, Italy; et al)

Arch Ophthalmol 127:1258-1265, 2009

Objectives.—To report intraoperative and 24-month refractive, topographic, tomographic, and aberrometric outcomes after corneal collagen cross-linking in progressive advanced keratoconus.

Methods.—Prospective, nonrandomized single-center clinical study involving 28 eyes. Main outcome measures included uncorrected and best spectacle-corrected visual acuities, sphere and cylinder refraction, topography, tomography, aberrometry, and endothelial cell count evaluated at baseline and follow-up at 1, 3, 6, 12, and 24 months after treatment. Topography was also recorded intraoperatively.

Results.—Two years after treatment, mean baseline uncorrected and best spectacle-corrected visual acuities improved significantly ($P = .048$ and $<.001$, respectively) and mean spherical equivalent refraction decreased significantly ($P = .03$). Mean baseline flattest and steepest meridians on simulated keratometry, simulated keratometry average, mean average pupillary power, and apical keratometry all decreased significantly ($P < .03$). Deterioration of the Klyce indices was observed in the untreated contralateral eyes but not in treated eyes. Total corneal wavefront aberrations Z_0 (piston), Z_2 (defocus), and Z_7 (III coma) decreased significantly ($P \leq .046$). Mean 12-month baseline pupil center pachymetry and total corneal volume decreased significantly ($P = .045$). Endothelial cell counts did not change significantly ($P = .13$).

TABLE 2.—Topographic Astigmatism as Measured With a Corneal Topographer[a]

Measurement	Pre-CXL With Epithelium	Pre-CXL Without Epithelium	Postoperative Follow-up, mo: 1	3	6	12	24	*P* Value[b]: Pre-CXL With and Pre-CXL Without Epithelium	Pre-CXL[c] and 24-mo Follow-up
Simulated keratometry, D									
Flattest meridian	46.10	47.49	46.56	46.30	45.45	45.44	45.43	.17	**.049**
Steepest meridian	50.37	53.59	51.62	50.86	49.89	49.58	49.02	**.03**	**.03**
Average	48.08	50.26	48.87	48.37	47.52	47.01	46.97	.06	**.03**
Cylinder	−4.27	−6.10	−5.06	−4.56	−4.44	−3.99	−3.80	**.01**	**.03**
Keratometry reading, D									
3 mm	−4.73	−5.35	−4.96	−4.94	−4.69	−4.19	−4.15	.39	.41
5 mm	−3.64	−4.36	−3.92	−3.68	−3.60	−3.27	−3.25	.21	.57

Abbreviations: CXL, corneal collagen cross-linking; D, diopters.
[a]Performed with the CSO EyeTop Topographer (Compagnia Strumenti Oftalmici, Florence, Italy).
[b]Significant differences are indicated in boldface.
[c]Indicates obtained with and without the epithelium intact.

Conclusions.—Two years postoperatively, corneal collagen crosslinking appears to be effective in improving uncorrected and best spectacle-corrected visual acuities in eyes with progressive keratoconus by significantly reducing corneal average pupillary power, apical keratometry, and total corneal wavefront aberrations.

▶ This is a small but encouraging study on the effects of collagen crosslinking for keratoconus. The authors describe for the first time the intraoperative topography after the epithelium has been removed (Table 2). This shows that the epithelium masks the steepness of the cornea and explains why topography obtained 1 month after the procedure shows an increase in steepness of the cornea. The patients in this prospective study did well overall, and there was no negative effect on endothelial cells. Another study this year from Koller et al discusses the complications from this procedure.[1] In an analysis of 117 patients, the complication rate was 2.9% (loss of 2 lines or more). Sterile infiltrates and scars were the most common causes of this. An additional 7.6% of the patients continued to progress despite crosslinking. They found that age over 35 years and keratometry greater than 58 D increased the complication rate. Thus, Koller et al recommended stricter inclusion criteria, which they felt would reduce the complication rate to 1%. Certainly, we eagerly await more data about the usefulness of this procedure and best candidates for this procedure.

K. M. Hammersmith, MD

Reference

1. Koller T, Mrochen M, Seiler T. Complication and failure rates after corneal crosslinking. *J Cataract Refract Surg*. 2009;35:1358-1362.

Late Varicella-Zoster Virus Dendriform Keratitis in Patients With Histories of Herpes Zoster Ophthalmicus

Hu AYH, Strauss EC, Holland GN, et al (David Geffen School of Medicine at UCLA, Los Angeles, CA; Univ of California, San Francisco)

Am J Ophthalmol 149:214-220, 2010

Purpose.—To describe the characteristics and course of late varicella-zoster virus (VZV) dendriform keratitis in patients with histories of herpes zoster ophthalmicus (HZO); to describe responses of corneal lesions to antiviral treatment; and to investigate risk factors for recurrence.

Design.—Retrospective case series.

Methods.—Included were patients known to have 1 or more episodes of dendriform lesions beginning at least 2 weeks after HZO in 2 academic practices. Epithelial lesions were evaluated for the presence of VZV DNA by a polymerase chain reaction assay. Demographic, medical, and ophthalmic data were collected for each episode. Responses to treatment with antiviral medications were evaluated. Cumulative risk of recurrence was determined using Kaplan-Meier analysis; potential risk factors for recurrence (age, systemic disease, lesion characteristics, corticosteroids) were evaluated using univariate Cox proportional hazard models.

Results.—We identified 20 patients (14 women; median age, 65 years) who met inclusion criteria. Dendriform lesions were pleomorphic with thickened, opaque epithelium. Seven patients had systemic diseases characterized by altered immune function. VZV DNA was identified in 15 of 16 cases tested, and all lesions responded to antiviral therapy. The 1-year incidence of first recurrence was 95.8 lesions per 100 person-years of follow-up. Patients had multiple recurrences, but risk of recurrence appeared to decrease over time. No statistically significant risk factors for recurrence were identified.

Conclusions.—Late dendriform lesions associated with HZO are foci of productive VZV infection. Lesions can be treated effectively with topical or systemic antiviral agents. Patients can have multiple recurrences of dendriform lesions despite treatment.

▶ This article presents data that challenges the way we have viewed varicella zoster keratitis. The authors present a study on 20 patients with late (more than 2 weeks following outbreak) dendriform lesions. These lesions were positive for zoster virus when evaluated by polymerase chain reaction (PCR) in 15 of the 16 patients tested, indicating an active infectious process. The authors treated these patients in a variety of ways but usually using an oral antiviral throughout the treatment period. This is counter to what we have traditionally been taught that oral antivirals are useful in varicella zoster virus only in the initial outbreak and that topical antivirals have little (to no) role in treating the epithelial disease. The fact that PCR is able to identify active virus has been shown in the past by Dr Pavan-Langston, but this furthers that body of evidence. The recurrence of epithelial disease is often seen and can be confusing and misdiagnosed as concurrent herpes simplex virus (HSV) infection. While there are morphological differences, these can be difficult to interpret. This study also shows that the patients with recurrent dendriform keratitis are more likely to be immunosuppressed, which has been the case in my practice. I have several patients (one with non-Hodgkin's lymphoma, one with an immune deficiency) whom I have kept on oral antivirals for extended periods of time, which has seemed to reduce recurrences. The way to treat these patients, however, is still unclear. We do not use topical trifluridine in these patients because of its toxic effects on an already compromised cornea. The authors did use some trifluridine, however. I have found good success with topical vidarabine ointment in treating these patients. We look forward to more data on this topic and, hopefully, some large studies that evaluate treatment strategies for these patients.

K. M. Hammersmith, MD

National Outbreak of *Acanthamoeba* Keratitis Associated with Use of a Contact Lens Solution, United States

Verani JR, for the *Acanthamoeba* Keratitis Investigation Team (Ctrs for Disease Control and Prevention, Atlanta, GA; et al)

Emerg Infect Dis 15:1236-1242, 2009

An outbreak of *Acanthamoeba* keratitis, a rare, potentially blinding, corneal infection, was detected in the United States in 2007; cases had been increasing since 2004. A case–control study was conducted to investigate the outbreak. We interviewed 105 case-patients from 30 states and 184 controls matched geographically and by contact lens use. Available contact lenses, cases, solutions, and corneal specimens from case-patients were cultured and tested by molecular methods. In multivariate analyses, case-patients had significantly greater odds of having used Advanced Medical Optics Complete Moisture Plus (AMOCMP) solution (odds ratio 16.9, 95% confidence interval 4.8–59.5). AMOCMP manufacturing lot information was available for 22 case-patients, but none of the lots were identical. Three unopened bottles of AMOCMP tested negative for *Acanthamoeba* spp. Our findings suggest that the solution was not intrinsically contaminated and that its anti-*Acanthamoeba* efficacy was likely insufficient. Premarket standardized testing of contact lens solutions for activity against *Acanthamoeba* spp. is warranted.

► Complete MoisturePlus was launched in the US market in late 2003, and the increase in the number of *Acanthamoeba* cases beginning in 2004 coincides with this launch. We noted an increased number of cases at Wills in 2004 and were the first to present this at the American Academy of Ophthalmology 2005 Annual Meeting.[1] It was at this time that we learned that there was a similar outbreak in the Chicago area. Dr Joslin and the group at the University of Illinois conducted a case-control study to identify the risk factors for the development of *Acanthamoeba* keratitis (AK).[2] They found that Complete MoisturePlus use was independently associated with AK among soft contact lens users. In March 2007, the Centers for Disease Control and Prevention (CDC) initiated a national outbreak investigation. Preliminary analysis of the first 46 cases found that the odds of having ever used Complete MoisturePlus solution were 20 times greater for *Acanthamoeba* case-patients than for controls. This knowledge was rapidly disseminated through *Morbidity and Mortality Weekly Report* (MMWR). Advanced Medical Optics (AMO) withdrew Complete MoisturePlus from the market on May 26, 2007.[3] The final analysis of the CDC data was published in 2009. This article further confirms the findings of the initial analysis and "identified use of a single contact lens solution as the primary risk factor for infection."

Further work by AMO and others has shown that the Complete MoisturePlus solution induced encystment at a much higher rate than other commercially available multipurpose contact lens solution. The presence of propylene glycol was shown to be an essential factor in inducing this encystment. The induction of encystment makes the *Acanthamoeba* organism more resistant to disinfection.

K. M. Hammersmith, MD

References

1. Thebpatiphat N, Hammersmith KM, Rocha FN, et al. *Acanthamoeba* keratitis; a parasite on the rise. *Cornea.* 2007;26:701-706.
2. Joslin CE, Tu EY, Shoff ME, et al. The association of contact lens solution use and *Acanthamoeba* keratitis. *Am J Ophthalmol.* 2007;144:169-180.
3. Centers for Disease Control and Prevention. *Acanthamoeba* keratitis multiple states, 2005–2007. *MMWR Morb Mortal Wkly Rep.* 2007;56:532-534.

Overall and cancer related mortality among patients with ocular inflammation treated with immunosuppressive drugs: retrospective cohort study

Kempen JH, Daniel E, Dunn JP, et al (Univ of Pennsylvania, Philadelphia; Johns Hopkins Univ, Baltimore, MD; et al)

BMJ 339:b2480, 2009

Context.—Whether immunosuppressive treatment adversely affects survival is unclear.

Objective.—To assess whether immunosuppressive drugs increase mortality.

Design.—Retrospective cohort study evaluating overall and cancer mortality in relation to immunosuppressive drug exposure among patients with ocular inflammatory diseases. Demographic, clinical, and treatment data derived from medical records, and mortality results from United States National Death Index linkage. The cohort's mortality risk was compared with US vital statistics using standardised mortality ratios. Overall and cancer mortality in relation to use or non-use of immunosuppressive drugs within the cohort was studied with survival analysis.

Setting.—Five tertiary ocular inflammation clinics.

Patients.—7957 US residents with non-infectious ocular inflammation, 2340 of whom received immunosuppressive drugs during follow up.

Exposures.—Use of antimetabolites, T cell inhibitors, alkylating agents, and tumour necrosis factor inhibitors.

Main Outcome Measures.—Overall mortality, cancer mortality.

Results.—Over 66 802 person years (17 316 after exposure to immunosuppressive drugs), 936 patients died (1.4/ 100 person years), 230 (24.6%) from cancer. For patients unexposed to immunosuppressive treatment, risks of death overall (standardised mortality ratio 1.02, 95% confidence interval [CI] 0.94 to 1.11) and from cancer (1.10, 0.93 to 1.29) were similar to those of the US population. Patients who used azathioprine, methotrexate, mycophenolate mofetil, ciclosporin, systemic corticosteroids, or dapsone had overall and cancer mortality similar to that of patients who never took immunosuppressive drugs. In patients who used cyclophosphamide, overall mortality was not increased and cancer mortality was non-significantly increased. Tumour necrosis factor inhibitors were associated with increased overall (adjusted hazard ratio [HR] 1.99, 95% CI 1.00 to 3.98) and cancer mortality (adjusted HR 3.83, 1.13 to 13.01).

Conclusions.—Most commonly used immunosuppressive drugs do not seem to increase overall or cancer mortality. Our results suggesting that tumour necrosis factor inhibitors might increase mortality are less robust than the other findings; additional evidence is needed.

▶ This study is one that results from the Systemic Immunosuppressive Therapy for Eye diseases (SITE) cohort study. The multicenter SITE study seeks to pool patients from 5 centers to give more power to our understanding of the treatment of ocular inflammation. This particular evaluation looks at an amazing 7957 patients, 2340 of whom were treated with immunosuppressive agents to answer whether there is increased overall and cancer-related mortality among those treated. The good news for our patients is that there was a similar overall and cancer-related mortality in patients who used immunosuppressive agents (azathioprine, methotrexate, mycophenolate mofetil, cyclosporine, systemic corticosteroids, and/or dapsone), and those who did not. There is a nonsignificant increase in cancer mortality in those who took cyclophosphamide. There were also some concerning findings regarding the biologics; however, the authors are cautious in interpreting these findings.

K. M. Hammersmith, MD

Practice patterns in the management of fungal corneal ulcers

Loh AR, Hong K, Lee S, et al (Univ of Pennsylvania School of Medicine, Philadelphia)

Cornea 28:856-859, 2009

Purpose.—The purpose of this study was to determine the practice patterns of ophthalmologists in the management of fungal corneal ulcers.

Methods.—In December 2007, a survey of 13 questions addressing the actual and preferred treatment of fungal ulcers was sent to the kera-net e-mail listserv facilitated by the Cornea Society.

Results.—Ninety-two respondents from North America, South America, Asia, Europe, and Australia participated by completing the electronic questionnaire. Natamycin was the most commonly used topical treatment for ulcers caused by filamentous fungi (96%) followed by amphotericin (75%) and voriconazole (63%). However, voriconazole was most often listed as the preferred topical treatment in an ideal world (79%) compared with 55% for natamycin. Approximately half of the respondents use combination topical therapy (56%) and the remainder monotherapy. The majority of respondents rescrape the epithelium at some time during the course of treatment, but the frequency of rescraping varied among the different topical treatments. The most common reasons cited for not using their preferred treatment were cost and a desire for further evidence to support preferred treatment.

Conclusion.—There appears to be significant variation in the management of fungal corneal ulcers. Although natamycin was the most commonly used treatment for ulcers caused by filamentous fungi, voriconazole was the most preferred as the ideal treatment. These results highlight the need for more evidence regarding the efficacy of the newer topical antifungals.

▶ This study demonstrates that the treatment of fungal keratitis has changed over the last few years. Topical voriconazole, which is not commercially available or Food and Drug Administration (FDA) approved, has become the preferred treatment for filamentous fungal keratitis. We have been using this medication over the last several years with good success. We used it on our first patient just before the national outbreak of *Fusarium* associated with Renu with MoistureLoc. Thus, we had an opportunity to try it out on many patients in a short period of time. It clearly seems clinically superior to natamycin. I think it would have been interesting to see what differences in treatment strategies were based on the type of practice, but I imagine the numbers were too low. I recently treated a patient, who works in health care, with Paecilomyces keratitis. He sought a second opinion after not responding to natamycin. As is common in the age of the Internet, he came with questions and articles regarding the use of topical and oral voriconazole. He was justifiably upset that his treating physician, a community-based cornea specialist at a respected practice, did not have knowledge on the use of voriconazole. This article makes me feel more confident that the word is out that voriconazole is a good treatment option.

K. M. Hammersmith, MD

Quality of Life in Keratoconus Patients After Penetrating Keratoplasty

Yildiz EH, Cohen EJ, Virdi AS, et al (Thomas Jefferson Univ, Philadelphia, PA)

Am J Ophthalmol 149:416-422, 2010

Purpose.—To determine vision-related quality of life (QoL) measured with the National Eye Institute Visual Function Questionnaire (NEI-VFQ) in keratoconus (KCN) patients who have undergone penetrating keratoplasty (PK) in 1 or both eyes and to compare the results of our study to those of historical controls.

Design.—Clinical-based, cross-sectional study.

Methods.—*Setting*: Wills Eye Institute, Cornea Service, Thomas Jefferson University, Philadelphia, Pennsylvania.

Study Population.—This study included 149 consecutive patients who had undergone PK for KCN.

Intervention.—Between June 1, 2008 and December 31, 2008, the NEI-VFQ was administered to 149 patients. The relationship between demographic and clinical factors and NEI-VFQ subscale scores was evaluated.

Main Outcome Measure.—Vision-related quality of life.

Results.—Eighty-three of 149 patients (55.7%) were male. Approximately half of the patients (76/149; 51.0%) had PK in both eyes. Visual acuity with current correction in the better eye was better than 20/40 in 80% of patients (119/149). Our sample had significantly lower (worse) NEI-VFQ scores compared to Collaborative Longitudinal Evaluation of Keratoconus (CLEK) historical control group for the subscales of role difficulties, dependency, driving, and peripheral vision. In general, scores of our sample were between scores of patients with age-related macular degeneration (AMD) category 3 and 4. Patients with visual acuity better than 20/40 (in the better eye) showed significantly higher scores in all subscales except color vision. There was a significant relationship between minimum time since the graft of 5 years or greater and NEI-VFQ overall score better than AMD category 3 ($P = .004$).

Conclusion.—Despite satisfactory results on visual outcome measures obtained after PK, vision-related QoL in KCN patients remains impaired.

▶ This study was undertaken after previous Collaborative Longitudinal Evaluation of Keratoconus (CLEK)-sponsored studies showed shocking low quality of life (QoL) in patients with keratoconus. While we were surprised that these patients had such poor QoL, we figured that if the patients who had undergone transplantation were separated, they would fare much better. However, we were saddened to find a slightly lower vision-related QoL in these patients as those in the previous study. This study is a cross-sectional study, so it does not evaluate the changes in QoL in an individual patient. That is a different but potentially important study to better assess the impact on individuals. This study does support that early surgical intervention likely does not improve QoL. Also, patients that did best were those who used a contact lens post-operatively. This supports our practice of fitting lenses as a first-line therapy and reserving surgery for those in whom fitting is not possible.

K. M. Hammersmith, MD

Recurrence rates of herpes simplex virus keratitis in contact lens and non-contact lens wearers

Mucci JJ, Utz VM, Galor A, et al (Cleveland Clinic, OH)

Eye Contact Lens 35:185-187, 2009

Objective.—To evaluate the recurrence rates of herpes simplex virus (HSV) keratitis in contact lens wearers compared with non-contact lens wearers.

Methods.—Retrospective cohort study. Charts of patients diagnosed with HSV keratitis seen at the Cleveland Clinic between January 2001 and December 2004 were reviewed.

Results.—One hundred seventeen patients were included in this study: 21 contact lens wearers and 96 non-contact lens wearers. Contact lens wearers were found to have a higher median recurrence rate (0.4 episodes/year) compared with non-contact lens wearers (0.2 episodes/year) ($P=0.02$). A multivariate regression evaluating factors predictive of the number of recurrences found that contact lens use remained a significant predictive variable ($P=0.02$) when accounting for patient demographic and disease factors and variable follow-up time.

Conclusions.—Patients with a history of HSV keratitis should be counseled about the potential increased risk of recurrence that may be associated with contact lens wear.

▶ When I read the title of this article, I was immediately interested. Whether or not contact lens wear increases recurrence rates in herpes keratitis is one of those incredibly relevant questions. This is a frequently asked question, and one that I do not feel I have a lot of good data to use for an answer. In general, I think most encourage against contact lens wear in the herpes patient as the microtrauma from lens wear and the increased level of pathogen exposure seems like a bad idea. But, then there are the patients with herpes-related scars, who need a lens to help with best-corrected visual acuity. This study seems to confirm these fears. The authors find a statistically significant increase in the number of recurrences in the contact lens wearer. However, a major disadvantage of this study is the combining of therapeutic and cosmetic contact lens wearers. It follows that those who had severe enough disease to cause corneal scarring and therefore, needed a rigid gas permeable lens for BCVA may have more recurrences. The baseline characteristics of the 2 groups need to be equalized, and a larger study would greatly enhance the findings.

K. M. Hammersmith, MD

Scleritis and Systemic Disease Association in a Community-Based Referral Practice

Raiji VR, Palestine AG, Parver DL (George Washington Univ, DC)
Am J Ophthalmol 148:946-950, 2009

Purpose.—To evaluate the association between scleritis and systemic disease in a non-university, non-tertiary referral practice and to describe our experience with scleritis treatment.

Design.—Retrospective chart review.

Methods.—The medical records of patients with scleritis between 2001 and 2007 were reviewed for associated systemic disease.

Results.—In our series of 86 patients with scleritis, 55 patients (64.0%) had isolated scleritis while 31 patients (36.0%) had associated

TABLE 3.—Scleritis Patient Characteristics Based on Systemic Disease Association in a Community-Based Referral Practice

Systemic Disease	Diffuse	Nodular	Necrotizing	Posterior	Female/Male	Bilateral
Rheumatoid arthritis (10)	2	5	3	0	7/3	5
Spondyloarthropathies (4)	0	3	1	0	2/2	1
IgA nephropathy (2)	0	2	0	0	0/2	0
Sarcoidosis (2)	1	1	0	0	2/0	2
Other autoimmune diseases (9)	1	6	1	1	8/1	7
HIV (2)	1	0	0	1	0/2	1
Herpes zoster (2)	0	2	0	0	2/0	0
Total (31)	5	19	5	2	21/10	16

HIV = human immunodeficiency virus.

systemic-disease. Twenty-six patients (83.9%) with systemic disease had diagnosed systemic disease at the time of initial scleritis presentation, while 5 patients (16.1%) were diagnosed following systemic work-up. Those diagnosed after systemic workup were more likely to have systemic vasculitic disease as opposed to a rheumatic or infectious disease. Patients with and without associated systemic disease were likely to require systemic therapy at similar rates (93.5% and 92.7%, respectively). Five patients with steroid-refractory scleritis were treated with infliximab (Remicade; Centocor Inc, Horsham, Pennsylvania, USA) and all responded without evidence of adverse effect. Seven patients were treated with mycophenolate mofetil (CellCept; Roche Laboratories, Nutley, New Jersey, USA), of which three improved.

Conclusions.—The association between scleritis and systemic disease in a community-based referral practice may be lower than in tertiary referral or university-based centers. Although thorough systemic disease evaluation is warranted in scleritis patients, most patients with associated systemic disease will have such a diagnosis prior to the development of scleritis. The need to institute aggressive systemic therapy cannot be predicted by the presence of an associated systemic disease. Infliximab and mycophenolate mofetil are useful additions to the scleritis practitioner's armamentarium for steroid-refractory scleritis (Table 3).

▶ This is a similar article to one of my selections a few years ago.[1] That study evaluated the underlying systemic disorders in patients with scleritis who presented to a tertiary care practice (Wilmer Eye Institute, Johns Hopkins University) and was essentially repeated here in a community-based referral practice. The findings are fairly similar. In the community-based study, 36% of the patients were found to have an associated systemic disease (44% in the Wilmer study). The initial evaluation resulted in a systemic diagnosis in 16% of these patients (14% at Wilmer). For those patients who I am sending for a work up for scleritis, I use these numbers to counsel them. I think it is helpful to tell them that in the absence of other systemic issues that would direct a diagnosis, only about 15% of the time will this work up result in the diagnosis of a related systemic disorder. We are, of course, obligated to look for other systemic diseases, but this helps reduce frustration that the patients seem to feel when their results end up normal (which they usually do). Another interesting finding is that patients with and without associated systemic disorders were likely to require systemic therapy at similar rates. So, it remains important to involve our rheumatologists in the management of these patients.

K. M. Hammersmith, MD

Reference

1. Akpek EK, Thorne JE, Qazi FA, et al. Evaluation of patients with scleritis for systemic disease. *Ophthalmology.* 2004;111:501-506.

5 Retina

Progression of Age-Related Macular Degeneration After Cataract Surgery

Dong LM, Stark WJ, Jefferys JL, et al (Stony Brook Univ School of Medicine, Baltimore, MD; Johns Hopkins Univ School of Medicine, Baltimore, MD)
Arch Ophthalmol 127:1412-1419, 2009

Objective.—To document age-related macular degeneration (AMD) progression after cataract surgery.

Methods.—Surgeons prospectively enrolled patients with nonneovascular AMD who were awaiting cataract surgery. Fluorescein angiography was performed preoperatively and at the postoperative week 1, month 3, and month 12 visits. Incidence of neovascular AMD development within 12 months after operation was the primary outcome measure.

Results.—A total of 108 subjects were enrolled. Of 86 eyes with preoperatively photographically confirmed nonneovascular AMD, 71 had gradable images by month 12. Neovascular AMD was observed in 9 of 71 eyes (12.7%; 95% confidence interval, 6.0%-22.7%). The progression rate between week 1 and month 12 decreased to 3 of 65 eyes (4.6%; 95% confidence interval, 1.0%-12.9%) after excluding 5 neovascular events identified on the postoperative week 1 visit and 1 case with missing photographs at this visit.

Conclusion.—The low incidence rate of neovascular AMD development between 1 week and 1 year after cataract surgery did not support the hypothesis that cataract surgery increases the risk of AMD progression. Several eyes appeared to have disease progression on postsurgery week 1 fluorescein angiograms, suggesting that many cases of presumed progression to neovascular AMD following cataract surgery may have been present prior to cataract surgery, but not recognized owing to lens opacity.

▶ This prospective study provides a nice complement to the recently published Age-Related Eye Disease Study (AREDS) report on the same clinical issue. The AREDS report found no link between cataract surgery and subsequent progression of age-related macular degeneration (ARMD). This report, while smaller in size has the advantage of sequential photos and fluorescein angiography to verify the findings. Of greatest value is the performance of angiograms just 1 week after cataract surgery. By comparing immediate preoperative and postoperative angiograms, we learn that in cases with visually significant cataracts it is quite possible that many cases of choroidal neovascularization cannot be easily identified before cataract removal, and the surgery very likely has unmasked rather than caused these more advanced cases. The similarity in the incidence of wet ARMD or progressive geographic atrophy between operated eyes and unoperated control eyes at the 1 year study supports the conclusion that cataract surgery does not substantially increase the risk of ARMD progression.[1]

J. F. Vander, MD

Reference

1. Chew EY, Sperduto RD, Milton RC, et al. Risk of advanced age-related macular degeneration after cataract surgery in the Age-Related Eye Disease Study: AREDS report 25. *Ophthalmology.* 2009;116:297-303.

Visual Acuity Outcomes after Cataract Surgery in Patients with Age-Related Macular Degeneration: Age-Related Eye Disease Study Report No. 27

Forooghian F, for the AREDS Research Group (Natl Eye Inst/Natl Insts of Health, Bethesda, MD; et al)

Ophthalmology 116:2093-2100, 2009

Objective.—To evaluate visual acuity outcomes after cataract surgery in patients with varying degrees of age-related macular degeneration (AMD).

Design.—Cohort study.

Participants.—A total of 4757 participants enrolled in the Age-Related Eye Disease Study (AREDS), a prospective, multicenter, epidemiological study of the clinical course of cataract and AMD and a randomized controlled trial of antioxidants and minerals.

Methods.—Standardized lens and fundus photographs, performed at baseline and annual visits, were graded by a centralized reading center using standardized protocols for severity of AMD and lens opacities. History of cataract surgery was obtained every 6 months. Analyses were conducted using multivariate logistic regression.

Main Outcome Measure.—The change in best-corrected visual acuity (BCVA) after cataract surgery compared with preoperative BCVA.

Results.—Visual acuity results were analyzed for 1939 eyes that had cataract surgery during AREDS. The mean time from cataract surgery to measurement of postoperative BCVA was 6.9 months. After adjustment for age at surgery, gender, type, and severity of cataract, the mean change in visual acuity at the next study visit after the cataract surgery was as follows: Eyes without AMD gained 8.4 letters of acuity ($P < 0.0001$), eyes with mild AMD gained 6.1 letters of visual acuity ($P < 0.0001$), eyes with moderate AMD gained 3.9 letters ($P < 0.0001$), and eyes with advanced AMD gained 1.9 letters ($P = 0.04$). The statistically significant gain in visual acuity after cataract surgery was maintained an average of 1.4 years after cataract surgery.

Conclusions.—On average, participants with varying severity of AMD benefited from cataract surgery with an increase in visual acuity postoperatively. This average gain in visual acuity persisted for at least 18 months.

▶ Earlier this year the Age-Related Eye Disease Study (AREDS) reported strong evidence that cataract surgery does not induce progression of macular degeneration, refuting concerns that have lingered for years about the safety of cataract removal in the presence of age-related macular degeneration (ARMD). This subsequent report attempts to address a logical follow-up question: Given that cataract surgery does not appear to make ARMD worse, how much does it help the patient see better? Other studies have shown a subjective improvement after cataract surgery in patients with ARMD, but good quality visual acuity data are harder to come by. The AREDS trial provides us with high quality visual acuity data. Although the trial was well designed and executed, its design makes answering this question a bit tricky. The decision to perform cataract surgery was not a randomized event, and presumably only patients determined to have a reasonable chance of visual improvement were operated upon. Furthermore, other measures of visual function, such as reading speed and glare sensitivity, may be more likely to improve than visual acuity in these patients, and this information was not reported. Nevertheless, even when using the parameter of visual acuity this trial confirms that for selected patients with advanced ARMD, cataract surgery may produce a measurable improvement. When combined with the previously noted safety data, it is reasonable to offer cataract surgery for these patients when otherwise appropriate.

For further reading on this subject I suggest an article by Chew et al.[1]

J. F. Vander, MD

Reference

1. Chew EY, Sperduto RD, Milton RC, et al. Risk of advanced age-related macular degeneration after cataract surgery in the Age-Related Eye Disease Study: AREDS Report 25. *Ophthalmology.* 2009;116:297-303.

Statin Use and the Incidence of Advanced Age-related Macular Degeneration in the Complications of Age-related Macular Degeneration Prevention Trial

Maguire MG, for the Complications of Age-related Macular Degeneration Prevention Trial (CAPT) Research Group (Univ of Pennsylvania, Philadelphia; et al)
Ophthalmology 116:2381-2385, 2009

Objective.—To evaluate the impact of statin use on the incidence of advanced age-related macular degeneration (AMD) and its components, choroidal neovascularization (CNV) and geographic atrophy (GA), among patients with bilateral large drusen.

Design.—Cohort study within a multicenter, randomized, clinical trial.

Participants.—Patients enrolled in the Complications of Age-related Macular Degeneration Prevention Trial (CAPT).

Methods.—Eligibility criteria for the clinical trial required that participants have ≥10 large (>125 μm) drusen and visual acuity ≥20/40 in each eye. Patients scheduled for their final CAPT visit after May 2005 were interviewed on their history of use of cholesterol-lowering medications, including statins. Trained readers identified CNV and end point GA (>1 Macular Photocoagulation Study disc area of GA) based on review of fluorescein angiograms and fundus photographs taken at annual follow-up visits and when patients reported symptoms. The risk ratio for participants developing CNV or developing GA associated with statin use was estimated with time-dependent Cox proportional hazards models.

Main Outcome Measures.—Development of advanced AMD, CNV, and end point GA.

Results.—Among 764 patients eligible for the interview, 744 (97.4%) patients completed the interview on medication use. Statin use was reported by 296 (39.8%) of those interviewed, with the majority, 187 (63.2%) of the 296, beginning use after enrollment in CAPT. Among 744 patients, advanced AMD developed in 332 (22.5%) eyes of 242 (32.5%) patients, CNV in 222 (15%) eyes of 176 (23.7%) patients, and GA in 114 (7.7%) eyes of 80 (10.8%) patients. With adjustment for other risk factors, the estimated risk ratio for eyes (95% confidence interval) associated with statin use was 1.15 (0.87–1.52) for advanced AMD, 1.35 (0.99–1.83) for CNV, and 0.80 (0.46–1.39) for GA.

Conclusions.—The CAPT data are not consistent with a strong protective effect (risk ratio, ≤0.85) of statins on the development of advanced AMD among patients with bilateral large drusen.

▶ There is considerable overlap between risk factors for developing coronary artery or peripheral vascular disease and age-related macular degeneration (ARMD). Recent evidence, as reviewed in this report, includes the role of complement factor H and elevation of C-reactive protein as predictors of these conditions. This report from the Complications of ARMD Prevention Trial (CAPT) failed to show any beneficial effect of statin use in altering the progression of ARMD. It is critical to realize that although this is a randomized clinical trial, the randomization was not regarding the use of statins. Patients entered into the trial with high-risk, dry ARMD based on ophthalmoscopic features. Statin use was based on the patient's medical needs and was independent of any study entry criteria. Surveys were used to determine statin use at the final CAPT visit. Presumably, patients with more significant cardiovascular risk factors were treated with statins. Based on the recent evidence of ARMD risk factors, it is likely that those patients treated with statins were also more likely to have a higher risk of ARMD progression than those not treated with statins. That there was no meaningful difference between the groups in terms of ARMD progression could in fact be an indication that statin use protected the higher risk patients to some degree. Furthermore, by the time patients were enrolled in CAPT, they already had significant dry ARMD. Earlier initiation of statin use might be protective and of great importance. These shortcomings are presented in the discussion section of the report and suggest that the conclusions described in the abstract do not tell the whole story. A randomized trial would be helpful, but problematic in light of the widespread use of statins in the population at risk.

For further reading on this subject I suggest articles by Delcourt et al,[1] and Klein et al.[2]

J. F. Vander, MD

References

1. Delcourt C, Michel F, Colvez A, et al. POLA Study Group. Associations of cardiovascular disease and its risk factors with age-related macular degeneration: the POLA study. *Ophthalmic Epidemiol.* 2001;8:237-249.
2. Klein R, Deng Y, Klein BE, et al. Cardiovascular disease, its risk factors and treatment, and age-related macular degeneration: Women's Health Initiative Sight Exam ancillary study. *Am J Ophthalmol.* 2007;143:473-483.

Subretinal Hemorrhages Associated with Age-Related Macular Degeneration in Patients Receiving Anticoagulation or Antiplatelet Therapy

Kuhli-Hattenbach C, Fischer IB, Schalnus R, et al (Klinikum der Johann Wolfgang Goethe-Universität, Frankfurt am Main, Germany; et al)

Am J Ophthalmol 149:316-321, 2010

Purpose.—To evaluate the incidence of and risk factors for subretinal hemorrhages in age-related macular degeneration (AMD) patients on anticoagulation or antiplatelet therapy.

Design.—Retrospective, observational case series.

Methods.—We retrospectively reviewed the medical and photographic records of 71 consecutive patients who sought treatment at our institution with acute subretinal hemorrhages complicating age-related macular degeneration. The size of the subretinal hemorrhage was measured in standardized Macular Photocoagulation Study disc areas. Data on the use of medications and medical indications for anticoagulation and antiplatelet therapy were obtained.

Results.—Overall, patients receiving antithrombotic therapy had a significantly larger subretinal hemorrhage size (mean, 9.71 disc areas) than patients not receiving anticoagulant or antiplatelet therapy (mean, 2.99 disc areas). Subgroup analysis revealed that both antiplatelet ($P < .0001$) and anticoagulant therapy ($P = .003$) were associated with a significantly larger bleeding size. Moreover, subgroup analysis among patients with arterial hypertension revealed that individuals receiving antithrombotic therapy had a statistically significantly larger hemorrhage size than hypertensive patients who did not receive anticoagulants or antiplatelet agents ($P < .0001$).

Conclusions.—Our results indicate that anticoagulants and antiplatelet agents are strongly associated with the development of large subretinal hemorrhages in AMD patients. Moreover, arterial hypertension is a strong risk factor for large subretinal hemorrhages in AMD patients receiving anticoagulants or antiplatelet agents. Physicians should be aware of an increased risk of extensive subretinal hemorrhage in AMD patients when deciding on the initiation and duration of anticoagulant and antiplatelet therapy.

▶ This retrospective study provides some useful information about submacular hemorrhages but, unfortunately, the discussion section takes the available data and draws broad conclusions not supported by the evidence provided. Intuitively, it makes sense that patients on an anticoagulant would have more problems with intraocular bleeding. The authors found that for patients with submacular hemorrhages, those using any anticoagulant tended to have larger hemorrhages. They conclude that the use of an anticoagulant increases the risk of "extensive bleeding." This conclusion may be true but the study results do not support this statement. Although this may seem a matter of semantics, the implications are important given the widespread use of anticoagulants in the age-related macular degeneration (ARMD) population. We don't know if initiating or maintaining anticoagulant use in a patient with ARMD increases the risk of submacular bleeding, and if it does, we have no idea as to the quantification of that risk. Many risk factors for ARMD are shared with systemic vascular disease, including hyperlipidemia, systemic inflammatory markers, and genetics. Patients with more severe ARMD may be the individuals most likely to have an anticoagulant prescribed. Given the abundant evidence that anticoagulants can be helpful for patients at risk for cardiovascular disease, to sound an alarm with so little evidence may well contribute to morbidity and mortality if the results are not properly put into perspective.

J. F. Vander, MD

A Prospective Randomized Evaluation of Topical Gatifloxacin on Conjunctival Flora in Patients Undergoing Intravitreal Injections

Moss JM, Sanislo SR, Ta CN (Stanford Univ Med Ctr, CA)
Ophthalmology 116:1498-1501, 2009

Purpose.—We sought to assess the efficacy of 3-day topical gatifloxacin use in combination with povidone-iodine (PVI) versus PVI alone in eliminating conjunctival bacterial flora in patients scheduled to undergo intravitreal (IVT) injection.

Design.—Prospective, randomized single-blind clinical trial.

Participants.—We included 129 patients scheduled to undergo 273 IVT injections at California Vitreoretinal Center at Stanford University.

Methods.—Study patients were randomized to self-administration of gatifloxacin drops for 3 days before injection, or no pretreatment antibiotics. Cultures were collected from the bulbar conjunctiva at the injection site and at the corresponding location in the fellow eye before PVI preparation. After topical PVI treatment and immediately before injection, a third culture was obtained at the injection site. Additionally, the injection needle was also cultured after the procedure.

Main Outcome Measures.—Incidence of positive bacterial samples collected from injection site conjunctiva and injection needles.

Results.—Three-day gatifloxacin use resulted in a significantly lower rate of SeptiChek (Becton Dickinson, Franklin Lakes, NJ) positive cultures compared with untreated controls (21% vs 48% respectively, $P = 0.005$). After topical PVI, the rate of positive bacterial cultures in gatifloxacin-treated and control eyes were similar (8% and 4%, respectively; $P = 0.324$).

Conclusions.—Although 3-day topical gatifloxacin use is effective in reducing the frequency of conjunctival bacterial growth relative to untreated eyes, antibiotic use confers no additional benefit in combination with PVI than eyes receiving PVI alone. This supports that topical PVI is an effective preinjection monotherapy for infection prophylaxis in the setting of IVT injections. Financial Disclosure(s): The authors have no proprietary or commercial interest in any materials discussed in this article.

▶ The use of povidone-iodine (PVI) is the one method of endophthalmitis prophylaxis clearly shown to reduce the rate of infection in a well-controlled clinical trial. For intravitreal injection prophylaxis, many strategies have been used, including preinjection use of topical antibiotics. This report demonstrates that topical antibiotics can reduce conjunctival flora, but that when compared with the overwhelming benefits of PVI, antibiotics don't make a meaningful contribution to endophthalmitis prophylaxis. Furthermore, repeated use of antibiotics might encourage development of resistance, and based on this report there is no justification for routine use of topical antibiotics before intravitreal injections.

J. F. Vander, MD

Verteporfin Photodynamic Therapy Combined With Intravitreal Bevacizumab for Neovascular Age-Related Macular Degeneration

Kaiser PK, for the Registry of Visudyne AMD Therapy Writing Committee (Cole Eye Inst, Cleveland, OH, et al)

Ophthalmology 116:747-755, 2009

Purpose.—To assess outcomes for patients with choroidal neovascularization (CNV) due to age-related macular degeneration (AMD) treated with verteporfin photodynamic therapy (PDT) and bevacizumab.

Design.—Retrospective, case series database study (registry).

Participants.—We included1196 patients with CNV due to AMD who received ≥1 combination treatment of 1.25 mg intravitreal bevacizumab within 14 days of verteporfin PDT.

Methods.—Retrospective analysis of baseline data with ongoing follow-up. Physicians from 45 clinical centers entered patient data at baseline and follow-up examinations, including subsequent treatments, into a secure, Web-accessed database. Snellen visual acuity (VA) was converted to logarithm of the minimum angle of resolution (logMAR) for statistical analyses.

Main Outcome Measures.—Change from baseline in VA and retreatment rates of any therapy after the initial combination treatment.

Results.—Of 1196 patients, 1073 patients had ≥6 months of follow-up. For these 1073 patients, mean baseline VA was 0.967 logMAR (approximate Snellen 20/185) and 56.3% of patients (604/1073) were treatment naïve. After their baseline combination treatment, patients received a mean of 0.6 additional verteporfin PDT retreatments and 2.0 bevacizumab retreatments over a mean follow-up period of 15.0 months. By 12 months, 82% of patients (578/701) had stable or improved vision (loss of <3 lines or a gain in VA), 36% (255/701) improved by ≥3 lines, and 17% (121/701) improved by ≥6 lines. By 12 months, patients gained approximately 1.2 lines (6 letters) of VA from baseline. Patients who were treatment naïve gained significantly more VA by month 12 (+8.4 letters) compared with those who had been previously treated (+2.4 letters; $P < 0.01$). Most serious adverse events (26/30) were judged by investigators as not related to any study treatment, although 3 ocular events were judged related to bevacizumab alone, and 1 ocular event was judged related to both bevacizumab and PDT.

Conclusions.—Combination therapy with PDT and bevacizumab led to vision benefit for most patients, particularly those who were treatment naïve at baseline. The number of retreatments was lower than published reports with either treatment delivered as monotherapy. Randomized clinical trials are underway to confirm these findings.

▶ The use of intravitreal vascular endothelial growth factor (VEGF) inhibitor injections has become widespread and, given the need for ongoing treatment in most cases, has become a major part of the typical retinal specialists efforts. Patient acceptance is generally high because of the impressive results obtained. Nevertheless, it would be highly desirable to find a method of treating choroidal neovascularization that would substantially diminish the burden of injections with an indeterminate endpoint. The combination of photodynamic therapy (PDT) and injections is an approach that is described in this report, and it is tempting to assume that this approach helps to diminish that treatment burden. That would be a mistake given the nature of the study methodology. This retrospective, multicenter collection of data consists of a variety of lesion types, clinical features, previous treatment usage, etc. As a result, it is not possible to say with any certainty that the combination approach is superior or even as good as injection monotherapy. Furthermore, it is possible that treatment with PDT could reduce final vision results due to the nature of the treatment.

Implementing this treatment strategy in clinical practice should wait until randomized trials can better advise us.

J. F. Vander, MD

A Variable-dosing Regimen with Intravitreal Ranibizumab for Neovascular Age-related Macular Degeneration: Year 2 of the PrONTO Study

Lalwani GA, Rosenfeld PJ, Fung AE, et al (Univ of Miami Miller School of Medicine, FL)

Am J Ophthalmol 148:43-58, 2009

Purpose.—To assess the long-term efficacy of a variable-dosing regimen with ranibizumab in the Prospective Optical Coherence Tomography (OCT) Imaging of Patients with Neovascular Age-Related Macular Degeneration (AMD) Treated with intraOcular Ranibizumab (PrONTO) Study, patients were followed for 2 years.

Design.—A 2-year prospective, uncontrolled, variable-dosing regimen with intravitreal ranibizumab based on OCT.

Methods.—In this open-label, prospective, single-center, uncontrolled clinical study, AMD patients with neovascularization involving the central fovea and a central retinal thickness (CRT) of at least 300 μm as measured by OCT were enrolled to receive 3 consecutive monthly intravitreal injections of ranibizumab (0.5 mg) [Lucentis; Genentech Inc, South San Francisco, California, USA]. During the first year, retreatment with ranibizumab was performed at each monthly visit if any criterion was fulfilled such as an increase in OCT-CRT of at least 100 μm or a loss of 5 letters or more. During the second year, the retreatment criteria were amended to include retreatment if any qualitative increase in the amount of fluid was detected using OCT.

Results.—Forty patients were enrolled and 37 completed the 2-year study. At month 24, the mean visual acuity (VA) improved by 11.1 letters ($P < .001$) and the OCT-CRT decreased by 212 μm ($P < .001$). VA improved by 15 letters or more in 43% of patients. These VA and OCT outcomes were achieved with an average of 9.9 injections over 24 months.

Conclusions.—The PrONTO Study using an OCT-guided variable-dosing regimen with intravitreal ranibizumab resulted in VA outcomes comparable with the outcomes from the phase III clinical studies, but fewer intravitreal injections were required.

▶ The Anchor and Marina trials showed the tremendous effectiveness of ranibizumab in preventing the vision loss of age-related macular degeneration (ARMD) and transformed the care of this condition. The cost and inconvenience of monthly injections for at least 2 years are obstacles to the widespread application of the drug. The Pronto data demonstrate that with close monitoring we may be able to come close to the same effectiveness with fewer injections. There are a few caveats to consider. First, the Pronto data are uncontrolled and the sample size is small. Second, even though patients don't necessarily need an injection at each visit, they still need monthly exams and optical coherence tomography (OCTs) to determine the completeness of their control. With this regimen, monthly OCTs are critical, whereas in a standardized regimen they are not. Furthermore, the uncertainty this protocol creates may actually worsen the anxiety patients experience because there is inevitably a good or bad report with each visit and that may well be more stressful over time. The best approach to wet ARMD may not be the same for every patient and the development of newer medications or treatment approaches may transform our care before long.

J. F. Vander, MD

Retinal pigment epithelial tears after single administration of intravitreal bevacizumab for neovascular age-related macular degeneration

Gelisken F, Ziemssen F, Voelker M, et al (Univ of Tuebingen, Germany)
Eye 23:694-702, 2009

Purpose.—To analyse retinal pigment epithelial (RPE) tears following single administration of intravitreal bevacizumab for neovascular age-related macular degeneration (AMD) during early follow-up.

Methods.—Interventional, retrospective, non-comparative case series included 397 patients (409 eyes) of the 746 consecutive patients that met the eligibility criteria. Standardized visual acuity testing, fluorescein angiography, and optical coherence tomography were performed. Data collected included status of the fellow eye, previous treatment, subtypes of choroidal neovascularization (CNV), size and composition of the lesion. Multiple linear regression modelling was used to explore the effect of baseline parameters on the RPE tears. Primary end point was occurrence of RPE tears within 6 weeks after therapy.

Results.—Fifteen of the 409 eyes (3.6%) developed RPE tear (95% confidence interval: 2.2–6.0, odds ratio: 26.3). The statistical modelling showed significant association between RPE tear and occult without classic CNV/predominantly haemorrhage *vs* predominantly/minimal classic CNV ($P = 0.019$), as well as medium or large (>4 disc area) *vs* small size of the total lesion ($P = 0.038$). Previous treatment and status of the fellow eye did not statistically influence the risk of RPE tears.

Conclusions.—An RPE tear can develop in up to 3.6% of eyes with neovascular AMD following single administration of intravitreal bevacizumab in a short-term follow-up. Medium and large lesion size and occult without classic and predominantly haemorrhagic subtype of CNV were important predictive factors. Preoperative assessment of the lesion characteristics may help in identifying the risk of individual patients with neovascular AMD before intravitreal bevacizumab treatment.

▶ Retinal pigment epithelial (RPE) tears in age-related macular degeneration (AMD) have been demonstrated as a part of the natural course of wet ARMD and part of the response to every popular form of treatment. This includes treatment with antivascular endothelial growth factor (VEGF) intravitreal injections. There are 2 important aspects of this study. The first is that given the short interval between injection and development of RPE tears, there is good reason to conclude that the treatment precipitated the tear. Of course it is possible that tears would have developed in many of these eyes anyway, but that remains unproven and, at the least, we should suspect that injection accelerates or concentrates the risk to the period of time shortly after injection. Second, the morphology of the neovascular lesion affects the prognosis, at least as it relates to the development of tears. Fluorescein, and sometimes indocyanine green angiography, are needed to properly assess the morphology, and given the substantial increase in risk described by the authors with certain lesion types, it is desirable to properly assess this before the first injection is given. In an era when nearly all wet ARMD is treated by initiating a course of injections, there is still a role for angiography, at least at baseline.

J. F. Vander, MD

A Multi-Year Analysis of Islet Transplantation Compared With Intensive Medical Therapy on Progression of Complications in Type 1 Diabetes

Warnock GL, Thompson DM, Meloche RM, et al (Univ of British Columbia, Vancouver, Canada)

Transplantation 86:1762-1766, 2008

Background.—We hypothesized that transplantation of islets into type 1 diabetics could improve outcomes of glucose metabolism, renal function, retinopathy, and neuropathy compared with intensive medical therapy.

Methods.—We conducted a prospective, crossover, cohort study of intensive medical therapy (group 1) versus islet cell transplantation (group 2) in 42 patients. All were enrolled in group 1 then 31 crossed over with group 2 when islet donation became available. Transplantation was performed by portal venous embolization of more than 12,000 islet equivalents/kg body weight under cover of immunosuppression with antithymocyte globulin, tacrolimus, and mycophenolate. Outcome measures were HbA1c, change in glomerular filtration rate (GFR), progression of retinopathy, and change in nerve conduction velocity. This report details interim analysis of outcomes after 34 ± 18 months (group 1) and 38 ± 18 months (group 2).

Results.—HbA1c (%) in group 1 was 7.5 ± 0.9 versus 6.6 ± 0.7 in group 2 ($P<0.01$). GFR (mL/min/month) declined in both groups (group 1 −0.45 ± 0.7 vs. group 2 −0.12 ± 0.7, $P=0.1$). Slope of the GFR decline in group 1 was significantly more than 0. Retinopathy progressed in 10 of 82 eyes in group 1 versus 0 of 51 in group 2 ($P<0.01$). Nerve conduction velocity (m/sec) remained stable in group 1 (47.8 ± 5 to 47.1 ± 5 m/sec) and group 2 (47.2 ± 4.5 to 47.7 ± 3.5).

Conclusion.—Islet transplantation yields improved HbA1c and less progression of retinopathy compared with intensive medical therapy during 3 years follow-up.

▶ Islet cell transplantation has not met initial expectations thus far. Insulin independence has not been consistently achieved, and problems with immunosuppressive side-effects and concerns about a negative impact on renal function are among the reasons for this disappointment. This study describes results that are a bit more promising–but only a bit. Almost 40% of patients required resumption of insulin usage, many required multiple transplantation sessions, and a few had significant adverse effects from their immunosuppressive regimen. Furthermore, the study design is not really a true prospective crossover model because a large percentage of patients were simply moved from standard intensive therapy to the transplant group in a nonrandomized fashion. There was no planned return to standard therapy, and this is really more an interventional study with an inadequate control group. Nevertheless, this report reveals that transplantation may improve glucose control and that improved control reduces the risk of retinopathy progression. Whether this method of glucose control will become clinically relevant for mainstream management of diabetes is uncertain.

J. F. Vander, MD

Development and Progression of Diabetic Retinopathy 12 Months after Phacoemulsification Cataract Surgery

Hong T, Mitchell P, de Loryn T, et al (Univ of Sydney, New South Wales, Australia)

Ophthalmology 116:1510-1514, 2009

Objective.—To assess whether phacoemulsification cataract surgery exacerbates the development and progression of diabetic retinopathy (DR) in a cataract surgical cohort.

Design.—Clinic-based cohort study.

Participants.—Patients aged 65+ years undergoing cataract surgery at an eye clinic in Sydney, Australia, between 2004 and 2006.

Methods.—Digital retinal photography was performed after pupil dilation preoperatively and at 1-, 6-, and 12-month postoperative visits. DR was assessed using the modified Early Treatment Diabetic Retinopathy Study (ETDRS) classification. Preoperative and 1-month postoperative (baseline) photographs were compared side-by-side with 12-month postoperative photographs. Odds ratios (ORs) and 95% confidence intervals (CIs) were calculated for DR progression in operated (pseudophakic) compared with nonoperated (phakic) eyes, adjusted for age, sex, diabetes duration, and preoperative glycosylated hemoglobin level.

Main Outcome Measures.—Incident DR was defined in eyes without DR at baseline in which DR was detected at 12-month postoperative visits. DR progression was defined as an increase of 1 or more ETDRS steps during the same period, including incident cases.

Results.—Of 1994 surgical patients recruited, 190 (9.53%) with diabetes and complete data and thus were included. There were 56 patients with unilateral surgery performed before baseline (mean postoperative duration 3.3 ± 3.3 years). The prevalence of DR at baseline was higher in these 56 pseudophakic eyes than in 324 phakic eyes (71.4% vs. 48.2%, respectively, adjusted OR 2.16; 95% CI, 1.16–4.03). Of the 190 patients, 169 were followed for 12+ months postoperatively; 278 eyes were pseudophakic, and 60 eyes remained phakic at 12 months. During the 12-month postoperative period, incident DR developed in 28.2% of pseudophakic eyes and 13.8% of phakic eyes (adjusted OR 2.65; 95% CI, 1.06–6.61). In a paired-eye comparison of 45 patients who remained unilaterally pseudophakic at 12 months and were at risk of DR progression, 35.6% of pseudophakic eyes exhibited DR progression compared with 20.0% of the fellow phakic eyes (adjusted OR 2.21; 95% CI, 0.85–5.71).

Conclusions.—Diabetic patients undergoing phacoemulsification cataract surgery appear to have a doubling of DR progression rates 12 months after surgery. This outcome, however, represents less progression than was previously documented with intracapsular and extracapsular cataract surgical techniques.

▶ The progression or development of diabetic retinopathy is multifactorial in origin. Important variables include expression of various molecules known to encourage angiogenesis and hyperpermeability such as vascular endothelial growth factor (VEGF). Intraocular inflammation, such as typically occurs after intraocular surgery, is known to increase concentrations of these substances. It is this mechanism that likely explains, at least in part, the finding that while retinopathy development or progression are less likely after small incision phacoemulsification, there is still a measurable increase in retinopathy development and progression after cataract surgery when compared with control eyes. The clinical implications of these facts are important in that diabetic patients must be apprised of this concern. Patients with bilateral cataracts are often scheduled for a second eye surgery within days or a few weeks of the first eye. This report suggests that diabetic patients might be better served by altering this strategy. Waiting a few months after the first eye is operated on might help to identify those uncommon individuals at particularly high risk of progression. Although this study did not address this point, it is likely that the fellow eye will behave similarly and it would be helpful to appreciate this before the second eye surgery has already been performed.

J. F. Vander, MD

Effect of Diabetic Retinopathy and Panretinal Photocoagulation on Retinal Nerve Fiber Layer and Optic Nerve Appearance

Lim MC, Tanimoto SA, Furlani BA, et al (Univ of California–Davis, Sacramento; Univ of São Paulo, Brazil)

Arch Ophthalmol 127:857-862, 2009

Objective.—To determine if panretinal photocoagulation (PRP) alters retinal nerve fiber layer (RNFL) thickness and optic nerve appearance.

Methods.—Patients with diabetes who did and did not undergo PRP and nondiabetic control subjects were enrolled in a prospective study. Participants underwent optical coherence tomography of the peripapillary retina and optic nerve. Stereoscopic optic nerve photographs were graded in a masked fashion.

Results.—Ninety-four eyes of 48 healthy individuals, 89 eyes of 55 diabetic patients who did not undergo PRP, and 37 eyes of 24 subjects with diabetes who underwent PRP were included in this study. Eyes that had been treated with PRP had thinner peripapillary RNFL compared with the other groups; this was statistically significantly different in the inferior ($P = .004$) and nasal ($P = .003$) regions. Optic nerve cupping did not increase with severity of disease classification, but the proportion of optic nerves graded as suspicious for glaucoma or as having nonglaucomatous optic neuropathy did ($P = .008$). These grading categories were associated with thinner RNFL measurements.

Conclusions.—Diabetic eyes that have been treated with PRP have thinner RNFL than nondiabetic eyes. Optic nerves in eyes treated with PRP are more likely to be graded as abnormal, but their appearance is not necessarily glaucomatous and may be related to thinning of the RNFL.

▶ Optic atrophy or optic disc changes suspicious for glaucoma often coexist with diabetic retinopathy. Whether the disc changes are primary, thereby requiring diagnostic evaluation and/or initiation of treatment such as drops for glaucoma, or secondary to diabetic retinopathy, or its treatment, is a dilemma frequently facing clinicians. This prospective cohort study demonstrates that disc changes are more likely in diabetic patients, particularly those treated with panretinal photocoagulation (PRP). Due to the study design, however, we can't definitively conclude that it is the application of PRP that precipitates the disc changes. It is possible that the same mechanism that precipitates progression of proliferative retinopathy (ie, ischemia) may also produce the disc and nerve fiber layer changes. Clarification of the mechanism for the disc changes would require a prospective evaluation of patients before and after placement of laser.

J. F. Vander, MD

Three-Year Follow-up of a Randomized Trial Comparing Focal/Grid Photocoagulation and Intravitreal Triamcinolone for Diabetic Macular Edema

Diabetic Retinopathy Clinical Research Network (DRCR.net) (Jaeb Ctr for Health Res, Tampa, FL)

Arch Ophthalmol 127:245-251, 2009

Objective.—To report 3-year outcomes of patients who participated in a randomized trial evaluating 1-mg and 4-mg doses of preservative-free intravitreal triamcinolone compared with focal/grid photocoagulation for treatment of diabetic macular edema.

Methods.—Eyes with diabetic macular edema and visual acuities of 20/40 to 20/320 were randomly assigned to focal/grid photocoagulation or 1 mg or 4 mg of triamcinolone. At the conclusion of the trial, 3-year follow-up data were available in 306 eyes.

Results.—Between 2 years (time of the primary outcome) and 3 years, more eyes improved than worsened in all 3 treatment groups. Change in visual acuity letter score from baseline to 3 years was +5 in the laser group and 0 in each triamcinolone group. The cumulative probability of cataract surgery by 3 years was 31%, 46%, and 83% in the laser and 1-mg and 4-mg triamcinolone groups, respectively. Intraocular pressure increased by more than 10 mm Hg at any visit in 4%, 18%, and 33% of eyes, respectively.

Conclusions.—Results in a subset of randomized subjects who completed the 3-year follow-up are consistent with previously published 2-year results and do not indicate a long-term benefit of intravitreal triamcinolone relative to focal/grid photocoagulation in patients with diabetic macular edema similar to those studied in this clinical trial. Most eyes receiving 4 mg of triamcinolone as given in this study are likely to require cataract surgery.

Trial Registration.—clinicaltrials.gov Identifier: NCT00367133.

▶ This article, like the one published in 2008 with 2-year follow-up information, reports on a trial that has produced high quality data but unfortunately has asked the wrong question. Patients with all patterns of diabetic macular edema (DME) were included so long as the fovea was involved. Experienced retinal physicians will all appreciate that not all forms of DME are created equal. Patients with primarily focal leakage and a well-preserved foveal avascular zone are not the same as patients with diffuse leakage and foveal ischemia. It is the latter group that fails to consistently respond favorably to focal laser and in which one might typically consider steroid injections as primary monotherapy.

Furthermore, the response to steroid injection is highly dependent on the interval between the time of injection and the time of evaluation. In this study, patients were evaluated 4 months after treatment. Often patients will show a waning of therapeutic benefit in this time frame.

If one concludes from this study that steroid injection is not the optimal primary treatment for DME as a whole, then that conclusion seems valid. If, however, one concludes that primary treatment is never valid, that might not be valid.

J. F. Vander, MD

A Randomized Trial Comparing the Efficacy and Safety of Intravitreal Triamcinolone With Observation to Treat Vision Loss Associated With Macular Edema Secondary to Central Retinal Vein Occlusion: The Standard Care vs Corticosteroid for Retinal Vein Occlusion (SCORE) Study Report 5

The SCORE Study Research Group (EMMES Corporation, Rockville, MD)
Arch Ophthalmol 127:1101-1114, 2009

Objective.—To compare the efficacy and safety of 1-mg and 4-mg doses of preservative-free intravitreal triamcinolone with observation for eyes with vision loss associated with macular edema secondary to perfused central retinal vein occlusion (CRVO).

Methods.—Multicenter, randomized, clinical trial of 271participants.

Main Outcome Measure.—Gain in visual acuity letter score of 15 or more from baseline to month 12.

Results.—Seven percent, 27%, and 26% of participants achieved the primary outcome in the observation, 1-mg, and 4-mg groups, respectively. The odds of achieving the primary outcome were 5.0 times greater in the 1-mg group than the observation group (odds ratio [OR], 5.0; 95% confidence interval [CI], 1.8-14.1; $P = .001$) and 5.0 times greater in 4-mg group than the observation group (OR, 5.0; 95% CI, 1.8-14.4; $P = .001$); there was no difference identified between the 1-mg and 4-mg groups (OR, 1.0; 95% CI, 0.5-2.1; $P = .97$). The rates of elevated intraocular pressure and cataract were similar for the observation and 1-mg groups, but higher in the 4-mg group.

Conclusions.—Intravitreal triamcinolone is superior to observation for treating vision loss associated with macular edema secondary to CRVO in patients who have characteristics similar to those in the SCORE-CRVO trial. The 1-mg dose has a safety profile superior to that of the 4-mg dose.

Application to Clinical Practice.—Intravitreal triamcinolone in a 1-mg dose, following the retreatment criteria applied in the SCORE Study, should be considered for up to 1 year, and possibly 2 years, for patients with characteristics similar to those in the SCORE-CRVO trial.

Trial Registration.—clinicaltrials.gov Identifier: NCT00105027.

▶ This is the first well-controlled randomized clinical trial to show level 1 evidence of a therapeutic benefit for the treatment of macular edema due to central retinal vein occlusion (CRVO). Intravitreal steroid injections produce a 5-fold increase in the rate of visual improvement. Unfortunately, this increase is from around 5% to 25%, meaning 75% of patients don't have a meaningful recovery with triamcinolone injections. The dosage of steroid used most widely is 4 mg/0.1 cc. This trial suggests that the therapeutic benefits of injections every 4 months seem to be comparable when using 1 mg and 4 mg, whereas there is a somewhat better safety profile, particularly concerning intraocular pressure increases, when using the lower dose. Of note, the data are much less useful for the second year since there was a large drop-off in compliance with follow-up visits in year 2. It is likely that cataract progression would be an ongoing issue for phakic patients, and that repeated injections might be necessary into the second year, and possibly beyond, but that information is not available in this report. Current interest in the use of intravitreal bevacizumab for this condition is substantial, although not studied in this work. For now, we can at least conclude that repeated intravitreal injection of 1 mg triamcinolone every 4 months for well-perfused macular edema due to CRVO is superior to observation.

J. F. Vander, MD

A Randomized Trial Comparing the Efficacy and Safety of Intravitreal Triamcinolone With Standard Care to Treat Vision Loss Associated With Macular Edema Secondary to Branch Retinal Vein Occlusion: The Standard Care vs Corticosteroid for Retinal Vein Occlusion (SCORE) Study Report 6

The SCORE Study Research Group (EMMES Corporation, Rockville, MD)

Arch Ophthalmol 127:1115-1128, 2009

Objective.—To compare the efficacy and safety of 1-mg and 4-mg doses of preservative-free intravitreal triamcinolone with standard care (grid photocoagulation in eyes without dense macular hemorrhage and deferral of photocoagulation until hemorrhage clears in eyes with dense macular hemorrhage) for eyes with vision loss associated with macular edema secondary to branch retinal vein occlusion (BRVO).

Methods.—Multicenter, randomized clinical trial of 411 participants.

Main Outcome Measure.—Gain in visual acuity letter score of 15 or more from baseline to month 12.

Results.—Twenty-nine percent, 26%, and 27% of participants achieved the primary outcome in the standard care, 1-mg, and 4-mg groups, respectively. None of the pairwise comparisons between the 3 groups was statistically significant at month 12. The rates of elevated intraocular pressure and cataract were similar for the standard care and 1-mg groups, but higher in the 4-mg group.

Conclusions.—There was no difference identified in visual acuity at 12 months for the standard care group compared with the triamcinolone groups; however, rates of adverse events (particularly elevated intraocular pressure and cataract) were highest in the 4-mg group.

Application to Clinical Practice.—Grid photocoagulation as applied in the SCORE Study remains the standard care for patients with vision loss associated with macular edema secondary to BRVO who have characteristics similar to participants in the SCORE-BRVO trial. Grid photocoagulation should remain the benchmark against which other treatments are compared in clinical trials for eyes with vision loss associated with macular edema secondary to BRVO.

Trial Registration.—clinicaltrials.gov Identifier: NCT00105027.

▶ The Branch Retinal Vein Occlusion (BRVO) study, reported over 20 years ago, established grid laser photocoagulation as the gold standard for managing macular edema due to BRVO. That remains the case today, as reaffirmed by the Standard Care versus Corticosteroid for Retinal Vein Occlusion (SCORE) study BRVO arm reported herein. Unlike for central retinal vein occlusion patients, use of intravitreal triamcinolone as monotherapy is not recommended. Visual acuity results are no better when using injections as opposed to laser, and safety issues such as glaucoma and cataract are noteworthy with steroid injections. There are some issues worth considering, however. A minority of patients improved in the trial, regardless of treatment strategy used. Laser was delayed in patients with edema and substantial macular hemorrhage. It is possible that intravitreal steroid injection at that point, followed by laser when clearance of blood permitted, would have produced superior visual results. Other combination strategies might also have given better results but were not within the scope of this trial. Also, alternative intravitreal medications, such as bevacizumab, were not tested and might have a role to play, either in a combination strategy or possibly as monotherapy. Until shown otherwise, primary placement of a macular grid, when not prevented by substantial macular hemorrhage, is the first line of treatment for most patients with perfused macular edema due to BRVO.

J. F. Vander, MD

Intravitreal Bevacizumab for Refractory Pseudophakic Cystoid Macular Edema: The Pan-American Collaborative Retina Study Group Results

Arevalo JF, Maia M, Garcia-Amaris RA, et al (Clinica Oftalmológica Centro Caracas, Venezuela; Universidade Federal de São Paulo, Brazil; et al)

Ophthalmology 116:1481-1487, 2009

Objective.—To determine the feasibility, safety, and clinical effect of intravitreal (IVT) bevacizumab (Avastin; Genentech, Inc., San Francisco, CA) in patients with refractory cystoid macular edema (CME) after cataract surgery.

Design.—Interventional, retrospective, multicenter study.

Participants.—Thirty-six eyes of 31 patients with refractory CME after cataract surgery and with a mean age of 68.2 years (range, 67–87 years).

Methods.—Patients were treated with at least 1 IVT injection of 1.25 or 2.5 mg bevacizumab. Patients were followed up for 12 months.

Main Outcome Measures.—Best-corrected visual acuity (BCVA) and central macular thickness (CMT) by optical coherence tomography (OCT).

Results.—Twenty-six eyes (72.2%) demonstrated improvement of BCVA (≥2 Early Treatment Diabetic Retinopathy Study [ETDRS] lines), and no eye experienced worsening of visual acuity (≥2 ETDRS lines). Mean baseline BCVA was 20/200 (0.96 logarithm of the minimum angle of resolution [logMAR] units), and the mean 12-month BCVA was 20/80 (0.62 logMAR units; $P < 0.0001$). Optical coherence tomography demonstrated that mean CMT at baseline was 499.9 μm (range, 298–784 μm) and decreased to a mean of 286.1 μm (range, 168–499 μm) at 12 months ($P < 0.0001$). Four (11%) eyes received 2 injections, 10 (27.8%) eyes received 3 injections, 10 (27.8%) eyes received 4 injections, 1 (2.8%) eye received 5 injections, and 1 (2.8%) eye received 6 injections. The mean number of injections was 2.7 (range, 1–6), and the mean interval between injections was 15.1 weeks (range, 4–45 weeks). No ocular or systemic adverse events were observed.

Conclusions.—Short-term results suggest that IVT bevacizumab is well tolerated in patients with refractory pseudophakic CME. Treated eyes had a significant improvement in BCVA and decrease in macular thickness by OCT at 12 months.

▶ As phacoemulsification techniques have improved, refractory pseudophakic cystoid macular edema (CME) has become relatively uncommon, particularly in eyes without complicating factors such as epiretinal membrane or uveitis. When corticosteroids or nonsteroidal anti-inflammatory drugs fail, however, it can leave patients severely impaired and disappointed. This retrospective report was prepared in response to a previous report by Spitzer et al that found no therapeutic effect of intravitreal bevacizumab for this problem. This article describes a significant benefit from injections given as often as 6 times over a 1-year period. Patients were determined to be refractory after at least 3 months of traditional therapy. Safety results were excellent. Given the variable clinical course and infrequency of the problem, it is difficult to perform a large randomized trial assessing therapy for CME. While the explanation for the discrepancy in results is unclear, it seems reasonable to consider intravitreal bevacizumab as a viable treatment option for similar patients.

For further reading on this subject I suggest an article by Spitzer et al.[1]

J. F. Vander, MD

Reference

1. Spitzer MS, Ziemssen F, Yoeruek E, Petermeier K, Aisenbrey S, Szurman P. Efficacy of intravitreal bevacizumab in treating postoperative pseudophakic cystoid macular edema. *J Cataract Refract Surg.* 2008;34:70-75.

Correlation between Metamorphopsia and Epiretinal Membrane Optical Coherence Tomography Findings

Watanabe A, Arimoto S, Nishi O (Nishi Eye Hosp, Osaka, Japan)
Ophthalmology 116:1788-1793, 2009

Purpose.—To examine the retinal morphologic features of metamorphopsia caused by epiretinal membrane (ERM) and to determine whether spectral-domain optical coherence tomography (SD-OCT) correlated with metamorphopsia.

Design.—Retrospective case series.

Participants.—This study included 19 eyes of 19 patients with ERM diagnosed by clinical ophthalmic findings and SD-OCT.

Methods.—The 19 eyes were classified into 3 groups based on Amsler chart results: no metamorphopsia (n = 4), local metamorphopsia (n = 8), and broad metamorphopsia (n = 7). The thickness of the 3 inner retinal layers: inner nuclear layer (INL), outer plexiform layer (OPL), and outer nuclear layer (ONL), on 5 horizontal SD-OCT cross-sections (1 line through the fovea, 2 regularly spaced lines superior to the fovea, and 2 regularly spaced lines inferior to the fovea) were measured using the electronic calipers of the SD-OCT system.

Main Outcome Measures.—Correlation between INL, OPL, and ONL thickness with metamorphopsia and visual acuity.

Results.—Metamorphopsia was detected in the same position as edematous areas of the INL with a thickness >50 μm. The maximum INL thickness was relatively significantly different between the subjects with no metamorphopsia and those with local or broad metamorphopsia (vs local, $P = 0.06$; vs broad, $P = 0.04$). Visual acuity significantly correlated with both maximum INL thickness ($A = -0.681$; $P = 0.001$) and maximum ONL thickness ($A = -0.708$; $P < 0.001$) in metamorphopsia.

Conclusions.—Metamorphopsia induced by ERM may be related to the edematous areas of the INL detected with SD-OCT. The classification of ERM based on INL thickness is a potentially useful indication for surgery (Fig 1).

▶ This study has implications beyond simply understanding the correlation between anatomic changes and changes with an Amsler grid. By demonstrating that thickening in the inner nuclear layer correlates with metamorphopsia and seems to be geographically correlated with the location of the metamorphopsia we might be able to make clinically useful predictions for patients with epiretinal membranes (ERM) (Fig 1 shows this correlation nicely). For example, in patients with ERM and cataract, if the preoperative optical coherence tomography (OCT) shows inner nuclear layer (INL) thickening then cataract surgery might unmask troublesome distortion, and therapeutic options for the ERM should be considered before cataract surgery occurs. If ERM surgery is being considered, the presence of internal limiting membrane (ILM) thickening might suggest a better prognosis in terms of symptomatic improvement. This latter point will require subsequent research to confirm that this OCT finding

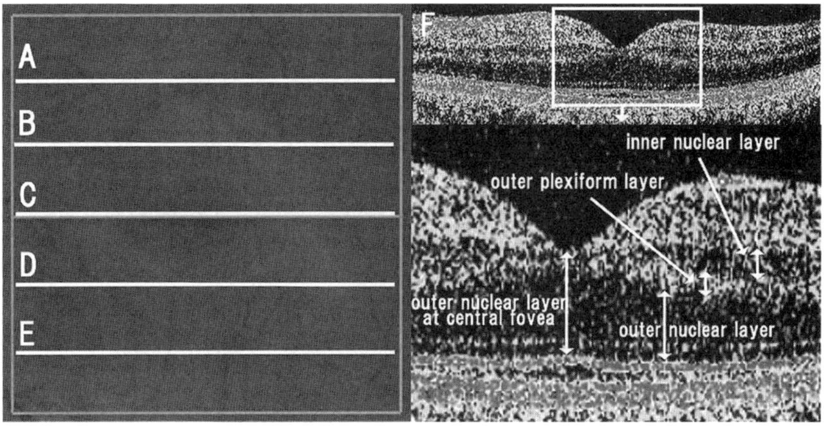

FIGURE 1.—Five horizontal B-scan cross-sections and thickness measurement of the inner retinal layer. Line C is a single horizontal B-scan cross-section through the fovea. Lines A, B and D, E are 4 horizontal B-scan cross-sections, placed at regular intervals superior (**A**, **B**) and inferior (**D**, **E**) to that of the horizontal line through the fovea. F, Measurements of the inner retinal layer on line C through the fovea performed using the electronic calipers. (Reprinted from Watanabe A, Arimoto S, Nishi O. Correlation between metamorphopsia and epiretinal membrane optical coherence tomography findings. *Ophthalmology.* 2009;116:1788-1793, with permission from the American Academy of Ophthalmology.)

improves with successful vitreous surgery. Although the sample size is small, this report suggests a potentially powerful use of OCT imaging.

J. F. Vander, MD

Lamellar Macular Holes: Tomographic Features and Surgical Outcome

Androudi S, Stangos A, Brazitikos PD (Aristotle Univ, Thessaloniki, Greece)
Am J Ophthalmol 148:420-426, 2009

Purpose.—To categorize tomographically the distinct entity of lamellar macular holes (MH) and present the surgical outcomes in our patient cohort.

Design.—Prospective observational and interventional study.

Methods.—All cases were clinically diagnosed initially with slit-lamp biomicroscopy and confirmed with the use of optical coherence tomography (OCT)-3. Cases either were observed or underwent surgical intervention with a 25-gauge pars-plana vitrectomy (PPV) technique. Follow-up was at least 12 months for all cases and ranged from 12 to 46 months. Main outcome measures included closure of the lamellar MH following surgical intervention; best-corrected visual acuity (BCVA) preoperatively and postoperatively for the cases that underwent surgery.

Results.—We identified 32 eyes of 30 patients with lamellar MH diagnosed by OCT-3. Lamellar MHs were classified into 3 different categories: 1) associated with macular epiretinal membrane (ERM) (20 eyes), 2) secondary to cystoid macular edema (8 eyes), and 3) attributable to

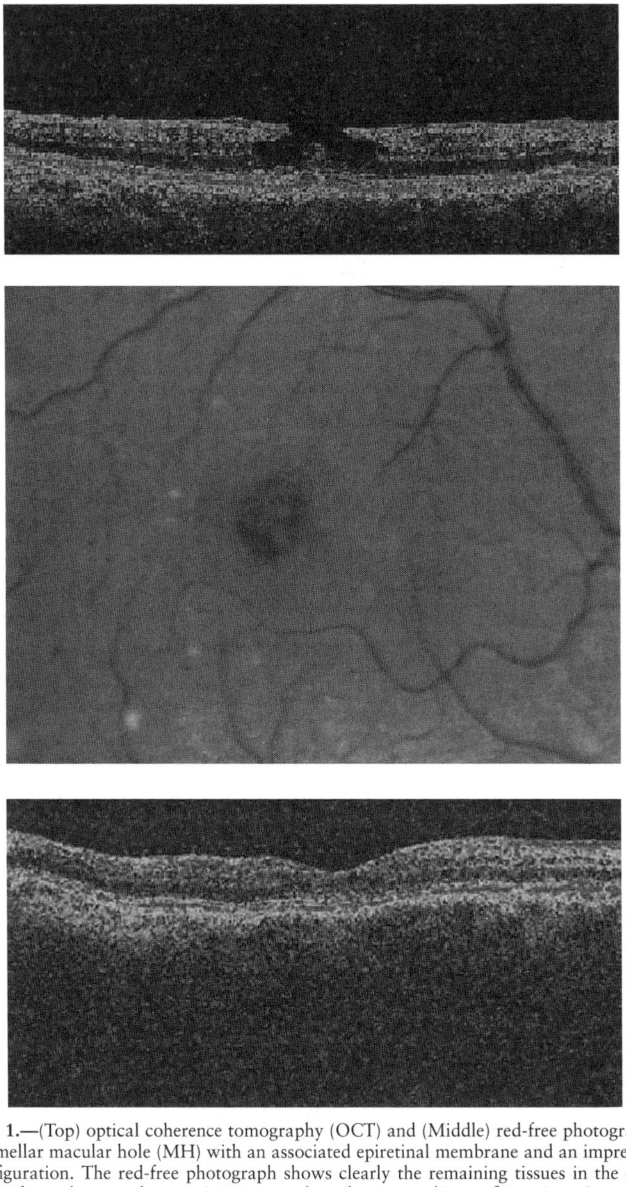

FIGURE 1.—(Top) optical coherence tomography (OCT) and (Middle) red-free photograph. Appearance of a lamellar macular hole (MH) with an associated epiretinal membrane and an impressive *omega-shaped* configuration. The red-free photograph shows clearly the remaining tissues in the center of the fovea that produces the very characteristic omega-shaped tomographic configuration. (Bottom) Postoperative tomographic appearance of the same patient showing normalization of the foveal contour. (Reprinted from Androudi S, Stangos A, Brazitikos PD. Lamellar macular holes: tomographic features and surgical outcome. *Am J Ophthalmol.* 2009;148:420-426, with permission from Elsevier Inc.)

partial-thickness macular avulsion after acute posterior vitreous detachment (PVD) (4 eyes). Visual acuity was less affected in cases with an associated ERM. Surgery included PPV and ERM removal (when present), followed by internal limiting membrane (ILM) removal and 16% C_3F_8 injection. Postoperatively, BCVA improved in 17 out of the 20 cases (85%) operated from the first group of patients; 3 cases retained the same BCVA preoperatively and postoperatively. Mean BCVA improvement in the first group was 2.6 Snellen lines, which was statistically significant ($P = .002$, paired t test).

Conclusions.—Surgical treatment of lamellar MH associated with an ERM may result in preservation or improvement of visual acuity, by relieving the tangential traction caused by the ERM (Fig 1).

▶ While it is widely appreciated that vitrectomy can be very helpful for patients with idiopathic macular holes, there is also considerable evidence that surgery for lamellar macular defects can also lead to visual recovery.[1] This report provides further guidance for case selection when contemplating surgical intervention. The report's flaws are considerable, including a relatively small sample size, nonrandomized intervention decision making, and variable follow-up periods. Nevertheless, the largest portion of the study population, patients with lamellar hole and optical coherence tomography (OCT), confirmed epiretinal membrane do have the potential for considerable visual recovery and that surgery should be considered for these patients. Whether intravitreal gas and face-down positioning are necessary is unclear. It is impossible to determine whether patients with cystoid macular edema (CME) and posterior vitreous detachment (PVD) related lamellar holes will also benefit from surgery given the very small sample sizes for these subgroups.

J. F. Vander, MD

Reference

1. Garretson BR, Pollack JS, Ruby AJ, Drenser KA, Williams GA, Sarrafizadeh R. Vitrectomy for a symptomatic lamellar macular hole. *Ophthalmology*. 2008; 115:884-886.

Value of internal limiting membrane peeling in surgery for idiopathic macular hole and the correlation between function and retinal morphology

Christensen UC (Glostrup Hosp, Denmark)

Acta Ophthalmol 87:1-23, 2009

Idiopathic macular hole is characterized by a full thickness anatomic defect in the foveal retina leading to loss of central vision, metamorphopsia and a central scotoma. Classic macular hole surgery consists of vitrectomy, posterior vitreous cortex separation and intraocular gas tamponade, but during the past decade focus has especially been on internal limiting membrane (ILM) peeling as adjuvant therapy for increasing closure rates. With increasing use of ILM peeling and indocyanine green (ICG) staining, which is used for specific visualization of the ILM, concerns about the safety of the procedure have arisen. At present, it is not known whether ICG-assisted ILM peeling potentially reduces the functional outcome after macular hole surgery.

The purpose of the present PhD thesis was to examine whether ICG-assisted ILM peeling offers surgical and functional benefit in macular hole surgery. We conducted a randomized clinical trial including 78 pseudophakic patients with idiopathic macular hole stages 2 and 3. Patients were randomly assigned to macular hole surgery consisting of (i) vitrectomy alone without instrumental retinal surface contact (non-peeling), (ii) vitrectomy plus 0.05% isotonic ICG-assisted ILM peeling or (iii) vitrectomy plus 0.15% trypan blue (TB)-assisted ILM peeling. Morphologic and functional outcomes were assessed 3, 6 and 12 months after surgery.

The results show that surgery with ILM peeling, for both stages 2 and 3 macular holes, is associated with a significantly higher closure rate than surgery without ILM peeling (95% versus 45%). The overall functional results confirm that surgery for macular hole generally leads to favourable visual results, with two-thirds of eyes regaining reading vision (≥20/40). Macular hole surgery can be considered a safe procedure with a low incidence of sight-threatening adverse events; the retinal detachment rate was 2.2%. Visual outcomes in eyes with primary hole closure were not significantly different between the intervention groups; however, for the stage 2 subgroup with primary macular hole closure, there was a trend towards a better mean visual acuity in the non-peeling group (78.2 letters) compared to the ICG-peeling group (70.9 letters), $p = 0.06$. Performing repeated macular hole surgery was associated with a significant reduction in functional outcome indicating that primary focus should be on closing the macular hole in one procedure.

Morphological studies of closed macular holes with contrast-enhanced optical coherence tomography (OCT) found thinning and discontinuity of the central photoreceptor layer matrix that were highly specific for predicting the likelihood of an eye having regained reading vision 12 months after macular hole surgery. Additionally, healing after macular hole surgery appeared to begin with the contraction of the inner aspect of the retina, forming a roof over a subfoveal fluid-filled cavity, and to end with a gradual restoration of the anatomy in the outer layers of the retina at the junction of the photoreceptor inner and outer segments. We found the more intact this structure was on contrast-enhanced OCT 3 months after macular hole surgery, the better the visual acuity after 12 months, whereas late rather than early resolution of subfoveal fluid had no impact on final visual outcome. The use ILM peeling and intraoperative dyes did not have any functionally important effects on postoperative macular structure.

Based on the above findings, we conclude that ILM peeling should be performed in all cases of full thickness macular hole surgery. The use of 0.05% intraoperative isotonic ICG with short exposure time appears to be a safe alternative in stage 3 macular hole surgery, whereas a slight reduction in functional potential cannot be excluded when performing 0.05% isotonic ICG-assisted ILM peeling in stage 2 macular hole surgery.

▶ Much of this report is a review of the pathogenesis of idiopathic macular hole and the evolution of treatment strategies for the condition. Buried within this text, however, is a nice randomized trial assessing the use of internal limiting membrane (ILM) peeling during primary hole repair. The initial randomization was between vitrectomy with no attempt at ILM peeling and vitrectomy with indocyanine green (ICG)-assisted ILM peeling. Of note, during the course of the trial, the data and safety monitoring committee found that the hole closure rate without ILM peeling was much lower and altered the randomization to ILM peeling using ICG or ILM peeling using trypan blue. By far, the most important factor determining anatomic success and visual recovery was successful closure of the hole during primary repair. Even for smaller stage 2 holes, the single most important factor is to close the hole with a single operation. Internal limiting membrane peeling enhances the likelihood of hole closure and should be used for all cases. No evidence of toxicity was found with ICG, supporting its widespread use in this application.

J. F. Vander, MD

Vitreous Penetration of Orally Administered Famciclovir

Chong DY, Johnson MW, Huynh TH, et al (Univ of Michigan, Ann Arbor, et al)
Am J Ophthalmol 148:38-42, 2009

Purpose.—To determine the vitreous penetration of penciclovir (Denavir; GlaxoSmithKline, Philadelphia, Pennsylvania, USA) after oral administration of the prodrug famciclovir (Famvir; Novartis Pharmaceuticals Corp, East Hanover, New Jersey, USA).

Design.—Prospective interventional case series.

Methods.—Ten patients undergoing elective pars plana vitrectomy at a single institution were enrolled to take 3 oral doses of famciclovir 500 mg the day preceding surgery and a fourth dose on the morning of surgery. Blood and undiluted vitreous samples were acquired from each patient during surgery. High-performance liquid chromatography was used to determine the concentration of penciclovir in each sample. Exclusion criteria included prior vitrectomy, compromised blood-retina barrier, renal or hepatic disease, human immunodeficiency virus infection, bone marrow or renal transplantation, pregnancy or breastfeeding, history of adverse reaction or allergy to famciclovir or penciclovir, and antiviral, probenecid, or cimetidine use within 1 month of surgery.

Results.—Ten eyes of 10 patients ranging in age from 26 to 82 were included. All patients had normal renal and hepatic function as determined by history and laboratory values. Mean serum penciclovir concentration ± standard deviation was 4.45 ± 1.31 μg/ml (range, 2.51 to 6.34 μg/ml). Mean vitreous penciclovir concentration was 1.21 ± 0.38 μg/ml (range,

0.39 to 1.88 μg/ml). Mean vitreous-to-serum concentration ratio of penciclovir was 0.28 ± 0.09 (range, 0.16 to 0.41).

Conclusions.—Oral administration of famciclovir results in vitreous concentrations of penciclovir within the inhibitory ranges for herpes simplex 1, herpes simplex 2, and varicella zoster virus. Oral famciclovir may be a reasonable alternative to intravenous acyclovir (Zovirax; GlaxoSmithKline) in the treatment of acute retinal necrosis, especially in cases of acyclovir resistance or patient inability to tolerate prolonged intravenous treatment.

▶ Although this study is modest in scale, it addresses an important clinical issue using a well-structured design. This is an important study because it supplies further evidence that the existing standard of care for acute retinal necrosis (ARN), which is hospitalization with intravenous medication, may be reasonably modified to an oral outpatient approach without sacrificing efficacy. An earlier pilot trial using this approach in the treatment of a small number of ARN patients demonstrated reasonable results, but it is reassuring to see the pharmacologic data to back that interpretation up.

J. F. Vander, MD

Feasibility Study of a Retinal Prosthesis: Spatial Vision With a 16-Electrode Implant

Caspi A, Dorn JD, McClure KH, et al (Second Sight Med Products, Inc, Sylmar; Doheny Eye Inst, Los Angeles, CA)

Arch Ophthalmol 127:398-401, 2009

Objective.—To demonstrate that an epiretinal prosthesis can produce patterned visual perception in patients blinded by photoreceptor degeneration who have no other treatment options.

Methods.—A totally blind subject with retinitis pigmentosa had a 16-electrode epiretinal prosthesis implanted. The implant is controlled wirelessly by an external computer or a head-mounted video camera. Spatial vision was assessed by measuring the subject's response to direct stimulation of patterns and by comparing the ability of the subject to identify the orientation of gratings with the system on and off.

Results.—In response to stimulation of 2 orthogonal rows of electrodes, the subject drew 2 lines with a mean (SEM) angle of 87.4° (1.8°) between them. With the system on, the subject identified the orientation of the grating target up to a spatial resolution that matches the spacing between the adjacent electrodes. In contrast, with the system off, the subject could not detect or identify the target's orientation.

Conclusion.—Synchronized stimulation of different retinal locations with an epiretinal prosthesis implanted long- term can produce spatial vision with an acuity level determined by the distance between the electrodes.

Trial Registration.—clinicaltrials.gov Identifier: NCT00279500.

▶ It is unusual for a case report describing only a single patient to find its way into a broad review of new and important information such as this series. This report is exceptional in that the development of the technology described, which is currently in its infancy, has the potential to transform care for an enormous number of profoundly visually impaired individuals. The placement of an epiretinal electronic prosthesis (see Fig 1 in the original article for the appearance of the prosthesis on the macular surface) is a complicated procedure, and the logistics of placing the prosthesis will undoubtedly evolve over time. More importantly, significant improvements in the materials, engineering, and production of the prosthesis must be made before this type of procedure can become widespread in its application. Nevertheless, it is remarkable that a patient with no light perception vision can demonstrate any degree of visual function as this subject did. Time will tell if epiretinal placement is optimal, whether other designs are superior or if an artificial retina ever becomes a legitimate therapeutic option.

J. F. Vander, MD

6 Oculoplastic Surgery

Rituximab Treatment of Patients with Severe, Corticosteroid-Resistant Thyroid-Associated Ophthalmopathy

Khanna D, Chong KKL, Afifiyan NF, et al (Univ of California at Los Angeles; Los Angeles Biomed Inst at Harbor-UCLA Med Ctr, Torrance, CA)

Ophthalmology 117:133-139, 2010

Purpose.—To study the effectiveness of anti-CD20 (rituximab [RTX]; Rituxan; Genentech, Inc., South San Francisco, CA) therapy in patients with severe, corticosteroid (CS)-resistant thyroid-associated ophthalmopathy (TAO).

Design.—Retrospective, interventional case series.

Participants.—Six consecutive subjects with severe, progressive TAO unresponsive to CS.

Methods.—Electronic medical record review of consecutive patients receiving RTX during the previous 18 months. Responses to therapy were graded using standard clinical assessment and flow cytometric analysis of peripheral lymphocytes.

Main Outcome Measures.—Clinical activity score (CAS), proptosis, strabismus, treatment side effects, and quantification of regulatory T cells.

Results.—Six patients were studied. Systemic CS failed to alter clinical activity in all patients (mean CAS ± standard deviation, 5.3 ± 1.0 before vs. 5.5 ± 0.8 during therapy for 7.5 ± 6.4 months; $P = 1.0$). However, after RTX treatment, CAS improved from 5.5 ± 0.8 to 1.3 ± 0.5 at 2 months after treatment ($P < 0.03$) and remained quiescent in all patients (CAS, 0.7 ± 0.8; $P < 0.0001$) at a mean follow-up of 6.2 ± 4.5 months. Vision improved bilaterally in all 4 patients with dysthyroid optic neuropathy (DON). None of the 6 patients experienced disease relapse after RTX infusion, and proptosis remained stable (Hertel measurement, 24 ± 3.7 mm before therapy and 23.6 ± 3.7 mm after therapy; $P = 0.17$). The abundance of T regulatory cells, assessed in 1 patient, increased within 1 week of RTX and remained elevated at 18 months of follow-up.

Conclusions.—In progressive, CS-resistant TAO, rapid and sustained resolution of orbital inflammation and DON followed treatment with RTX.

▶ The search for the ideal treatment for thyroid-associated ophthalmopathy (TAO) remains elusive. As we slowly learn more about the factors causing TAO we are finding more potential treatments for TAO. This article looks at

6 patients with severe TAO treated with rituximab after their disease continued to progress with corticosteroid treatment.

This is a retrospective study looking at the results of rituximab treatment of active TAO. These patients had progressive TAO despite multiple modalities of treatment, including corticosteroids, orbital decompression, orbital radiation, or immunosuppressant therapy. Being a retrospective study, not all patients were treated the same before rituximab, but all were considered to be steroid failures. The patients all received 2 infusions of rituximab 2 weeks apart according to the protocol for treatment of rheumatoid arthritis.

The results in these 6 patients were quite impressive. All corticosteroid treatment was tapered so no patient was on corticosteroids 4 weeks after the first rituximab infusion. There was improvement in the clinical activity score (CAS) noted within 4 weeks of the first rituximab treatment. The improvement was maximum by 8 weeks and remained stable for the average follow-up of 6.2 months. Four patients had optic nerve compression, and all 4 had resolution of the optic neuropathy by 2 months postinfusion. Proptosis did not improve, and 4 patients demonstrated progression of their strabismus. These findings are very similar to what happens in TAO patients successfully treated with orbital radiation and/or corticosteroids. Even when the disease burns out and quiets on its own there is not much improvement in the proptosis or strabismus.

A small but potentially important finding in the one patient tested was the increase in T regulatory cells after rituximab. The increase of T regulatory cells has been shown to reflect response to treatment in rheumatoid arthritis patients. This could be a future marker for treatment success in treatment of TAO.

This article continues to explore the treatment of TAO. The results are very promising, but we must be cautious since this is a small study; the patients had very different courses of treatment before and even soon after rituximab infusions, and as always TAO is a disease that will burn out with time, so uncontrolled studies can be deceptive. In the mean time this may be a reasonable treatment for a patient with TAO who has failed other accepted treatment modalities and continues to worsen.

I believe the ultimate treatment for TAO will be medical, and as we learn more about the disease we are beginning to target our treatment. Our current mode of waiting for TAO to quiet and then surgically correct the damage is less than ideal. If we can stop the inflammatory process and prevent the fibrosis and scarring associated with TAO, treatment would be much easier for patients and physicians. This article is hopefully just the beginning of innovative medical treatment trials for TAO. As the authors note, we need further controlled studies to better define where rituximab fits in our treatment of TAO. More importantly, we need to find more and earlier ways to prevent the disease process.

R. B. Penne, MD

Prevalence of canaliculitis requiring removal of SmartPlugs

Hill RH 3rd, Norton SW, Bersani TA (SUNY Upstate Med Univ, Syracuse, NY)

Ophthal Plast Reconstr Surg 25:437-439, 2009

Purpose.—To report the first accurate prevalence of canaliculitis associated with the use of the SmartPlug.

Methods.—All patients from a single private ophthalmology practice who received SmartPlugs from 2002 to 2007 were identified. All patients from the private ophthalmology practice that developed canaliculitis secondary to SmartPlug insertion were referred to a single private ophthalmic plastic and reconstructive surgery office. A retrospective review of those 17 patients was performed.

Results.—From 2002 to 2007, a total of 235 patients were identified from a single private ophthalmology practice with a total of 402 SmartPlugs inserted. Of those 235 patients, 17 developed canaliculitis and were referred to a single private ophthalmic plastic and reconstructive surgery office. The prevalence of canaliculitis per patient was 7.23%. The prevalence of canaliculitis per SmartPlug inserted was 4.73%. The average time from SmartPlugs insertion to onset of symptoms was 3 years. All affected patients required canaliculotomy and plug removal.

Conclusions.—This is the first study reporting the prevalence of canaliculitis associated with the use of the SmartPlug. All affected patients required surgical intervention, after which many continued to have dry eye and one required bilateral Jones tubes. Ophthalmologists using the SmartPlug for the treatment of dry eye syndrome should carefully weigh the risks and benefits of their use.

► We continue to see a significant number of cases of canaliculitis secondary to SmartPlugs. This is the first study that outlines the prevalence of canaliculitis secondary to SmartPlugs.

There were a number of interesting facts in this retrospective study. The incidence of the problem was found to be 4.73% per plug placed. The other finding was the time of onset of symptoms from plug placement was an average of 3 years, but varied from 5 months to 6 years. All 17 of the patients with canaliculitis secondary to SmartPlug required plug removal for their symptoms to resolve. Once removed, many patients are asymptomatic. This study did not comment on the state of the lacrimal passage after plug removal. In my experience, most are blocked or significantly narrowed if not blocked. Because the plug was usually placed to treat dry eye, the patient does well with this blockage.

This was a somewhat unique opportunity to capture the number of patients with canaliculitis secondary to SmartPlug placement because there is only one practice where these patients can go for treatment. Even so, this is an underestimation of the incidence of the problem. Because every patient who had a plug placed was not contacted, there are a number of reasons the incidence may be higher. Patients may have seen someone out of the area for a canaliculitis either because they moved from the area or wanted another opinion. There are also some patients who will develop canaliculitis in the future.

The authors conclude that future, routine use of SmartPlugs should be discontinued. At Wills Eye Institute, we have been teaching that for the past 3 to 4 years. There may be rare exceptions where intracanalicular plugs are the only option. In these patients, the risk of problems with these plugs needs to be clearly outlined, and even then they are still used. Most of the patients will not have problems, but they need to know there is a 5% or more chance they will.

R. B. Penne, MD

Thyroid-Associated Ophthalmopathy after Treatment for Graves' Hyperthyroidism with Antithyroid Drugs or Iodine-131

Träisk F, the Thyroid Study Group of TT 96 (Karolinska Inst, Stockholm, Sweden; et al)

J Clin Endocrinol Metab 94:3700-3707, 2009

Context.—Previous randomized trials have suggested an association between radioiodine treatment for Graves' hyperthyroidism and thyroid-associated ophthalmopathy (TAO).

Objectives.—The aim of the study was to compare the occurrence of worsening or development of TAO in patients who were treated with radioiodine or antithyroid drugs.

Design.—We conducted a randomized trial (TT 96) with a follow-up of 4 yr.

Patients, Setting, and Intervention.—Patients with a recent diagnosis of Graves' hyperthyroidism were randomized to treatment with iodine-131 (163 patients) or 18 months of medical treatment (150 patients). Early substitution with T_4 was given in both groups.

Main Outcome Measure.—Worsening or development of TAO was significantly more common in the iodine-131 treatment group (63 patients; 38.7%) compared with the medical treatment group (32 patients; 21.3%) ($P < 0.001$).

Results.—The risk for *de novo* development of TAO was greater in patients treated with iodine-131 (53 patients) than with medical treatment (23 patients). However, worsening of TAO in the 41 patients who had ophthalmopathy already before the start of treatment was not more common in the radioiodine group (10 patients) than in the medical group (nine patients). Smoking was shown to influence the risk of worsening or development of TAO, and smokers treated with radioiodine had the overall highest risk for TAO. However, in the group of smokers, worsening or development of TAO was not significantly associated with the choice of treatment for hyperthyroidism.

Conclusions.—Radioiodine treatment is a significant risk factor for development of TAO in Graves' hyperthyroidism. Smokers run the highest

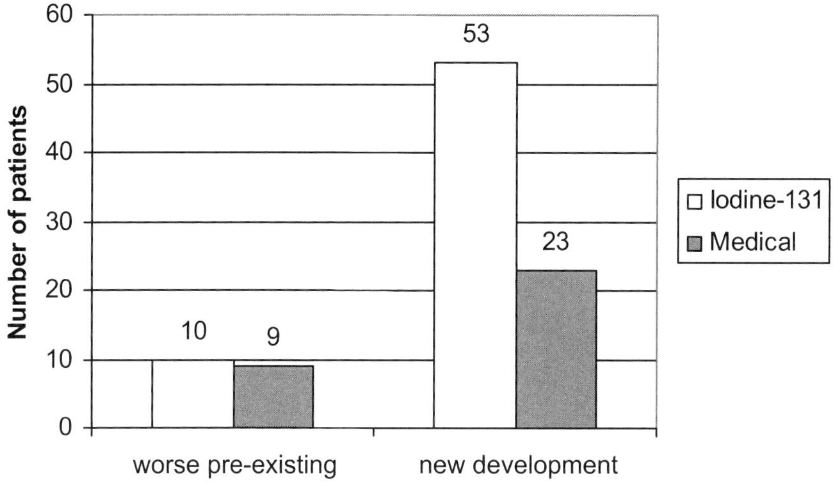

FIGURE 1.—Number of patients with worsening of preexisting TAO [10 of 22 patients (45%) in group I; and nine of 19 patients (47%) in group M] and *de novo* development of TAO [53 of 141 patients (38%) in group I; and 23 of 131 patients (18%) in group M] at any time during follow-up. (Reprinted from Träisk F, Tallstedt L, Abraham-Nordling M, et al. Thyroid-associated ophthalmopathy after treatment for Graves' hyperthyroidism with antithyroid drugs or iodine-131. *J Clin Endocrinol Metab.* 2009;94:3700-3707, with permission from The Endocrine Society.)

risk for worsening or development of TAO irrespective of treatment modality (Fig 1).

▶ This is a prospective, randomized study that looks again at the question of whether patients with Graves' hyperthyroidism are at a higher risk of developing thyroid-associated ophthalmopathy (TAO) when treated with iodine-131 versus medical treatment. This has been a question for years, and recent studies have suggested that patients receiving iodine-131 have a higher risk of developing TAO. A criticism of past studies has been that the iodine-131 group often develops a period of hypothyroidism after treatment, and some thought that this hypothyroidism might have been the reason for the higher rate of TAO development. These patients treated with iodine-131 received thyroid hormone replacement early to avoid large variations in the thyroid levels.

This study confirms that patients receiving iodine-131 are at higher risk of developing TAO than those treated medically. It also confirmed that smokers are at higher risk of developing TAO, and smokers receiving iodine-131 are at the highest risk. One interesting finding was that patients who smoked as a group had an equally high chance of developing TAO or worsening of their TAO whether in the iodine-131 or medical treatment group.

This is important information to discuss with patients as they make decisions on how best to treat their hyperthyroidism. There are options for patients to try and decrease this risk such as systemic steroid. Discussing the risks of treatment options and potential ways of modulating these risks is an important educational task for ophthalmologists.

R. B. Penne, MD

Inadvertent evisceration of eyes containing uveal melanoma

Eagle RC Jr, Grossniklaus HE, Syed N, et al (Thomas Jefferson Univ, Philadelphia, PA)

Arch Ophthalmol 127:141-145, 2009

Objectives.—To report an important complication of ocular evisceration therapy for blind, painful eyes that has been unreported in the literature, and to stress the need for careful preoperative evaluation to exclude occult neoplasms prior to therapy.

Design.—Multicenter, retrospective, nonrandomized clinicopathological case series of patients found to have previously unsuspected uveal malignant melanoma during histopathological examination of blind, painful eyes treated by evisceration.

Results.—Histopathological examination of evisceration specimens disclosed previously unsuspected uveal melanoma in 7 patients who were treated for blind, painful eyes. Inflammation caused by necrosis of the tumor and other ocular tissues led to misdiagnosis as endophthalmitis, orbital cellulitis, or idiopathic orbital inflammation in several cases. Preoperative imaging was not performed in 3 cases and failed to detect tumors in the remaining 4 cases. Failure of necrotic tumors to enhance contributed to misdiagnosis.

Conclusions.—The presence of a malignant intraocular neoplasm should be excluded prior to evisceration of any blind eye or blind, painful eye, particularly with opaque media. Necrosis-related inflammation can confound the clinical diagnosis of occult lesions, as can failure of necrotic tumors to enhance on imaging studies.

▶ The report of 7 patients who had an evisceration done when they had an intraocular melanoma has raised multiple concerns and questions. Because the article was released, there have been multiple discussions about the article both in journals and at meetings.

There has long been debate over whether enucleation or evisceration is the better surgical procedure. The advantages of evisceration have been that it is a simpler, less-invasive procedure that can often be done with sedation. It is less invasive into the orbit and may result in better long-term orbital stability. Enucleation has always been the procedure of choice for intraocular tumors. This paper questions the ability to always detect a tumor in a blind painful eye, and suggests enucleation is the safest way to treat a blind painful eye.

I agree that if we cannot detect a tumor in a blind painful eye, then we cannot safely do eviscerations on a routine basis. I would argue that this article does not prove that. Of the 7 patients, 3 had no attempt at any imaging to detect a tumor. Three others had only a CT scan done. The details of the CT study are not given. I would argue that a CT scan is not the best way to detect an intraocular tumor, especially in an eye that is not anatomically normal. That leaves one case where a B-scan was done and the tumor was not detected. What the B-scan showed, and whether this may have been missed preoperatively, we do not know. I would argue that one reported case out of the many thousands that was not detected should not be a reason to abandon the use of evisceration. If thousands of patients undergo general anesthesia for an enucleation instead of local for an evisceration statistically, there will be at least one person who dies from general anesthesia. Is that better?

What this article does very well is bring to everyone's mind the risk of missing an intraocular tumor when doing evisceration surgery. This needs to be discussed with the patient, and the appropriate preoperative evaluation needs to be done to rule out an intraocular tumor. If the retina cannot be seen, then this eye should have a good B-scan ultrasound. The authors are correct that if the tumor is missed, the surgeon will be blamed for any future metastatic disease despite the fact that there is 50% risk of metastasis even if an enucleation was done.

R. B. Penne, MD

Early Versus Late Repair of Orbital Blowout Fractures

Ben Simon GJ, Syed HM, McCann JD, et al (David Geffen School of Medicine at UCLA, Los Angeles, CA)

Ophthalmic Surg Lasers Imaging 40:141-148, 2009

Background and Objective.—To compare early and late surgical repair of orbital blowout floor fractures.

Patients and Methods.—A retrospective, comparative interventional case series reviewed medical records of 50 consecutive patients who underwent unilateral orbital floor fracture repair in a 4-year period. Comparative analysis was performed between patients operated on within 2 weeks of injury and those operated on at a later stage.

Results.—Assault, motor vehicle accidents, and sports injuries were the most common causes of injury. Surgery was performed due to inferior rectus muscle entrapment and limitations in up gaze in 20 (40%) patients or to prevent enophthalmos in cases with significant bony orbital expansion in 30 (60%) patients. After surgery, enophthalmos improved an average of 0.8 mm. Limitation in ocular motility improved after surgery but was statistically significant only in up gaze. Patients who underwent early repair (within 2 weeks) achieved less improvement in enophthalmos versus patients who underwent late repair (delta enophthalmos of 0.2 ± 1.1 vs 1.3 ± 1.9 mm, respectively; $P = .02$).

Conclusion.—In these patients, postoperative vertical ductions and postoperative enophthalmos improved after fracture repair. Surgery was associated with a low rate of postoperative complications. No apparent difference in surgical outcome was seen between early (within 2 weeks) and late surgical repair (Table 3).

► This is a retrospective study of 50 consecutive patients who underwent orbital floor fracture repair. The purpose was to compare the results of motility and enophthalmos in early fracture repair (within 2 weeks of trauma) versus late repair (1 month to 3.5 years after trauma).

TABLE 3.—Preoperative and Postoperative Vertical Ductions in Patients Operated on for Orbital Blowout Fracture at the Jules Stein Eye Institute in a 4-Year Period[a]

	Muscle Entrapment (n = 20)				No Muscle Entrapment (n = 30)			
	Up		Down		Up		Down	
Motility	Preop	Postop	Preop	Postop	Preop	Postop	Preop	Postop
0	0	10	13	13	16	22	23	24
−1	6	5	2	3	4	4	5	3
−2	8	2	4	2	8	2	2	3
−3	5	2	1	2	2	2	0	0
−4	1	1	0	0	0	0	0	0

Preop = preoperative; Postop = postoperative; 0 = normal motility; −1 = mild restriction; −2 = moderate; −3 = severe; −4 = no motility.

[a]Patients are divided into those with inferior rectus muscle entrapment and those without inferior rectus muscle entrapment (the number of patients in each category is shown in the table). Motility was graded on a scales of 0 to −4 , with 0 indicating normal motility and −4 indicating no motility.

This study is somewhat confusing because of the mention of multiple different groups. There is the early repair group of 27 patients and the late repair group of 23 patients. There is also discussion about 20 patients with evidence of entrapment who had surgery for this entrapment, but it is not clear whether all 20 were in the early repair group. Likewise, 30 patients had surgery for enophthalmos, but how many were in the early and late group is not defined.

The conclusion of this study is interesting. There was no significant difference in the surgical results looking at motility and enophthalmos between the 2 groups (Figs 3,4,5, and 6 in the original article, and Table 3). The fact that motility improved equally in both groups is surprising to me. An article by Delcanto[1] in 2008 showed no difference between surgical repair before 2 weeks and repair 15 days to 29 days after trauma. This article has patients as far out as 3.5 years. I would think that most patients with significant restriction were repaired within 2 weeks, but there can be reasons that patients do not present until well after 2 weeks with their problem. It can be seen in Fig 6 in the original article that there were a number of patients repaired later that had improvement in their motility.

Comparing enophthalmos between the 2 groups is more difficult as most patients repaired before 2 weeks still have swelling, and the true amount of enophthalmos has not yet manifested. Thus, it is not surprising that these patients had less enophthalmos preoperative and also had less improvement in their enophthalmos. Although not mentioned in this article, patients with motility limitation often have smaller fractures, so they would be in a group repaired early because of the motility but also less likely to have significant enophthalmos because of the small fracture.

There are a lot of areas in this study that are open to speculation. What can be taken from this article is that surgical repair of fractures, even years after the fracture, can improve motility. The fact that enophthalmos can be improved late is not anything new. It is important to emphasize that any fracture with significant motility limitations secondary to entrapment (Fig 1 in the original article) should be repaired within 2 weeks if possible. Also, any white-eyed blowout fracture needs to be repaired emergently.

R. B. Penne, MD

Reference

1. Del Canto AJ, Linberg JV. Comparison of orbital fracture repair performed within 14 days versus 15 to 29 days after trauma. *Ophthal Plast Reconstr Surg*. 2008;24: 437-443.

Graves' Orbitopathy Activation after Radioactive Iodine Therapy with and without Steroid Prophylaxis

Vannucchi G, Campi I, Covelli D, et al (Univ of Milan, Italy; et al)
J Clin Endocrinol Metab 94:3381-3386, 2009

Context.—The reactivation of Graves' orbitopathy (GO) after radioiodine (RAI) for Graves' disease (GD) is a known effect, and its clinical relevance is controversial. Prevention of RAI-induced GO activation is possible in at-risk patients with oral glucocorticoids (OGC).

Objectives.—The aim of the study was to analyze the effects of RAI on GO with or without prophylactic steroids based on known risk factors and to compare the effectiveness of prophylaxis with iv glucocorticoids (IVGC) and OGC.

Design.—We conducted a retrospective study in which patients were assessed before and 1-12 months after RAI.

Patients and Setting.—A total of 113 patients were included in the study; 83 underwent RAI without prophylactic steroids for the absence of risk of activation, and 30 were treated with either OGC (n = 21) or IVGC (n = 9).

Main Outcome Measures.—We analyzed the prevalence of GO activation with or without steroid prophylaxis and the difference in the prevalence of GO activation after OGC or IVGC.

Results.—GO activation was observed in 7.2% of patients without and 33.3% of patients with steroid prophylaxis ($P < 0.0001$), for an overall prevalence of 14.6%. GO activation occurred in 47.6% of patients treated with OGC but in none of the nine patients treated with IVGC ($P < 0.0001$). Disease activation was more prevalent in males ($P < 0.02$) and in older patients ($P < 0.04$) with a shorter duration of GD ($P < 0.01$) and time from GO onset ($P < 0.01$).

Conclusions.—GO may occur after RAI in approximately 15% of patients also in the absence of signs of active GO. Prophylactic OGC did not prevent GO activation in a large proportion of patients, compared to IVGC (Table 1).

▶ This article does not answer questions as much as it brings up additional questions concerning the development of Graves' orbitopathy (GO) during

TABLE 1.—Clinical and Biochemical Characteristics of the Patients Undergoing RAI Therapy for Hyperthyroidism Without (Group A) and with (Group B) Steroid Prophylaxis

	Group A	Group B	*P* value	Group B		*P* value
				OGC	IVGC	
No. of patients	83	30		21	9	
Sex (males/females)	16/67	7/23	0.6	5/16	2/7	1
Age (yr)	45.2 ± 1.5	50 ± 2.2	0.12	47.9 ± 2.6	53.2 ± 4.5	0.2
No. of smokers (%)	31 (37.3)	14 (46.7)	0.5	11 (52)	3 (33.3)	0.4
CAS	0.6 ± 0.1	1.4 ± 0.3	0.01[a]	1 ± 0.3	2.1 ± 0.4	0.04[a]
Serum FT3 levels (pmol/liter)	6.7 ± 0.5	8.1 ± 1.4	0.2	8.1 ± 1.4	7.7 ± 0.7	0.8
Serum TRAb levels (mU/liter)	6.2 ± 1.2	10.9 ± 3.5	0.2	12.6 ± 6.5	9.1 ± 2.2	0.2
Dose of RAI (MBq)	561.6 ± 12	508.6 ± 23	0.06	480 ± 30	572.2 ± 28	0.07

All values are reported as mean ± SE or number (%).
[a]Mann-Whitney test.

the treatment of hyperthyroidism with radioactive iodine (RAI). This issue has long been debated, and we still have no definitive answer. This study does however provide other variables regarding how to prevent the development of active GO when patients undergo RAI therapy.

This was a retrospective review and there were 2 groups of patients (Table 1). The patients considered to be at risk of developing active GO were treated with corticosteroids; those not at risk were not treated. The group at risk was further divided into those who received oral steroids and those who received intravenous (IV) steroids. The group not considered at risk still had a 7.2% risk of activation of GO. The group at risk who received steroids still had a 33% risk of developing active GO. The surprising thing was that none of the 9 patients who received IV steroids had activation of their GO despite being in the at risk group.

We now have even more of a need for a controlled study looking at RAI treatment and the activation of GO. This study suggests that oral steroids, which I have considered protective, are really not protective and that IV steroid treatment may be required to be protective. For now this is one more point of discussion to have with patients in their treatment of Graves' disease. Unfortunately, we still have no definitive answers.

R. B. Penne, MD

Balloon Catheter Dilation and Nasolacrimal Duct Intubation for Treatment of Nasolacrimal Duct Obstruction After Failed Probing

Pediatric Eye Disease Investigator Group (Jaeb Ctr for Health Res, Tampa, FL)
Arch Ophthalmol 127:633-639, 2009

Objective.—To compare the outcomes of balloon catheter dilation and nasolacrimal intubation as treatment for congenital nasolacrimal duct obstruction after failed probing in children younger than 4 years.

Methods.—We conducted a prospective, nonrandomized, multicenter study that enrolled 159 children aged 6 months to younger than 48 months who had a history of a single failed nasolacrimal duct probing and at least 1 of the following clinical signs of nasolacrimal duct obstruction: epiphora, mucous discharge, or increased tear lake. One hundred ninety-nine eyes underwent either balloon catheter nasolacrimal duct dilation or nasolacrimal duct intubation. Treatment success was defined as absence of epiphora, mucous discharge, or increased tear lake at the outcome visit 6 months after surgery.

Results.—Treatment success was reported in 65 of 84 eyes (77%; 95% confidence interval, 65%-85%) in the balloon catheter dilation group compared with 72 of 88 eyes (84% after adjustment for intereye correlation; 74%-91%) in the nasolacrimal intubation group (risk ratio for success for intubation vs balloon dilation, 1.08; 0.95-1.22).

Conclusion.—Both balloon catheter dilation and nasolacrimal duct intubation alleviate the clinical signs of persistent nasolacrimal duct obstruction in a similar percentage of patients.

▶ This article was originally designed to be a much larger, randomized study. A problem with recruitment limited the size and prevented this from being a randomized study. The study still does have value in that it confirms a previous study that found similar success with balloon catheter dilation and lacrimal intubation after failed probing for congenital nasolacrimal duct obstruction.

This then leaves the decision of which procedure to use up to the physician and parents. The cost of the balloon is higher than tubes, but because this cost is rarely paid by the patient's parents it is not a factor. I personally prefer the balloon for use after failed probing. I find that lacrimal intubation can sometimes be difficult. The biggest reason is that during the 6 weeks to 8 weeks with tubes in place, the tube can cause complications and can also become displaced. Finally, removal of the tubes is generally stressful and mentally traumatic for the child and the family when done in the office. Rarely it can be done in the OR, which is less stressful, but brings the cost and risk of another anesthesia. The bottom line is that either procedure is appropriate and around 80% successful.

R. B. Penne, MD

Prospective randomised comparison of external dacryocystorhinostomy with and without silicone intubation

Saiju R, Morse LJ, Weinberg D, et al (Tilganga Eye Centre, Kathmandu, Nepal; Univ of Vermont College of Medicine, Burlington; Univ of Utah, Salt Lake City)
Br J Ophthalmol 93:1220-1222, 2009

Background/Aims.—The aim of the study was to compare surgical outcomes of external dacryocystorhinostomy (DCR) with and without silastic intubation for treatment of primary uncomplicated nasolacrimal duct obstruction (NLDO).

TABLE 3.—Surgical Outcomes: Postoperative Follow-up

Follow-up Time	n	Total*	With Tubes*	Without Tubes*	p Value
1 week	94	98 (92/94)	98 (43/44)	98 (49/50)	0.93
6 weeks	84	96 (81/84)	98 (41/42)	95 (40/42)	1.0
6 months	47	98 (46/47)	96 (26/27)	100 (20/20)	0.33
Overall	52	88 (46/52)	90 (26/29)	87 (20/23)	0.77
Overall (including dropouts)†		94 (94/100)	93 (41/44)	95 (53/56)	0.77

*Values are % (n/n).
†Dropouts classified as a success as of last visit.

Design.—The study was a prospective randomised trial conducted at the Tilganga Eye Centre (Kathmandu, Nepal).

Methods.—One-hundred consecutive patients with uncomplicated primary NLDO were randomly assigned into two groups (44 underwent DCR with silastic intubation and 56 underwent DCR without intubation). Patients were re-assessed at 1 week, 6 weeks and 6 months after surgery. Success was defined objectively by irrigation of the puncta without regurgitation and subjectively by the absence of epiphora or discharge.

Results.—The success rate at 6 months was 90% for DCR with silastic intubation and 87% for DCR without silastic intubation. There was no statistically significant difference between the two groups ($p = 0.77$). No complications were encountered in either group. Silicone tubes increased surgical cost by 20% at the Tilganga Eye Centre.

Conclusion.—DCR without silastic intubation is less expensive than DCR with silastic intubation in primary uncomplicated NLDO, and has a similar success rate. DCR with silastic intubation may create increased burden for patients in the form of more post-surgical follow-up visits. In cases of uncomplicated primary NLDO, the use of silastic intubation in DCR may be unnecessary (Table 3).

▶ This is a simple, randomized, prospective study looking at the value of silicone tube placement during dacryocystorhinostomy (DCR) surgery. The conclusion is simple, but it was surprising to me. There was no statistically significant difference in the surgical outcome in the group with tubes versus those without silicone tubes. Both groups fell near the general success rate that we quote for DCR surgery of 90%.

This study was of moderate size, and only those patients who completed the 6-month follow-up were included in the final statistics. The patients included were only those with simple straightforward dacryostenosis. Thus, these findings do not apply to more complicated cases.

For me, this is an important article. It is well done and I see no reason to doubt the results. If that is the case, then there is no reason to place tubes during a DCR on patients with simple dacryostenosis. I currently place tubes in all my DCR surgeries and have been my entire career. As outlined in the article, they are not only a direct cost (around $80) but indirectly there is cost in longer OR time, office visits, time to take out the tube, and rarely complications related to the tube. I will start trying to do surgery without tube placement in select patients at first and see my results. It is important to realize this only applies to simple dacryostenosis and not to complicated cases with infections, scarring, or previous surgery.

R. B. Penne, MD

Survey of oculoplastic surgeons regarding clinical use of tear production tests

Espinoza GM, Israel H, Holds JB (Saint Louis Univ, MO)

Ophthal Plast Reconstr Surg 25:197-200, 2009

Purpose.—To determine by a survey of ophthalmic plastic surgeons with specific expertise in blepharoplasty surgery the perceived role of Schirmer testing and other evaluation features in determining patient predisposition to postoperative dry-eye complaints.

Methods.—A literature review of tear production tests was performed. An anonymous survey was mailed to all members of the American Society of Ophthalmic Plastic and Reconstructive Surgery. The survey included questions on practice patterns, the role of different objective tests, and the occurrence of postblepharoplasty dry-eye or exposure complaints.

Results.—Forty-eight percent (263 of 544) of those surveyed responded. All responding physicians perform a clinical history and examination to preoperatively evaluate for dry eye, 36% perform no additional tear production tests, 33% perform a test if indicated by signs or symptoms, 29% always perform a test, and 1% perform a test only if multiple procedures were planned. Schirmer testing with anesthetic is the predominant test used by physicians who perform tear production tests (89%), followed by Schirmer test without anesthetic (10%), and phenol red thread test (1%). Nevertheless, 74% of physicians felt that Schirmer testing should not be a medical standard of care in evaluating blepharoplasty patients.

Conclusions.—The preoperative evaluation of blepharoplasty patients may be severely limited in specialties that perform Schirmer testing or other tear production tests without the benefit of a directed clinical history and slit lamp examination. Current tear production tests are unreliable in detecting dry eye. The ideal approach to the evaluation of the blepharoplasty patient remains controversial.

▶ The usefulness of tear function tests in the diagnosis of dry eye has long been questioned. For the eyelid surgeon, both ophthalmic and nonophthalmic, the question is what is the best way to predict which patients will develop dry eye symptoms after eyelid surgery. This article does not answer which test is best, but it does shed light on the current practice pattern of oculoplastic surgeons when it comes to tear production tests.

This was a survey of oculoplastic surgeons. All surgeons indicated that they perform a clinical history and exam preoperatively. The survey found that 29% always perform a tear production test preoperatively, 33% perform it if indicated, and 36% never perform it. The tear production test of choice is Schirmers test in 99%. However, 74% indicated they did not think Schirmers testing should be the medical standard of care in blepharoplasty surgery.

The problem is there is no test that accurately predicts which patient will develop dry eye symptoms after eyelid surgery. Clinical exam with a slit lamp and history are the most helpful, but it still remains unpredictable who will develop dry eye symptoms. I continue to do Schirmer testing, but acknowledge all of the above. It is a subjective number and, although changing, still seems to be something looked for in medical legal situations. More importantly, I tell every patient I do ptosis or blepharoplasty surgery on that they may develop dry eye symptoms after surgery, even if they do not appear dry preoperatively.

R. B. Penne, MD

Intratarsal Keratinous Cysts of the Meibomian Gland: Distinctive Clinicopathologic and Immunohistochemical Features in 6 Cases

Jakobiec FA, Mehta M, Iwamoto M, et al (Massachusetts Eye and Ear Infirmary, Bostan; et al)

Am J Ophthalmol 149:82-94, 2010

Purpose.—To describe 6 patients representing a new entity of Meibomian gland keratinous cysts.

Design.—Retrospective, interventional, clinicopathologic study.

Methods.—Review of clinical histories and findings, histopathologic evaluations, and immunohistochemical studies of the cysts' linings with monoclonal antibodies directed against cytokeratins and cell surface epithelial markers.

Results.—Six patients with an average age of 62.5 years had noninflamed, upper eyelid nodules fixed to the tarsus. Eyelid eversion revealed a white–yellow nodular bulge in 3 cases, a bluish coloration in 2 cases, and a translucent appearance in 1 case. The cysts were lined by undulating squamous epithelium possessing an inner eosinophilic cuticle that produced a peculiar refractile, strand-like intracavitary keratin. Immunostaining for cytokeratin 17 and carcinoembryonic antigen showed strongly positive results in the Meibomian gland cysts and, by comparison, negative results in cutaneous epidermal cysts. Multiple recurrences occurred after incomplete excisions.

Conclusions.—After chalazia and sebaceous cell tumors, Meibomian gland keratinous cysts seem to be the third most common primary intratarsal lesion. Anterior fixation to the tarsus and posterior protrusion beneath the palpebral conjunctiva without inflammation suggest the diagnosis. Histopathologic and immunohistochemical evaluations can distinguish unequivocally the current entity from common epidermal cysts. The optimal treatment consists of an en bloc excision of the cyst with a tarsectomy, or else wide excision with intratarsal cautery of any remnants of the cellular lining.

▶ This article describes 6 patients with intratarsal keratinous cysts (Table 1 in the original article). Identification of these lesions is important because they are often mistaken for a chalazion and the treatment approach is different. These lesions are not common. I see this 2 to 3 times a year. The key is recognition. Externally, they are slightly different than most chalazions with a more discrete firm nodule without any inflammation. It appears the cyst is on top of the tarsus as opposed to being within the tarsus in the case of a chalazion. The most important difference is when the lid is flipped the tarsal changes are distinctive (Table 2 and Fig 1 in the original article). I have always noted a white or yellow-white spot in the tarsus. In this article, they describe 2 cases with a bluish change noted in the tarsal plate.

The reason recognition is so important is because of the difference in the surgical approach. Chalazions just need to be incised and the contents curetted where these cysts need to be completely excised or they will recur. I have had success using a transcutaneous approach, excising the entire cyst, removing tarsus at the base, and then cauterizing the surrounding tissue. I believe a similar approach from the tarsal side would work, but visualizing the cyst wall and being sure it is completely excised I find more difficult working against the obicularis and skin than against the tarsus. I have never needed to do a full thickness pentagon eyelid excision for these lesions.

This article makes us aware of this rare lesion. The key to diagnosis is to flip the lid in all quiet chalazions before excision. When these classic tarsal changes are present, complete excision of the cyst is required rather than drainage of the chalazion. This is more extensive and more instruments are needed, but it can still be done in the office.

R. B. Penne, MD

One-Snip Punctoplasty and Canalicular Curettage Through the Punctum: A Minimally Invasive Surgical Procedure for Primary Canaliculitis

Lee MJ, Choung H-K, Kim NJ, et al (Seoul Natl Univ Hosp, Korea; Seoul Natl Univ Boramae Hosp, Korea; Seoul Natl Univ Bundang Hosp, Korea)

Ophthalmology 116:2027-2030, 2009

Purpose.—To evaluate treatment results of canalicular curettage through the punctum after 1-snip punctoplasty for primary canaliculitis.

Design.—Retrospective, interventional case series.

Participants.—Thirty patients with primary canaliculitis who were treated at Seoul National University Hospital between February 2005 and January 2008.

Methods.—All patients underwent 1-snip punctoplasty and canalicular curettage through the punctum, and granules or concretions were removed. After the procedure, oral and topical antibiotics were used for

TABLE 1.—Presenting Symptoms and Clinical Signs of the Patients

	No. of Patients (%)
Presenting symptoms	
Mucous discharge	18 (60.0)
Epiphora	13 (43.3)
Conjunctival injection	5 (16.7)
Pus from the punctum	5 (16.7)
Medial canthal pain	2 (6.7)
Eyelid swelling	1 (3.3)
Clinical signs	
Pus or concretion from punctum	27 (90.0)
Punctal and canalicular swelling	16 (53.3)
Punctal and canalicular erythema	16 (53.3)

3 weeks. Demographic data and clinical presentations of the patients were analyzed. The resolution of symptoms and inflammatory signs and complications were evaluated 3 weeks after the procedure.

Main Outcome Measures.—Resolution rate of the canaliculitis and complications after the procedure.

Results.—There was a female predominance in the study group (23:7). Common symptoms of canaliculitis included discharge, tearing, and pus or concretions from the punctum. During the procedure, concretions, granules, or discharges were drained in all patients. In 25 (83.3%) of 30 patients, the symptoms and signs of canaliculitis completely resolved 3 weeks after 1 treatment. Two patients (6.7%) required additional curettage. Symptomatic canalicular strictures developed in 2 patients.

Conclusions.—Materials were removed easily from the canaliculus using a 1-snip punctoplasty and curettage through the punctum. This procedure, combined with systemic and topical antibiotic therapy, can be a highly effective treatment for primary canaliculitis (Table 1).

▶ This article is a retrospective look at 30 patients treated for canaliculitis with a 1-snip punctoplasty. The signs and symptoms of canaliculitis (Table 1) are outlined in the article and important to note. My experience is that canaliculitis is one of the most common causes of chronic conjunctivitis. The results were very good, with 28 of 30 patients having resolution of the infection and 2 patients required a second curettage.

The procedure as described (Fig 1 in the original article) is simple but effective, and is exactly what I do for my patients. Complications are rare. Most patients who have canaliculitis are so happy to be rid of the chronic irritation and discharge that they rarely complain of any problem after the procedure. This article excluded patients with canaliculitis secondary to punctal plugs, but I can say that this procedure is equally effective to remove a plug that is causing a canaliculitis. It is well worth reading this and tucking it away for reference when this type of procedure is needed in the office.

R. B. Penne, MD

Infection rates in outpatient eyelid surgery

Lee EW, Holtebeck AC, Harrison AR (Univ of Minnesota, Minneapolis)

Ophthal Plast Reconstr Surg 25:109-110, 2009

Purpose.—The authors used the database of eyelid surgeries performed at the Phillips Eye Institute in Minneapolis, MN, to help determine the infection rate in outpatient eyelid surgery.

Methods.—The authors retrospectively reviewed the reported cases of infections after all eyelid surgeries performed between January 1, 1999 and December 31, 2004 at the Phillips Eye Institute in Minneapolis, MN.

Results.—Of a total of 2,227 patients who underwent oculoplastic procedures, there was only one reported infection (0.04%).

Conclusions.—The infection rate in outpatient eyelid surgery is extremely low.

▶ The incidence of eyelid infections after eyelid surgery is very low. This article looks at that issue in a single surgical facility over 5 years. The conclusion is that the rate of infection is very low and is 0.04% for eyelid surgery. They also conclude that the use of prophylactic oral antibiotics is unnecessary in eyelid surgery.

I agree with the articles' conclusions, but I am somewhat concerned with the way the results were gathered. The finding of an infection was based on quarterly quality surveys filled out by surgeons. I can attest to the fact that in a busy practice if you have someone with a postoperative mild infection that you treat successfully with antibiotics, you may not remember that patient when surveyed 3 to 4 months later. Thus, there is a very good chance that the infection incidence is under-reported by design. There is no mention of whether the patient may have been placed on oral antibiotic after surgery. The patients were from multiple surgeons and the charts were not reviewed for this study. Thus, some of the patients included in the study may have actually been taking oral antibiotics.

This article studies eyelid surgery, however, in the discussion, there is mention of, and recommendations for, use of antibiotics in DCR surgery. It is important to realize that eyelid and DCR are very different surgeries when it comes to infection risk. Eyelids are done under sterile conditions, whereas a DCR is open to the nose and is not sterile. I disagree with the conclusion that DCRs do not need systemic antibiotics. The reference they site[1] did not advocate any systemic antibiotics but rather selective use of systemic antibiotics instead of routine use. In their study, 9% of patients received systemic antibiotics to achieve the 1% infection rate.

In summary, I agree that topical antibiotic alone is adequate for routine eyelid surgery. The question of when to use systemic antibiotics remains a question and is not properly addressed in this article.

R. B. Penne, MD

Reference

1. Yazici B, Meyer DR. Selective antibiotic use to prevent postoperative wound infection after external dacryocystorhinostomy. *Opththal Plast Reconstr Surg*. 2002; 18:331-335.

Histologic Safety Margin in Basal Cell Carcinoma of the Eyelid: Correlation with Recurrence Rate

Auw-Haedrich C, Frick S, Boehringer D, et al (Albert-Ludwigs-Univ, Freiburg, Germany)

Ophthalmology 116:802-806, 2009

Objective.—To examine the correlation between the minimum histologic safety margin (HSM) and recurrence rate of periorbital basal cell carcinomas (BCC).

Design.—Cohort study.

Participants.—One hundred one patients with 101 BCCs treated surgically between 1997 and 1999 at the eye hospital in Freiburg were enrolled in this study. Mean follow-up was 7 years (range, 104 days to 9.7 years).

Methods.—The tumors' minimum HSM was measured retrospectively in photographs of hematoxylin and eosin–stained paraffin slides using the digital picture analysis system AnalySIS of Soft Imaging System Inc, and/or calculated according to the tumor-free section number. Statistical analysis was performed using the Kaplan–Meier method and the log-rank test.

Main Outcome Measures.—Histologic margins of solid and fibrous BCC and recurrence rate.

Results.—Seven of the 101 patients experienced tumor recurrence (6.93%) after a mean follow-up of 34.7 months (range, 3–83) according to Kaplan–Meier analysis. The patients were assigned to 1 of 3 groups: (I) those without HSM (n = 11), 3 recurrences (27.27%); (II) those with HSM <0.2 mm (n = 18), 3 recurrences (16.67%); and (III) those with HSM >0.2 mm (n = 72), 1 recurrence (1.39%). The difference in recurrences between those groups with HSM and HSM = 0, as well as between the HSM >0.2 mm-group and HSM <0.2 mm-group were statistically significant ($P = 0.01$; $P = 0.03$).

Conclusions.—Extremely small HSMs are likely to prevent recurrences. At critical and visually easily accessible tumor sites (e.g., adjacent to the lacrimal puncta) a re-resection in solid BCCs with tumor-positive margins may not be mandatory, provided the surgical site is clinically inspected regularly. This conclusion does not apply to fibrous BCC (Tables 1 and 2).

▶ This was a retrospective study that looked at the distance between the surgical margin and the edge of the basal cell carcinoma in eyelid tissue. This was a unique opportunity, as frozen sections or Mohs' surgery was not used at this hospital. The basal cell carcinoma was excised and then the eyelid repair

TABLE 1.—Synopsis of All Recurrences: Histologic Subtype, Histologic Safety Margin (HSM), Interval Between Excision and Recurrence (Time) and Location

Case	Histologic Subtype	HSM (mm)	Time (mos)	Location
1	Fibrosing	0.68	55	Lower lid
2	Fibrosing	0.08	3	Medial canthus
3	Fibrosing	0.00	7	Lower lid
4	Fibrosing	0.08	83	Lower lid
5	Fibrosing	0.14	21	Lateral canthus
6	Solid	0.00	66	Lower lid
7	Solid	0.00	8	Medial canthus

TABLE 2.—All Cases Classified in 3 Categories According to Histologic Safety Margin (HSM) and Recurrence Rates

	HSM = 0	HSM < 0.2 mm	HSM > 0.2 mm
Solid BCC (case number)	10	15	59
Solid BCC with recurrence	2 (20%)	0	0
Fibrous BCC (case number)	1	3	13
Fibrous BCC with recurrence	1 (100%)	3 (100%)	1 (8%)

BCC = basal cell carcinoma.

was delayed until the pathology had been evaluated. Once the permanent pathology was evaluated, the eyelid was either closed or re-excised and closed. This allowed for evaluation of the pathology and determination of the distance between the margin and the basal cell carcinoma.

The findings were an overall recurrence rate of 6.93%. The rate of recurrence was really related to the type of basal cell. The solid basal cells (SBC) had an overall recurrence rate of just 2.38%, and both of these were in tumors that had a positive margin. There were 10 SBC with a positive margin, and only 20% had recurrence. In contrast, the fibrous basal cell (FBC) tumors had an overall recurrence rate of 29.41%. All FBC with positive margins or margins less than 0.2 mm recurred. In margins greater than 0.2 mm, the rate of recurrence was much lower at 8%.

These results emphasize the need for greater margins in FBC, and that not all SBC with positive margins will recur. I believe this is a case for the value of Mohs' surgery, especially in FBC tumors.

R. B. Penne, MD

Effectiveness of canalicular laceration repair using monocanalicular intubation with Monoka tubes

Lee H, Chi M, Park M, et al (Korea Univ, Seoul; Gachon Univ, Incheon, Korea; Kong Eye Ctr, Seoul, Korea)

Acta Ophthalmol 87:793-796, 2009

Purpose.—This study aimed to evaluate the clinical efficacy of canalicular laceration repair using monocanalicular intubation with Monoka tubes.

Methods.—A total of 36 single lacerated canaliculi were repaired using monocanalicular intubation with Monoka tubes, without mucosal anastomosis of the canaliculi, and were retrospectively reviewed. Demographic information, injury locations, associated ocular injuries, complications and outcomes were analysed.

Results.—Mean patient age was 34 years (range 1–64 years). Tubes were removed at a mean of 4.2 months (range 3–6 months). There were 26 lower canalicular lacerations (72%) and 10 upper canalicular lacerations (28%). Overall, 34 of 36 cases (92%) showed improvement in symptoms and exhibited positivity on the dye disappearance test at 4–12 months after the procedure (mean 7.8 months). In total, 21 patients (58%) achieved complete success, 13 patients (36%) achieved partial success and two patients (6%) suffered surgical failure. Complications were seen in five cases and included two early tube protrusions, two punctal slits and one punctal granuloma.

Conclusions.—Monocanalicular intubation with Monoka tubes leads to successful outcomes without significant complications and offers an alternative to bicanalicular intubation in the treatment of monocanalicular lacerations (Table 3).

▶ This article looks retrospectively at 36 patients who had canalicular lacerations repaired with a Monoka monocanalicular tube. The results were impressive, with only 2 (6%) having failure based on symptomatic tearing and complete obstruction on irrigation. There were very few complications (see Table 3).

These results are very good. It certainly gives credibility to the use of a monocanalicular tube for the repair of a monocanalicular laceration. The use of a Monoka tube rather than a mini-Monoka tube is the one difference from

TABLE 3.—Associated Ocular Injury in Patients with Canalicular Injury

Ocular injury	No. of cases (%)
Traumatic hyphaema	7 (33%)
Subconjunctival haemorrhage	5 (24%)
Retinal oedema	4 (19%)
Orbital wall fracture	3 (14%)
Traumatic optic neuropathy	1 (5%)
Traumatic cataract	1 (5%)
Total	21 (100%)

what I routinely do for canalicular lacerations. The Monoka tube has a metal probe on the end, which needs to be passed into and retrieved from the nose. The mini-Monoka tube does not have to be located in the nose. Often locating the tube in the nasal cavity can be a difficult part of the case, especially if the surgery is done where a nasal endoscope is not available. This makes the mini-Monoka easier to use in my experience. Doing this may be part of why the success rate was so high in this study. Locating the tube assures that the entire lacrimal system is patent.

I do not routinely irrigate patients with a single canalicular laceration unless they are complaining of tearing. For that reason, I really don't know how often there is anatomic success with a mini-Monoka tube. I do know that it is rare that a patient has symptomatic epiphora after repair. I will continue to use a mini-Monoka tube for repair of most monocanalicular lacerations.

R. B. Penne, MD

Informing patients: oculoplastic surgery and the internet

Zaidi FH, Jones CA (Maidstone Hosp, England, UK)
Eye 23:2090-2093, 2009

Aims.—Oculoplastic surgery has received little attention compared with other subspecialties in terms of how the internet influences patient expectations. Blepharoplasty resembles a model for oculoplastic operations. We aimed to assess the quality of information accessed by patients on blepharoplasty using the internet as a resource.

Methods.—After surveying doctors and lay persons, the word 'blepharoplasty' and related terms were studied using an advanced keyword search. This scanned average monthly search volume over a recent 12-month period. The three most popular search terms that were found were entered into the Google search engine. Criteria published in the *Journal of the American Medical Association* for qualifying information from the internet were used in the analysis, yielding a possible score from 0 to a maximum of 4.

Results.—Of the 150 websites that were studied, these criteria were fully applied to 101 websites. Only 2.5% of sites scored favourably on all four criteria; 6.5% scored three points; 10% scored two points; 41% scored one point; 40% of sites scored zero for objective quality. Superior scores were achieved by online encyclopaedias ('medipedias'), peer-reviewed journals, online abstracts, and book chapters. The websites of professional bodies scored poorly. The lowest scored were private clinics and National Health Service (NHS) hospital websites.

Conclusions.—Using the internet, the quality of information obtained for oculoplastic surgery seems far inferior to other subspecialties within ophthalmology as well as non-ophthalmic specialties. These findings are

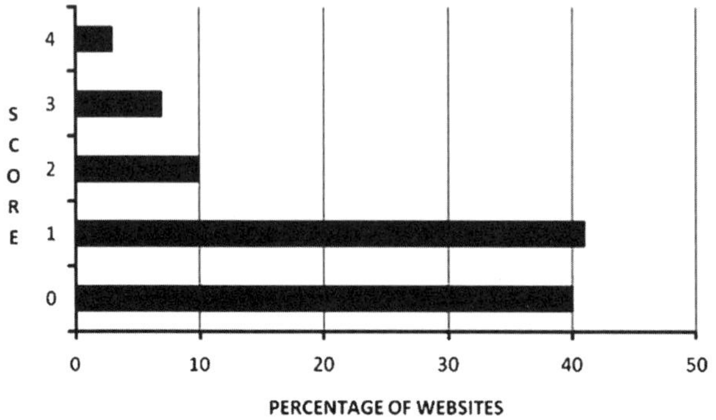

FIGURE 1.—Quality of websites scored using criteria published in *JAMA*. (Reprinted from Zaidi FH, Jones CA. Informing patients: oculoplastic surgery and the internet. *Eye*. 2009;23:2090-2093.)

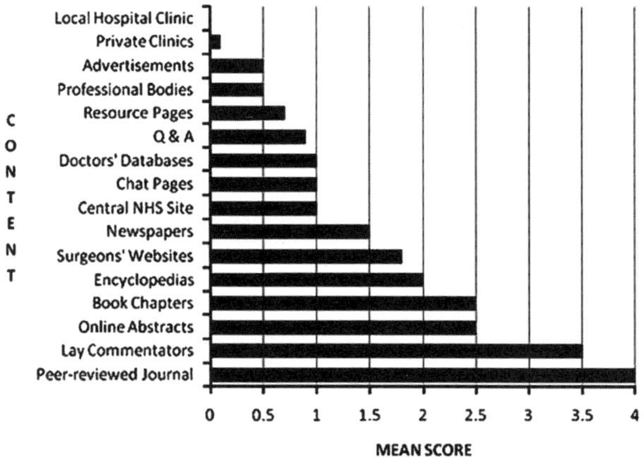

FIGURE 2.—Breakdown of quality of information on the basis of website content: mean scores for different types of website. The maximum mean score for quality is 4.0 and the minimum score is 0. (Reprinted from Zaidi FH, Jones CA. Informing patients: oculoplastic surgery and the internet. *Eye*. 2009;23:2090-2093.)

specifically relevant to surgeons carrying out blepharoplasty and of general relevance to ophthalmic plastic surgeons (Figs 1 and 2).

▶ Everyone has patients who use the World Wide Web as their information source about their medical condition or proposed treatment. This article looks at the quality of information available on the Internet when patients sought information about blepharoplasty. Blepharoplasty is a common surgery in oculoplastics and would represent something for which information should be able to be found easily. The conclusion is that the information is overall not of high quality, with only 2.5% of the sites found on a search achieving a score of 4 of 4 (Figs 1 and 2), and 40% scored 0 of 4.

This study confirms the large amount of poor and inaccurate information on the Internet about medical conditions. The 3 groups that scored the best (score of 2 through 4 of 4) were either not aimed at the lay public, such as peer-reviewed journals or book chapters, or had questionable accuracy, such as layperson-authored and referenced articles. Medical encyclopedias scored the best overall.

This article is a reminder of the large amount of poor and inaccurate information that is available on the Internet. As the authors note, this can be a source of unrealistic expectations and an unhappy patient. Physicians need to assume that patients will access this source of poor information and provide written information of their own to their patients or address the potential inaccuracy of the Internet when they discuss medical procedures and treatments.

R. B. Penne, MD

"Sutureless" Repair of Orbital Floor and Rim Fractures

Lane KA, Bilyk JR, Taub D, et al (Children's Hosp of Philadelphia, PA; Wills Eye Inst, Philadelphia, PA; Jefferson Univ Hosp, Philadelphia, PA)
Ophthalmology 116:135-138, 2009

Purpose.—To report on the surgical outcomes of patients undergoing orbital fracture repair without periosteal or conjunctival closure.

Design.—Retrospective interventional case series.

Participants.—Eighty-two patients (85 eyes) who underwent transconjunctival repair of isolated floor (n = 38) or complex orbital fracture (n = 47) without conjunctival closure.

Methods.—A transconjunctival incision below the tarsus provides preseptal access to the inferior orbital rim, after which the periosteum is incised for exploration and repair of orbital floor fractures. Forced ductions are performed after release of entrapped tissue and placement of an orbital floor implant, and the conjunctiva is reapproximated with forceps and draped into the inferior fornix.

Main Outcome Measures.—Incidence of postoperative complications, including orbital implant exposure, infection, and migration.

Results.—Patients were followed for an average of 318 days postoperatively (range 82–978 days). One patient experienced a pyogenic granuloma at the conjunctival incision that resolved with steroid drops. Other complications included lateral canthal dystopia or pyogenic granuloma at the lateral canthotomy site, when used. There were no cases of postoperative implant exposure, infection, or migration.

Conclusions.—Forgoing closure of the periorbita and conjunctiva after transconjunctival orbital floor and rim fracture repair is associated with a low incidence of postoperative complications. This technique is applicable in the repair of both isolated floor fractures and complex orbital fractures.

▶ This is a retrospective review of patients who had orbital fracture repair without conjunctival closure. A total of 85 eyes were included, and there were no significant complications. There was one pyogenic granuloma. Importantly, there was no infection or implant exposure in any of these studied patients.

In the current atmosphere of no-stitch small incision surgery, this approach fits right in. As the authors state, this is not better than standard conjunctival closure, but shows that the extra time and suture material are not necessary in orbital fracture repair cases. I have not closed lower eyelid transconjunctival blepharoplasty incisions for years. Since this study came out, I have not closed my orbital fracture incisions in many cases, and I have not had any problem. I do still close the conjunctiva if the repair is more extensive or incision is larger than normal.

R. B. Penne, MD

7 Pediatric Ophthalmology

Postoperative outcomes in children with intermittent exotropia from a population-based cohort

Ekdawi NS, Nusz KJ, Diehl NN, et al (Mayo Clinic and Mayo Foundation, Rochester, MN)

J AAPOS 13:4-7, 2009

Purpose.—To describe the long-term surgical outcomes in a population-based cohort of children with intermittent exotropia.

Methods.—The medical records of all children (<19 years) who were diagnosed with intermittent exotropia as residents of Olmsted County Minnesota, from January 1, 1975, through December 31, 1994, and managed with surgery were retrospectively reviewed.

Results.—Of 184 patients with intermittent exotropia, 61 (33%) underwent surgery at a mean age of 7.6 years (range, 3.2 to 23 years). Twelve of the 61 children (19.7%) underwent a second surgery (10 for recurrent exotropia and 2 for consecutive esotropia), and no patient received 3 or more surgeries during a mean follow-up of 10 years from the first surgery. The final postoperative measurements were recorded in 56 of 61 patients (92%) at a mean of 7.4 years (range, 0 to 18 years) after the first surgery: 31 of the 56 (55%) were within 9^{Δ} of orthotropia at distance and 25 of 55 (45%) had better than 60 seconds of stereopsis. The Kaplan-Meier rate of developing $\geq 10^{\Delta}$ of misalignment after the first surgery was 54% by 5 years, 76% by 10 years, and 86% by 15 years.

Conclusions.—In this population-based study of surgery in children with intermittent exotropia, although only 1 in 5 received a second surgery, after a mean follow-up of 8 years, approximately half were successfully aligned and 45% had high-grade stereopsis.

▶ A clinical factor that may help to predict successful postoperative outcomes in children with intermittent exotropia (IXT) is the duration in time in which indications are present and surgical procedure is performed. This information is not available in this retrospective study. The patients in this study were homogenous and may not represent the general population of the United States in terms of race or ethnicity. A well-designed prospective study on the long-term follow-up of children with IXT following surgery is necessary to avoid the problems of a retrospective study.

L. B. Nelson, MD, MBA

The relationship between preoperative alignment stability and postoperative motor outcomes in children with esotropia

Pediatric Eye Disease Investigator Group (Jaeb Ctr for Health Res, Tampa, FL)
J AAPOS 13:335-338, 2009

Purpose.—To examine the effect of preoperative alignment stability on postoperative motor outcomes in children who underwent surgery for esotropia.

Methods.—One hundred sixty-seven subjects (68 with infantile esotropia and 99 with acquired esotropia) aged less than 6 years had surgery after completing 18 weeks of follow-up as part of an observational study. Preoperative alignment was classified as stable, uncertain, or unstable, based on measurements taken at baseline and every 6 weeks for 18 weeks. Distance alignment measured by prism and alternate cover test was compared among stability classification groups at 6 weeks and 6 months after surgery.

Results.—Among subjects with infantile esotropia, median 6-week postoperative deviation was 2^{Δ}, 6^{Δ}, and 2^{Δ} for subjects with stable, uncertain, and unstable preoperative alignment, respectively ($p = 0.73$ for stable vs unstable). Median 6-month postoperative deviation was 1^{Δ}, 9^{Δ}, and 1^{Δ} for stable, uncertain, and unstable, respectively ($p = 1.00$ for stable vs unstable). Among subjects with acquired esotropia, median 6-week postoperative deviation was 6^{Δ}, 4^{Δ}, and 4^{Δ} for subjects with stable, uncertain, and unstable preoperative alignment, respectively ($p = 0.69$ for stable vs unstable). Median 6-month postoperative deviation was 8^{Δ}, 4^{Δ}, and 6^{Δ} for stable, uncertain, and unstable, respectively ($p = 0.22$ for stable vs unstable).

Conclusions.—Postoperative alignment at 6 weeks and 6 months appears similar in children with stable versus unstable preoperative esotropia. Nevertheless, our finding should be interpreted with caution due to small sample size.

▶ Strabismus surgeons may delay surgery for childhood esotropia until the alignment stabilizes. Yet, how often is there an instability of alignment before surgical intervention and how long on average does it have to reach stability are presently not well defined. Bias may have occurred because the examiners in the study were not masked to the preoperative stability status of the children with esotropia in determining the outcome measurement of alignment. Other variables (eg, such as whether amblyopia was present in these children) that may have altered the results were not taken into account.

L. B. Nelson, MD, MBA

A child with bilateral orbital cellulitis one day after strabismus surgery

Basheikh A, Superstein R (McGill Univ, Montreal, Quebec, Canada; The Montreal Children's Hosp, Quebec, Canada)

J AAPOS 13:488-490, 2009

Orbital cellulitis is a rare complication of strabismus surgery. We report a case of a 4-year-old boy with bilateral orbital cellulitis after uneventful surgery to correct esotropia. Concomitant sinusitis was the likely source of infection. To our knowledge, this is the first case of bilateral orbital cellulitis following strabismus surgery.

▶ Periocular infections, including orbital cellulitis and endophthalmitis, following strabismus surgery are rare and potentially serious. The authors recommend doing a thorough preoperative history with attention to signs and symptoms of sinusitis. However, the ability to ascertain a clear history of recent sinusitis may be difficult. The authors also recommend the routine instillation of a single dose of povidone-iodine at the conclusion of strabismus surgery. However, whether povidone-iodine is more effective than an antibiotic or antibiotic-steroid combination remains undetermined.

L. B. Nelson, MD, MBA

Associations between near work, outdoor activity, and myopia among adolescent students in rural China: the Xichang Pediatric Refractive Error Study report no. 2

Lu B, Congdon N, Liu X, et al (Joint Shantou International Eye Ctr of Shantou Univ and Chinese Univ of Hong Kong, Guangdong, China)

Arch Ophthalmol 127:769-775, 2009

Objective.—To study the associations between near work, outdoor activity, and myopia among children attending secondary school in rural China.

Methods.—Among a random cluster sample of 1892 children in Xichang, China, subjects with an uncorrected acuity of 6/12 or less in either eye (n = 984) and a 25% sample of children with normal vision (n = 248) underwent measurement of refractive error. Subjects were administered a questionnaire on parental education, time spent outdoors, and weekly time spent engaged in and preferred working distance for a variety of near-work activities.

Results.—Among 1232 children with refraction data, 998 (81.0%) completed the near-work survey. Their mean age was 14.6 years (SD, 0.8 years), 55.6% were girls, and 83.1% had myopia of −0.5 diopters or less (more myopia) in both eyes. Time and diopter-hours spent on near activities did not differ between children with and without myopia. In regression models, time spent on near activities and time outdoors were unassociated with myopia, adjusting for age, sex, and parental education.

Conclusions.—These and other recent results raise some doubts about the association between near work and myopia. Additional efforts to identify other environmental factors associated with myopia risk and that may be amenable to intervention are warranted.

▶ In an attempt to prevent or slow the progression of myopia, pharmacologic, refractive, and behavior strategies have been attempted. Near work has been reported by several investigators to increase the risk of myopia development and progression. Studies have suggested that reducing visual tasks at near fixation might result in less myopia development in children. More than any other factor, genetics play a dominant role in the development and progression of myopia. As many ophthalmologists have found, the number of children with myopia do not have a greater time spent at near-work activities compared with those children who do not develop myopia.

L. B. Nelson, MD, MBA

Astigmatism in the Early Treatment for Retinopathy of Prematurity Study: Findings to 3 Years of Age

Davitt BV, Dobson V, Quinn GE, et al (Saint Louis Univ School of Medicine, MO; Univ of Arizona, Tucson; Univ of Pennsylvania Health System, Philadelphia; et al)

Ophthalmology 116:332-339, 2009

Purpose.—To examine the prevalence of astigmatism (≥1.00 diopter [D]) and high astigmatism (≥2.00 D) at 6 and 9 months corrected age and 2 and 3 years postnatal age, in preterm children with birth weight of less than 1251 g in whom high-risk prethreshold retinopathy of prematurity (ROP) developed and who participated in the Early Treatment for Retinopathy of Prematurity (ETROP) Study.

Design.—Randomized, controlled clinical trial.

Participants.—Four hundred one infants in whom prethreshold ROP developed in one or both eyes and who were randomized after they were determined to have a high risk (≥15%) of poor structural outcome without treatment using the Risk Management of Retinopathy of Prematurity (RM-ROP2) program. Refractive error was measured by cycloplegic retinoscopy. Eyes with additional retinal, glaucoma, or cataract surgery were excluded.

Intervention.—Eyes were randomized to receive laser photocoagulation at high-risk prethreshold ROP (early treated [ET]) or to be conventionally managed (CM), receiving treatment only if threshold ROP developed.

Main Outcome Measures.—Astigmatism and high astigmatism at each visit. Astigmatism was classified as with-the-rule (WTR; 75°–105°), against-the-rule (ATR; 0°–15° and 165°–180°), or oblique (OBL; 16°–74° and 106°–164°).

Results.—The prevalence of astigmatism in ET and CM eyes was similar at each test age. For both groups, there was an increase in prevalence of astigmatism from approximately 32% at 6 months to approximately 42% by 3 years, mostly occurring between 6 and 9 months. Among eyes that could be refracted, astigmatism was not influenced by zone of acute-phase ROP, presence of plus disease, or retinal residua of ROP. Eyes with astigmatism and high astigmatism most often had WTR astigmatism.

Conclusions.—By age 3 years, nearly 43% of eyes treated at high-risk prethreshold ROP developed astigmatism of ≥1.00 D and nearly 20% had astigmatism of ≥2.00 D. Presence of astigmatism was not influenced by timing of treatment of acute-phase ROP or by characteristics of acute-phase or cicatricial ROP. These findings reinforce the need for follow-up eye examinations in infants with high-risk prethreshold ROP.

▶ While retinopathy of prematurity (ROP) remains of major concern in premature children, significant refractions are frequently associated findings in these children with and without ROP. Since the prevalence of astigmatism increases with age, it is necessary that these children are carefully and routinely followed up for the possible development of this refractive error. Early treatment of significant and or asymmetric astigmatism will give these children the best chance for a good visual outcome.

L. B. Nelson, MD, MBA

Diplopia and Fluoroquinolones

Fraunfelder FW, Fraunfelder FT (Oregon Health & Science Univ, Portland)
Ophthalmology 116:1814-1817, 2009

Purpose.—To report a possible association between fluoroquinolones and diplopia.

Design.—Database study.

Participants.—A total of 171 subjects were studied.

Methods.—Spontaneous reports from the National Registry of Drug-Induced Ocular Side Effects, World Health Organization, and Food and Drug Administration were collected on fluoroquinolones and diplopia.

Main Outcome Measures.—Data garnered from the spontaneous reports include the type of fluoroquinolone, age, gender, adverse drug reaction (ADR), dosage, duration of therapy until onset of ADR, concomitant drugs, other systemic disease, and dechallenge and rechallenge data.

Results.—A total of 171 case reports of diplopia associated with fluoroquinolones were reported, including 76 men, 91 women, and 4 case reports in which the gender was not specified. The median age was 51.6 years. Dosage varied between the different fluoroquinolone drugs, with the median dosage within the range recommended in the package insert for each different fluoroquinolone. Median time from beginning of therapy to appearance of the ADR was 9.6 days (range 1 day to 5 months). Seventeen subjects also had concomitant tendinitis, 49 patients were 60 years or older, 1 patient had renal cysts, and 4 patients were taking systemic anti-inflammatory steroids. There were 53 positive dechallenge and 5 positive rechallenge case reports.

Conclusions.—According to World Health Organization criteria, the relationship between fluoroquinolone therapy and diplopia is "possible." This causality assessment is based on the time relationship of drug administration and ADR development, the multiple positive dechallenge and rechallenge reports, and the plausible mechanism by which diplopia could occur: possible tendinitis of the extraocular muscles.

▶ Fluoroquinolones have become much more popular in recent years for a variety of ophthalmological conditions. Like any medication topically or systemically applied, side effects can develop. While the true incidence of diplopia associated with fluoroquinolones is unknown, it certainly should be considered in any patient with a recent onset of diplopia. If a patient complains of recent diplopia and is on a fluoroquinolone, the medication should be discontinued. If the diplopia persists beyond a week or 2, further neurological intervention should be undertaken.

L. B. Nelson, MD, MBA

Evaluation of refraction in a statistically significant sample: changes according to age and strabismus

Chiesi C, Chiesi L, Cavallini GM (Modena & Reggio Emilia Univ, Italy)

J Pediatr Ophthalmol Strabismus 46:266-272, 2009

Purpose.—To assess possible refractive changes according to age and strabismus in a statistically significant cohort.

Methods.—A population-based sample of 12,534 subjects 0.5 to 20 years old, examined between 2004 and 2006, was tested. Each subject received a complete orthoptic examination, including spherocylindrical streak retinoscopy in cycloplegia. Patients were divided into those with orthophoria (7,784) and those with strabismus (4,750), and the latter group was further divided into those with esodeviation (3,026) and those with exodeviation (1,724). A statistical analysis of the spherical equivalent, astigmatism, and anisometropia was performed with an independent samples t test or one-way analysis of variance.

Results.—The percentage of patients with a mean spherical equivalent within ±1 and ±2 standard deviations was greater than 68% and 95%, respectively. The mean spherical equivalent of the total sample was 1.62 diopters (D) (±2.88). The mean spherical equivalent was 1.10 ± 2.94 D in the orthophoria group, 3.22 ± 2.29 D in the esodeviation group, and 1.13 ± 2.50 D in the exodeviation group (one-way analysis of variance; P =.000). Age-related changes in the mean spherical equivalent showed a clear and steady myopic shift, reaching mean myopic refraction at 12 to 14 years in both the total sample and the orthophoria and exodeviation groups. It assumed a more constant trend, with no myopic swing, in the esodeviation group ($P = .000$). Mean astigmatism was less in patients with less than 1.00 D anisometropia (0.83 ± 0.92 D) than in those with 1.00 D or greater anisometropia (1.42 ± 1.18 D) (t test; $P = .0001$).

Conclusion.—Both the age-related trend in the spherical equivalent and the high hyperopic values of the distribution peak in patients with esodeviation confirm the importance of the hypermetropic refractive component. The statistically significantly higher incidence of astigmatism in patients with 1.00 D or greater ametropia highlights its incidence in amblyopia.

▶ In the perfect eye, the refractive power of the cornea and resting lens is just enough to focus light rays from a distant object onto the retinal plane. This condition whereby the length of the eye precisely matches the power of the cornea and lens, emmetropia, rarely exists or persists. It is generally accepted that the refraction of patients with accommodative esotropia averages +4.75 D, with a range of +3.00 to +10.00 D, whereas patients with intermittent exotropia have refractive errors similar to those of the general population. The authors confirmed that patients with esodeviation tend to share a higher initial degree of hyperopia than the general population, and the hyperopia tended to increase in the first year of life. Also confirmed that those patients with exodeviations have similar refractive errors to those with orthophoria. This finding contributes to the low incidence of amblyopia in patients with intermittent exotropia. The management of refractive errors and its relation to strabismus and amblyopia conditions is probably the most common problem faced by pediatric ophthalmologists in their practices and needs to be carefully documented and followed in children.

L. B. Nelson, MD, MBA

Is the Incidence of Infantile Esotropia Declining?: A Population-Based Study From Olmsted County, Minnesota, 1965 to 1994

Louwagie CR, Diehl NN, Greenberg AE, et al (Mayo Clinic and Mayo Foundation, Rochester, MN)

Arch Ophthalmol 127:200-203, 2009

Objective.—To investigate the incidence of infantile esotropia from a defined population in the United States over a 30-year period. Recent reports from the United Kingdom have suggested that strabismus or strabismus surgery is occurring less frequently today than in previous years.

Methods.—The medical records of all patients diagnosed with infantile esotropia within Olmsted County, Minnesota, from January 1, 1965, through December 31, 1994, were retrospectively reviewed.

Results.—The birth prevalence of infantile esotropia during the 30-year period was 25 (95% confidence interval, 21–29) per 10 000, or 1 in 403 live births. Although there were slightly more cases of infantile esotropia in the earlier years (45 from 1965–1974, 51 from 1975–1984, and 34 from 1985–1994), the change in incidence over time was not statistically significant (P = .32). The mean number of surgeries performed on each patient in this cohort was similar during the 30-year study: 1.8 for those diagnosed from 1965 to 1974, 1.9 for 1975 to 1984, and 1.6 for 1985 to 1994.

Conclusions.—The incidence of infantile esotropia in this population has not significantly changed from 1965 through 1994. Moreover, the rate of surgical intervention over these years is similar for this patient population.

▶ While esodeviations are the most common type of strabismus in children, infantile esotropia is not the most common form of esotropia in childhood. In the past, infantile esotropia was considered the most common type of esodeviations, probably because central nervous system disorders and/or acquired nonaccommodative esotropia were included. Some pediatric ophthalmologists believe that infantile esotropia is less common now than in the past. However, with the increase in the number of pediatric ophthalmologists over the years the same number of infantile esotropia patients has been spread out to more ophthalmologists.

L. B. Nelson, MD, MBA

Levodopa/carbidopa in the treatment of amblyopia

Dadeya S, Vats P, Malik KP (Guru Nanak Eye Ctr, Delhi, India)

J Pediatr Ophthalmol Strabismus 46:87-90, 2009

Purpose.—To evaluate the role of levodopa/carbidopa in the treatment of amblyopia.

Methods.—Thirty patients with strabismic amblyopia between the ages of 3 and 12 years were part of this double-blind, randomized study. Patients were divided into two groups. Group A received 0.50 mg + 1.25 mg of levodopa/carbidopa per kilogram body weight three times daily after meals, with a protein rich drink, whereas Group B received placebo. Both groups received full-time conventional occlusion until a visual acuity of 6/6 was achieved or for a maximum of 3 months.

Results.—The authors observed more than two lines improvement in visual acuity that was greater in the levodopa group (15 of 15) than in the placebo group (9 of 15) ($P < .005$). Furthermore, improvement in visual acuity of more than two lines was greater in patients younger than 8 years (100%) than in patients older than 8 years of age (60%) (P =.0026). There was also no significant reversal of the improved visual acuity in up to 6 months of follow-up.

Conclusion.—Levodopa/carbidopa improves visual acuity in patients with amblyopia and maintains improved visual acuity, especially in patients younger than 8 years.

▶ Amblyopia is one of the most common ocular disorders in childhood. Occlusion therapy is still the mainstay of treatment. However, poor compliance is a major obstacle in successfully testing amblyopic patients. While levodopa has been shown to improve visual acuity in amblyopic patients, it is not known how long the effect lasts or whether it is reversible. Prospective double-blind studies comparing levodopa with other methods of treatment of amblyopia are necessary.

L. B. Nelson, MD, MBA

Long-term follow-up of congenital esotropia in a population-based cohort

Louwagie CR, Diehl NN, Greenberg AE, et al (Mayo Clinic and Mayo Foundation, Rochester, MN)

J AAPOS 13:8-12, 2009

Purpose.—To report the long-term outcomes of a population-based cohort of children diagnosed with congenital esotropia during a 30-year period.

Methods.—The medical records of all patients diagnosed with congenital esotropia as residents of Olmsted County, MN, from January 1, 1965, through December 31, 1994, were retrospectively reviewed.

Results.—A total of 130 children were diagnosed during the 30-year period at a median age of 7.4 months with a mean deviation of 30^{Δ}. During a median follow-up of 11.9 years, 126 patients underwent a mean of 1.8 strabismus surgeries. The risk for undergoing a second surgery was significantly greater in patients with a larger presenting angle ($p = 0.017$) and a younger age at first surgery ($p = 0.006$). The Kaplan-Meier rate of having a second surgery was 51% at 10 years and 66% at 20 years. For those with 6 weeks or more of follow-up from the final surgery, last examined at a mean age of 15.1 years, 42 of 94 (45%) were within 8^{Δ} of orthotropia and 30 of 98 had some level of stereopsis ($\leq$3000 arcsec).

Conclusions.—In this population-based study of children with congenital esotropia, a second surgery was necessary in half the patients after 10 years and was more likely in those patients with a larger presenting angle and a younger age at first surgery. Approximately half of the patients were within 8^{Δ} of orthotropia and one-third had measurable stereopsis after a mean of 10.9 years of follow-up.

▶ During the 30-year period that the authors retrospectively reviewed surgical results of congenital esotropia, strabismus surgical approaches have evolved.

Bias may have been introduced into this study since the study population is homogeneous and does not match the general population of the United States in terms of race or ethnicity. This study was retrospective in that the patients were managed by a variety of physicians who may have introduced inconsistencies in measurement that wouldn't have been introduced had the measurements been performed by 1 individual trained in pediatric ophthalmology. Since congenital esotropia is usually present by 6 months of age, and the shorter duration for surgical intervention gives the best postoperative results, the fact that the mean age at first surgery was 19 months makes this study questionable.

L. B. Nelson, MD, MBA

Optical Treatment Reduces Amblyopia in Astigmatic Children Who Receive Spectacles Before Kindergarten

Dobson V, Clifford-Donaldson CE, Green TK, et al (Univ of Arizona, Tucson)
Ophthalmology 116:1002-1008, 2009

Objective.—To examine the effect of spectacle correction of astigmatism during preschool on best-corrected recognition visual acuity (VA), grating VA, and meridional amblyopia (difference between acuity for vertical versus horizontal gratings) once the children reach kindergarten.

Design.—Comparative case series.

Participants.—Seventy-three astigmatic (right eye ≥1.50 diopters [D] cylinder) Native American (Tohono O'odham) children 5 to 7 years of age. All had with-the-rule astigmatism. In 28 children, the astigmatism was simple myopic, compound myopic, or mixed (M/MA), and in 45 children, it was simple or compound hyperopic (HA).

Intervention.—Thirty-nine children (Treated Group) had spectacle correction of refractive error, prescribed for full-time wear, in preschool (0.8–2.4 years before testing). Thirty-four children (Untreated Group) had no prior correction.

Main Outcome Measure.—Comparison of Treated versus Untreated Groups for mean best-corrected right-eye recognition VA, measured with the Early Treatment Diabetic Retinopathy Study (ETDRS) chart and the Lea Symbols chart, for grating VA, measured with modified Teller acuity card stimuli, and for meridional amblyopia, based on grating acuity results.

Results.—Mean ETDRS VA was significantly better in the Treated Group (20/37) than in the Untreated Group (20/48; $P < 0.003$), but the difference between mean Lea Symbols VA in the Treated Group (20/33) and in the Untreated Group (20/38) was not significant. No significant Treated versus Untreated Group differences were found for either vertical or horizontal grating acuity. Meridional amblyopia differed between the M/MA group, which showed better acuity for vertical than for horizontal gratings, and the HA group, which showed better acuity for horizontal than for vertical gratings. However, in neither the M/MA group nor the

HA group was there a significant difference in magnitude of meridional amblyopia in the Treated versus the Untreated Group.

Conclusions.—Spectacle correction during the preschool years results in a significant improvement in best-corrected letter recognition acuity in astigmatic children by the time they reach kindergarten. However, grating acuity was not improved and magnitude of meridional amblyopia was not reduced in children who had received early spectacle correction.

▶ Astigmatic errors of 1.50 diopters or greater can result in amblyopia, especially when there is an asymmetry. This amount of astigmatic error should be given to a child certainly before kindergarten and preferably as early in childhood as it is detected. Unfortunately, many children who have a moderate amount of astigmatic error are asymptomatic and are not detected unless they have a visual screen test. It was not surprising that the authors did not find that the magnitude of meridional amblyopia was not reduced in children who had received early spectacle correction.

L. B. Nelson, MD, MBA

Predictive factors of surgical outcome in oculomotor nerve palsy

Cabrejas L, Hurtado-Ceña FJ, Tejedor J (Hosp Ramón y Cajal, Madrid, Spain)

J AAPOS 13:481-484, 2009

Purpose.—To investigate the outcomes and predictive factors of surgical treatment of oculomotor nerve palsy.

Methods.—Records of patients requiring eye muscle surgery for oculomotor nerve palsy in our institution were retrospectively reviewed. Age, sex, etiology, deviation, completeness of involvement, time between onset and surgery, botulinum toxin treatment, and number of surgical procedures were recorded as potential predictive factors. Muscle function, presence of diplopia, and torticollis were also recorded. The main outcome measure was motor function. Secondary outcome measures were presence of diplopia, torticollis, and limitation of muscle function.

Results.—Surgery was required in 22 patients, of whom motor success was obtained in 14 (63.6%). Frequency of diplopia and torticollis were significantly reduced by surgery. After multivariate regression analysis, longer time between onset and surgery ($p = 0.03$) and larger initial deviation ($p = 0.05$) were significantly associated with poorer postsurgical results in terms of motor function.

Conclusions.—Longer time from onset to surgery and larger eye deviation are negative prognostic factors of postsurgical motor success for oculomotor nerve palsy.

▶ One of the most difficult strabismus disorders to correct is oculomotor nerve palsy. Often there is a vertical and horizontal component, and when it occurs in an adult it is accompanied by diplopia. Since there can be some improvement in oculomotor nerve palsies, usually there is a waiting period of approximately 6 months from its onset before surgery is contemplated. It is not surprising that the authors found the longer time from onset to surgery and larger eye deviations are negative prognostic factors for postoperative motor success. Long-term secondary overactions and contraction of both the antagonistic muscle and supporting structures surrounding the muscle are probably the contributing factors to the authors' findings.

L. B. Nelson, MD, MBA

Prevalence and sex differences of psychiatric disorders in young adults who had intermittent exotropia as children

McKenzie JA, Capo JA, Nusz KJ, et al (Mayo Clinic and Mayo Foundation, Rochester, MN)

Arch Ophthalmol 127:743-747, 2009

Objective.—To evaluate the prevalence and sex differences of mental disorders diagnosed among young adults who had intermittent exotropia (IXT) as children.

Methods.—The medical records of all children (<19 years) diagnosed as having IXT as residents of Olmsted County, Minnesota, from January 1, 1975, through December 31, 1994, and their randomly selected nonstrabismic birth- and sex-matched controls (1:1) were retrospectively reviewed.

Results.—A mental health disorder was diagnosed in 97 (53.0%) of the 183 patients with childhood IXT followed to a mean age of 22 years compared with 55 (30.1%) controls ($P < .001$). Patients with IXT were 2.7 (95% confidence interval, 1.7-4.1) times more likely to develop a psychiatric illness than controls. A mental health disorder was diagnosed in 63% (41 of 65) and 47% (56 of 118) of males and females with IXT, respectively, compared with 33% (22 of 66) and 28% (33 of 117) of male and female controls, respectively. Additionally, males with IXT had a greater use of psychotropic medication ($P = .003$), psychiatric emergency department visits ($P < .001$), psychiatric hospital admissions ($P = .04$), suicide attempts ($P = .004$), and suicidal ideation ($P = .002$) than controls, and females with IXT had more suicidal ideation ($P = .02$) than controls.

Conclusions.—Children diagnosed as having IXT, especially males, are more likely to develop mental illness by the third decade of life compared with children without strabismus.

▶ Psychosocial aspects of patients with strabismus have been previously described by a number of investigators. Therefore, it should not be surprising that there would be psychiatric disorders in young adults who had intermittent exotropia (IXT) as children. It is unclear from this study whether early surgery to eliminate the IXT had an effect on the possibility of developing mental illness in an adult. As the authors pointed out, this study was performed in an ethnically homogeneous population of a single geographic area and may not be representative of other population groups.

L. B. Nelson, MD, MBA

Topical anesthesia in strabismus surgery: a review of 101 cases

Seijas O, Gómez de Liaño P, Merino P, et al (Gergorio Marañon Univ Hosp, Madrid, Spain)

J Pediatr Ophthalmol Strabismus 46:218-222, 2009

Purpose.—To analyze the results over a 10-year period with a different type of strabismus surgery performed with topical anesthesia, to describe the differences in technique compared with surgery performed with general anesthesia, and to detail current indications and technical changes made according to the experience accrued during these years.

Methods.—A total of 101 patients undergoing strabismus surgery with topical anesthesia in a single hospital were analyzed. These patients were randomly selected from a total of 567 patients who had undergone extraocular muscle surgery in the past 10 years.

Results.—A good result was obtained (squint angle < 10 prism diopters and absence of diplopia) in 95% of patients immediately after surgery and in 85% at final follow-up (mean follow-up: 3.1 years). The mean operating time for each muscle was 29 minutes. Surgery was well tolerated in every patient. Conversion to general anesthesia was not necessary in any case. Atropine was used in three patients (3%) because of induction of the vagal reflex.

Conclusion.—Topical anesthesia in strabismus surgery is a useful technique in the treatment of extraocular muscle pathology, with few limitations. Appropriate monitoring by an anesthetist is vital to ensure adequate control of pain and possible side effects and to enable conversion to general anesthesia. The oculocardiac reflex is infrequent. For experienced strabismus surgeons, the total surgical time is comparable with topical and general anesthesia.

▶ While topical anesthesia has become the preferred method of choice in cataract surgery for many ophthalmologists, it remains an integrated technique in strabismus surgery. While I applaud the authors for their success in using topical anesthesia in strabismus surgery, this technique often causes considerable discomfort. The authors' use of propofol to supplement the topical anesthesia probably was one of the reasons they were successful in performing strabismus surgery. I have not found that topical use of lidocaine gel before surgery causes keratitis. Subtenon's infusion of local anesthesia has been the preferred method for strabismus surgery by many pediatric ophthalmologists without the need for intubation. It does not seem to cause as much discomfort as topical anesthesia does.

L. B. Nelson, MD, MBA

8 Neuro-ophthalmology

"Cloud-like Enhancement" Is a Magnetic Resonance Imaging Abnormality Specific to Neuromyelitis Optica

Ito S, Mori M, Makino T, et al (Chiba Univ, Japan)

Ann Neurol 66:425-428, 2009

Neuromyelitis optica (NMO) is presumably mediated by an autoantibody against aquaporin-4 densely expressed at the blood-brain barrier. In 18 patients with NMO, brain magnetic resonance imaging (MRI) findings were systematically reviewed. Brain MRI abnormalities were found for 89% of the patients, and the most prominent feature was "cloud-like enhancement," multiple patchy enhancing lesions with blurred margin, found in 90% of the patients with positive contrast enhancement. In NMO, brain MRI abnormalities are frequent, and cloud-like enhancement appears to be an MRI finding specific to NMO, possibly caused by primary involvement of the blood-brain barrier by the autoantibodies.

▶ Neuromyelitis optica (NMO) is being diagnosed with more and more frequency because of the identification of autoantibodies against aquaporin-4. Although this disease mimics the phenotype of multiple sclerosis, the patients do not respond to the current therapeutic agents used for multiple sclerosis (MS). Differentiation between NMO and MS is always difficult. The current study analyzes postcontrast brain MRIs and reports a different enhancing pattern in NMO lesions (see Fig in the original article). All patients with NMO were positive for NMO antibodies and all patients with MS were seronegative for MS antibodies. This simple and straightforward study and its results will aid clinicians in recognizing patients with NMO as opposed to MS.

R. C. Sergott, MD

Anti-aquaporin-4 antibody-positive optic neuritis

Takagi M, Tanaka K, Suzuki T, et al (Niigata Univ, Japan; Dokkyo Med Univ Koshigaya Hosp, Saitama, Japan)

Acta Ophthalmol 87:562-566, 2009

Purpose.—It has recently been reported that the anti-aquaporin-4 antibody (AQP4-Ab) can be a specific marker of neuromyelitis optica. We present three cases of optic neuritis (ON) where the patients tested positive for AQP4-Ab, but showed no neurological signs.

Methods.—Sera were obtained from 32 Japanese patients with ON and no other neurological abnormalities (mean age 46 ± 20 years). AQP4-Ab was detected by indirect immunofluorescence staining using human-AQP4-transfected HEK 293 cells.

Results.—AQP4-Ab was positive in three female patients (aged 9, 64 and 82 years). Their illness was characterized by bilateral severe optic nerve involvement, insufficient visual recovery, and autoimmune abnormalities (such as positive antinuclear antibody). Two of these patients experienced recurrent episodes of ON. In at least two episodes, the intracranial portion of the optic nerve showed significant inflammation on magnetic resonance imaging.

Conclusions.—These cases indicate that some ON patients have an immunological pathogenesis similar to that seen in neuromyelitis optica. In addition, examination for AQP4-Ab positivity in the initial phase of ON is important in predicting the prognosis, including the possibility of the development of transverse myelitis.

▶ This article demonstrates the value of completely evaluating patients when their signs, symptoms, and clinical course are atypical. For years we have categorized patients with isolated optic neuritis as clinically isolated syndromes, and clearly some of those go on to develop multiple sclerosis (MS) by McDonald and/or Poser criteria. However, a particularly troubling group of patients are those with bilateral optic neuritis, incomplete recovery, recurrent attacks, and normal MRIs and neurological examinations.

This straightforward, well-done study addresses just that issue, and the investigators have found that some of these patients are serologically positive for anti-aquaporin-4-antibody, a marker for neuromyelitis optica (NMO). NMO in its classic, and supposedly most common form, attacks both the optic nerves as well as the cerebral cortex and spinal cord. Based on this study, I will now be obtaining NMO antibodies on all patients with bilateral inflammatory optic neuropathies and MRI scans that do not show MS lesions. The results of this study will enable us to make more accurate diagnoses in a group of patients whose disease has not obeyed the "rules" of diagnosing remitting/relapsing MS.

R. C. Sergott, MD

Association of anti-aquaporin-4 antibody-positive neuromyelitis optica with myasthenia gravis

Uzawa A, Mori M, Iwai Y, et al (Chiba Univ, Chuo-ku, Japan)

J Neurol Sci 287:105-107, 2009

We describe 2 patients who developed anti-aquaporin-4 antibody-positive neuromyelitis optica (NMO) following the development of anti-acetylcholine receptor antibody-positive myasthenia gravis (MG). A literature review of 13 similar cases in addition to the present 2 cases of NMO with MG showed predominance among Asian women and frequent development of NMO following thymectomy for MG. Moreover, in one of our patients, serial assays of anti-aquaporin-4 antibody and anti-acetylcholine receptor antibody were performed. Accumulating evidence for the coexistence of NMO and MG suggests that a common immunopathogenesis of NMO and MG may exist, and the association of NMO with MG may be more frequent than hitherto believed.

▶ The readers can now see that neuromyelitis optica (NMO) is a very hot topic this year in neuro-ophthalmology because the Nobel prize–winning discovery of the aquaporin channels (Peter Agre, Johns Hopkins University) and now the discovery of antibodies to aquaporin-4 in NMO have opened up a completely new area of clinical research.

In this concise but clinically useful report, the authors describe 2 patients who developed NMO after thymectomy for myasthenia gravis. The authors report that 13 other similar cases have been described in the literature, with an apparently increased incidence in Asian women.

The work alerts clinicians to this association, which is of obvious clinical value, and suggests that myasthenia and NMO may share some common pathogenetic properties through Th2 immune cells.

R. C. Sergott, MD

Central and Peripheral Visual Impairment and the Risk of Falls and Falls with Injury

Patino CM, for the Los Angeles Latino Eye Study Group (Univ of Southern California, Los Angeles)

Ophthalmology 117:199-206, 2010

Objective.—To evaluate whether central (CVI) and peripheral visual impairment (PVI) are independent risk factors for falls and falls with injury 4 years later.

Design.—Population-based, prospective cohort study.

Participants.—A population-based sample of 3203 adult Latinos.

Methods.—Baseline presenting binocular central distance acuity was measured and impairment was classified as mild (20/40–20/63) or moderate/severe (≤20/80). Peripheral visual impairment was classified as mild (-6 dB < mean deviation < -2 dB in worse eye), moderate/severe (mean deviation ≤ -6 dB in worse eye).

Main Outcome Measures.—Falls and falls with injury in the past 12 months were assessed by self-report at the 4-year follow-up visit.

Results.—Out of 3203 individuals, 19% reported falls and 10% falls with injury 4 years after the baseline examination; participants with falls were more likely to be ≥60 years of age, be female, report lower income, have >2 comorbidities, report alcohol use, report wearing bifocal glasses, and report obesity. Among those who reported falls, 7% had CVI (visual acuity >20/40) compared with 4% who did not report falls; and 49% had PVI (mean deviation < -2 dB) compared with 39% of those who did not report falls (both $P < 0.0001$). After adjusting for confounders, moderate to severe CVI and PVI were associated with increased risk for falls (odds ratio [OR], 2.36; 95% confidence interval [CI], 1.02–5.45; $P_{trend} = 0.04$; and OR, 1.42; 95% CI, 1.06–1.911 $P_{trend} = 0.01$, respectively) and with falls with injury (OR, 2.76; 95% CI, 1.10–7.02; $P_{value} = 0.03$; and OR, 1.40; 95% CI, 0.94–2.05 $P_{trend} = 0.04$, respectively).

Conclusions.—Both CVI and PVI were independently associated with increased risk for falls and falls with injury 4 years after the initial examination in a dose–response manner. Although vision-related interventions for preventing falls have mainly focused on correcting CVI, this study suggests that targeting both central and peripheral components may be necessary to effectively reduce rates of falls and falls with injury related to vision loss.

▶ Most past clinical research work with falling has concentrated on central visual impairment. This well-designed prospective cohort study examined a population of 3203 Latinos and found a significant correlation between falling and both central and peripheral visual impairment.

Part of the future ophthalmologic, general medical, and rehabilitation care of patients with visual field loss will need to include strategies for adapting daily activities to this disability.

R. C. Sergott, MD

Chromatic Pupil Responses: Preferential Activation of the Melanopsin-mediated versus Outer Photoreceptor-mediated Pupil Light Reflex

Kardon R, Anderson SC, Damarjian TG, et al (Univ of Iowa; et al)

Ophthalmology 116:1564-1573, 2009

Objective.—To weight the rod-, cone-, and melanopsin-mediated activation of the retinal ganglion cells, which drive the pupil light reflex by varying the light stimulus wavelength, intensity, and duration.

Design.—Experimental study.

Participants.—Forty-three subjects with normal eyes and 3 patients with neuroretinal visual loss.

Methods.—A novel stimulus paradigm was developed using either a long wavelength (red) or short wavelength (blue) light given as a continuous Ganzfeld stimulus with stepwise increases over a 2 log-unit range. The pupillary movement before, during, and after the light stimulus was recorded in real time with an infrared illuminated video camera.

Main Outcome Measures.—The percent pupil contraction of the transient and sustained pupil response to a low- (1 cd/m^2), medium- (10 cd/m^2), and high-intensity (100 cd/m^2) red- and blue-light stimulus was calculated for 1 eye of each subject. From the 43 normal eyes, median and 25th, 75th, 5th, and 95th percentile values were obtained for each stimulus condition.

Results.—In normal eyes at lower intensities, blue light evoked much greater pupil responses compared with red light when matched for photopic luminance. The transient pupil contraction was generally greater than the sustained contraction, and this disparity was greatest at the lowest light intensity and least apparent with bright (100 cd/m^2) blue light. A patient with primarily rod dysfunction (nonrecordable scotopic electroretinogram) showed significantly reduced pupil responses to blue light at lower intensities. A patient with achromatopsia and an almost normal visual field showed selective reduction of the pupil response to red-light stimulation. A patient with ganglion cell dysfunction owing to anterior ischemic optic neuropathy demonstrated global loss of pupil responses to red and blue light in the affected eye.

Conclusions.—Pupil responses that differ as a function of light intensity and wavelength support the hypothesis that selected stimulus conditions can produce pupil responses that reflect phototransduction primarily mediated by rods, cones, or melanopsin. Use of chromatic pupil responses may be a novel way to diagnose and monitor diseases affecting either the outer or inner retina.

▶ Simple, straightforward explanations always provide the best insights into neuro-ophthalmology. The authors studied a group of patients with neuroretinal visual loss by assessing their pupillary responses to long wavelength light (red) and short wavelength light (blue).

While the authors used sophisticated pupillometer techniques as outcome metrics, some very practical applications may emerge from this study. A patient with primary rod dysfunction demonstrated significantly reduced responses to blue light. In contrast, a patient with achromatopsia demonstrated a reduced pupillary response to red light. Finally, a patient with ischemic optic neuropathy demonstrated reduced pupillary responses to both red and blue lights. Assessing the pupillary response with different colors and wavelengths of light may prove useful in the future to identify the site of pathological damage in cases of cryptic visual loss. In summary, the hope is that a chromatic light pupil test will differentiate outer retinal dysfunction (rod and cone damage) from inner retinal ganglion cell loss (optic neuropathy).

R. C. Sergott, MD

Functional Visual Loss in Idiopathic Intracranial Hypertension

Ney JJ, Volpe NJ, Liu GT, et al (Univ of Pennsylvania School of Medicine, Philadelphia; et al)

Ophthalmology 116:1808-1813, 2009

Objective.—To identify and describe patients with idiopathic intracranial hypertension (IIH) with concurrent functional visual loss (FVL).

Design.—Observational, retrospective case series.

Participants.—Seventeen patients with IIH and FVL.

Methods.—Clinical features were collected retrospectively. Data from 281 cases of IIH were analyzed for concurrence of FVL.

Main Outcome Measures.—Occurrence of FVL diagnosed at presentation or on subsequent follow-up.

Results.—Seventeen patients had FVL and IIH. Of the 17 patients with FVL and IIH, 11 (65%) had FVL on presentation, with the remaining 6 patients developing FVL after initial presentation. Two patients in this cohort had documented recurrence of their IIH. There were several common patterns of FVL. All 17 patients had functional visual fields, with 82% having tubular fields and 71% exhibiting nonphysiologic constriction on perimetry testing. Seventy-six percent of patients had nerve/field mismatch showing no atrophic disc changes. Eighty-eight percent of patients had significant psychiatric, psychosocial, or other medical comorbidities. The majority of patients were managed surgically at some point in their clinical history, with 53% having nerve decompression, shunt, or both. Three patients had optic nerve sheath fenestrations after the diagnosis of FVL.

Conclusions.—Results suggest a high prevalence of FVL in IIH with a potential association with psychiatric illness and psychosocial stressors requiring careful consideration before surgical intervention.

▶ This article reinforces the observation that patients with true pathophysiological findings may also demonstrate nonphysiological findings. This scenario presents major challenges for even the most experienced clinician.

Although the article has shortcomings of retrospective design and nonuniform examination techniques, the association of functional visual loss with real visual loss in pseudotumor cerebri is valid. We have found that automated visual field examinations are especially prone to produce artifacts of severely constricted visual fields as the result of long testing time and high false-negative errors—either intentionally or unintentionally on the part of the patient. In our opinion, Goldmann visual fields are much more accurate for distinguishing physiologically and nonphysiologically constricted visual fields.

R. C. Sergott, MD

Natural History of Leber's Hereditary Optic Neuropathy: Longitudinal Analysis of the Retinal Nerve Fiber Layer by Optical Coherence Tomography

Barboni P, Carbonelli M, Savini G, et al (Studio Oculistico d'Azeglio, Bologna, Italy; Fondazione G.B. Bietti-IRCCS, Roma, Italy; et al)

Ophthalmology 117:623-627, 2010

Purpose.—To investigate by optical coherence tomography (OCT) the topographic pattern and temporal sequence of fiber loss in the peripapillary retinal nerve fiber layer (RNFL) of patients with Leber's hereditary optic neuropathy (LHON) in a longitudinal follow-up.

Design.—Cohort study.

Participants.—Six eyes of 4 patients with molecularly defined LHON were enrolled before the subacute period of visual loss.

Methods.—Subjects were studied by StratusOCT (Carl Zeiss Meditec, Inc., Dublin, CA) during a 9-month follow-up starting from the presymptomatic stage of the disease. Examinations were carried out at 4 different time points: presymptomatic stage, time of visual loss, and 3 and 9 months later.

Main Outcome Measures.—Peripapillary RNFL thickness for each quadrant of the optic nerve. Statistical comparisons were performed by ordinary analysis of variance with Dunnett's post-test.

Results.—A significant increase of RNFL thickness was detected in the temporal and inferior quadrants between the presymptomatic stage and the disease onset ($P < 0.05$). The 360-degree average and the superior and nasal quadrants showed a nonstatistically significant increase of thickness at this time. In the 360-degree average ($P < 0.01$), superior ($P < 0.01$), nasal ($P < 0.05$), and inferior ($P < 0.01$) quadrants, RNFL thickening showed statistically significant changes between the presymptomatic stage and the 3-month follow-up. At 3 months, a nonsignificant reduction of RNFL thickness was detected in the temporal quadrant. A significant reduction of RNFL was detected in all but the nasal quadrants between the presymptomatic stage and the 9-month Follow-up.

Conclusions.—The RNFL thickness increase first appeared at the temporal and inferior quadrants. Conversely, at 3 months the thickening fibers were more evident in the superior and nasal quadrants. These findings are consistent with the established preferential early involvement of the papillomacular bundle in LHON. We also demonstrated the previously unrecognized simultaneous early involvement of the inferior quadrant. The late involvement of both superior and nasal quadrants suggests a dynamic evolution of the acute stage that continues for 3 months and may represent a therapeutic window of opportunity.

▶ Despite the identification of numerous mutations in mitochondrial DNA, Leber's hereditary optic neuropathy (LHON) remains an untreatable cause of significant visual loss. This study used time domain optical coherence tomography (OCT) technology, which has provided some interesting insights, but verification with spectral domain technology will have to be done. In addition, we would have preferred seeing the evaluation of macular contour, thickness, and volume. The authors' discovery of a 3-month period of evolution of these changes is the most important and intriguing finding of this study.

R. C. Sergott, MD

Optic neuropathy in patients with glioblastoma receiving bevacizumab

Sherman JH, Aregawi DG, Lai A, et al (Univ of Virginia, Charlottesville; UCLA Med Ctr, Los Angeles, CA; et al)

Neurology 73:1924-1926, 2009

Bevacizumab, a monoclonal antibody targeting vascular endothelial growth factor, was recently approved for treatment of glioblastoma. Initial data indicate increased response rates and progression-free survival compared to historical controls. Despite these promising data, we have identified several cases of severe optic neuropathy in patients with glioblastoma treated with bevacizumab.

▶ The authors from several very well-respected centers report the association of optic neuropathy in patients treated with bevacizumab for glioblastoma. While not seen in patients treated for nonbrain tumor indications, this association appears to require dose-independent radiation to the optic apparatus suggesting a priming effect for optic nerve injury. The patients in this report received standard chemoradiation, with radiation to the optic apparatus generally considered within tolerance level. While the authors indicate that the visual loss was severe, we are left wondering how severe the visual acuity and visual field loss was. As is commonly the case, visual side effects of many medications are not realized before drug approval but after larger numbers of patients are exposed to the medication. Visual side effects do not necessarily limit the use of medications but require an appropriate risk/benefit discussion.

R. C. Sergott, MD

Optical Coherence Tomography in Clinically Isolated Syndrome: No Evidence of Subclinical Retinal Axonal Loss

Outteryck O, Zephir H, Defoort S, et al (Université Lille Nord de France; et al)
Arch Neurol 66:1373-1377, 2009

Background.—Optical coherence tomography has emerged as a new tool for quantifying axonal loss in multiple sclerosis (MS). A reduction in retinal nerve fiber layer (RNFL) thickness is correlated with Expanded Disability Status Scale score and brain atrophy.

Objective.—To investigate RNFL and macular volume measurements using optical coherence tomography in the clinically isolated syndrome population.

Design.—Prospective case series.

Settings.—Neurologic clinics at the university hospitals of Lille and Strasbourg (France).

Participants.—Fifty-six consecutive patients with clinically isolated syndrome (18 with optic neuritis and 38 without optic neuritis) and 32 control subjects.

Main Outcome Measures.—Macular volume and RNFL thickness.

Results.—Mean (SD) overall RNFL thickness (98.98 [10.26] μm) and macular volume (6.86 [0.32] μm^3) in the clinically isolated syndrome population were not significantly different compared with the controls (98.71 [9.08] μm and 6.92 [0.38] μm^3, respectively). No link was noted between atrophy of the RNFL or macula and conversion to MS at 6 months.

Conclusions.—Optical coherence tomography does not reveal retinal axonal loss at the earliest clinical stage of MS and does not predict conversion to MS at 6 months.

▶ I have major problems with this study and do not understand how it could have been published. The authors studied 56 patients with optic neuritis, but we are given no information about the severity of their visual loss or visual field defect or confirmatory findings of an acute unilateral optic neuropathy. The bigger problem is an inadequate control group. The study population consisted of 56 patients while only 32 patients comprised the control group, which is referred to as a nonmatched healthy population. Proper controls for optical coherence tomography (OCT) studies must be age and gender matched as well as exclude patients with over 6 diopters of myopia or hyperopia. We also have no data about the test/retest variability at the center where the study was performed. I believe that these issues explain why these authors' findings are diametrically opposed to all other published studies.

R. C. Sergott, MD

Optical coherence tomography is less sensitive than visual evoked potentials in optic neuritis

Naismith RT, Tutlam NT, Xu J, et al (Washington Univ, Saint Louis, MO)
Neurology 73:46-52, 2009

Objectives.—Determine the utility of optical coherence tomography (OCT) to detect clinical and subclinical remote optic neuritis (ON), its relationship to clinical characteristics of ON and visual function, and whether the retinal nerve fiber layer (RNFL) thickness functions as a surrogate marker of global disease severity.

Methods.—Cross-sectional study of 65 subjects with at least 1 clinical ON episode at least 6 months prior. Measures included clinical characteristics, visual acuity (VA), contrast sensitivity (CS), OCT, and visual evoked potentials (VEP).

Results.—Ninety-six clinically affected optic nerves were studied. The sensitivity of OCT RNFL after ON was 60%, decreasing further with mild onset and good recovery. VEP sensitivity was superior at 81% ($p = 0.002$). Subclinical ON in the unaffected eye was present in 32%. VEP identified 75% of all subclinically affected eyes, and OCT identified <20%. RNFL thickness demonstrated linear correlations with VA ($r = 0.65$) and CS ($r = 0.72$) but was unable to distinguish visual categories <20/50. RNFL was thinner with severe onset and disease recurrence but was unaffected by IV glucocorticoids. OCT measurements were not related to overall disability, ethnicity, sex, or age at onset. The greatest predictor for RNFL in the unaffected eye was the RNFL in the fellow affected eye.

Conclusions.—Visual evoked potentials (VEP) remains the preferred test for detecting clinical and subclinical optic neuritis. Optical coherence tomography (OCT) measures were unrelated to disability and demographic features predicting a worse prognosis in multiple sclerosis. OCT may provide complementary information to VEP in select cases, and remains a valuable research tool for studying optic nerve disease in populations.

▶ This is a very interesting study with several important observations that will prompt more investigations. While optical coherence tomography (OCT) has stimulated intense research in multiple sclerosis (MS), we are still trying to define exactly where it fits with other assessments of vision in MS patients as well as other measures of disease severity. Ultimately, I believe that these assessments will be complimentary and will also show better correlation as we move from time domain to spectral domain OCT and also as we advance to multifocal visual evoked potential (VEP) from whole field VEP.

R. C. Sergott, MD

Retinal microvascular abnormalities and cognitive decline: The ARIC 14-year follow-up study

Lesage SR, Mosley TH, Wong TY, et al (Univ of Maryland, Baltimore; Univ of Mississippi Med Ctr, Jackson; Univ of Melbourne, Australia; et al)

Neurology 73:862-868, 2009

Background.—Because retinal and cerebral arterioles share similar pathologic processes, retinal microvascular changes are expected to be markers of cerebral small vessel disease (SVD). To better understand the role of SVD in cognitive function, we investigated the relationship between retinal microvascular abnormalities and longitudinal changes in cognitive function in a community-based study.

Methods.—A total of 803 participants underwent 4 cognitive assessments between 1990–1992 and 2004–2006, using the Word Fluency (WF) test, Digit Symbol Substitution (DSS), and Delayed Word Recall as well as retinal photography in 1993–1995. Covariate adjusted random effects linear models for repeated measures were used to determine the associations of cognitive change with specific retinal vascular abnormalities.

Results.—Individuals with retinopathy showed declines in executive function and psychomotor speed, with 1) an average decline in WF of −1.64 words per decade (95% confidence interval [CI] −3.3, −0.02) compared to no decline in those without retinopathy +0.06 (95% CI −0.6, 0.8) and 2) a higher frequency of rapid decliners on the DSS test.

Conclusion.—Signs of retinal vascular changes, as markers of the cerebral microvasculature, are associated with declines in executive function and psychomotor speed, adding to the growing evidence for the role of microvascular disease in cognitive decline in the elderly.

▶ There is growing interest in neuro-ophthalmology in correlating various markers of optic nerve retinal structure and function with cognitive issues. This important work has been stimulated by the realization that multiple sclerosis has a major cognitive neurodegenerative component. In addition, we are finding fascinating retinal and optic nerve abnormalities in diseases like Alzheimer and Parkinson with obvious cognitive components. This study with impeccable methodology adds further evidence that what we see in the retina, retinal blood vessels, and optic nerves mirrors significant pathological processes in the brain.

R. C. Sergott, MD

Saccade testing to distinguish between non-organic and organic visual-field restriction

Zinkernagel MS, Pellanda N, Kunz A, et al (Kantonsspital, St Gallen, Switzerland)
Br J Ophthalmol 93:1247-1250, 2009

Aim.—The authors described and tested a simple bedside procedure to detect non-organic visual-field loss.

Methods.—Prospective comparative observational case series of 16 patients with non-organic visual-field loss and 15 patients with organic visual-field loss were examined. Saccade patterns provoked by a stimulus outside the claimed visual field were assessed by a masked observer.

Results.—Whereas, in organic visual-field defects, eye movements as noted by the observer were in small and erratic searching patterns towards the visual-field defect in all patients (15/15), most patients with non-organic visual-field loss (14/16) were able to jump directly to the presented red cap in one directional large saccade, although the stimulus was outside their stated visual field. The sensitivity of the saccade test in detection of non-organic visual-field loss by a masked observer was 87% (95% CI 60% to 97%) and the specificity was 100% (95% CI 75% to 100%). The positive predictive value for non-organic visual-field loss of the saccade test was 100%, and the negative predictive value was 90%.

Conclusions.—The saccade test is a quick and reproducible examination to use and is largely independent of the patient's willingness for cooperation. The authors believe that the test will be of value to clinicians on bedside evaluation when non-organic visual-field loss is suspected.

▶ Any test that helps clinicians distinguish between organic and nonorganic visual loss has value. The authors have developed an interesting bedside procedure that depends upon the patient believing that their eye movements are being tested and not their ability to see. Figs 1 and 2 in the original article nicely summarize how to perform the test.

R. C. Sergott, MD

The role of optical coherence tomography in the detection of pituitary adenoma

Johansson C, Lindblom B (Sahlgrenska Univ Hosp/Mölndal Hosp, Sweden)
Acta Ophthalmol 87:776-779, 2009

Purpose.—To analyse retinal nerve fibre layer (RNFL) thickness in eyes with compression of the optic chiasm by a pituitary adenoma. RNFL thickness was analysed with optical coherence tomography (OCT) and compared to visual field measurements using high-pass resolution perimetry (HRP).

Methods.—Sixteen eyes from eight patients with pituitary adenoma were studied. All had bitemporal visual field depression caused by compression of the optic chiasm. Patients were submitted to an ophthalmic examination more than 14 months after surgery (seven patients had undergone trans-sphenoidal and one trans-cranial adenomectomy). The examination included HRP, fundus photography and measurement of the peripapillar RNFL thickness using OCT.

Results.—In spite of temporal visual field depression, not all eyes showed reduced RNFL thickness by OCT. This was also true for some eyes in which RNFL was judged to be reduced on fundus photographs. Contrary to our expectations, RNFL thickness in the nasal quadrant was normal in nine of the 16 eyes. Corresponding figures for the superior, inferior and temporal quadrants were eight, six and five, respectively. The overall RNFL thickness, as measured by OCT, did not correlate well with neural capacity, which is an index of remaining retino-cortical neural channels in HRP.

Conclusion.—RNFL thickness as measured with OCT was reduced in most, but not all, eyes with temporal field depression caused by chiasmal compression. The pattern of RNFL loss did not correlate well with the visual field defect. Sensitivity of RNFL thickness measurement in OCT was low. The method has limited value in the diagnosis of pituitary tumour compression.

▶ Our experience mirrors the findings in this report—optical coherence tomography (OCT) is not helpful in the diagnosis of lesions compressing the optic nerve chiasm. However, we have found that OCT is extraordinarily helpful in providing clinicians and patients with an assessment of patients' ability to improve after surgery. Therefore, there is a definite role for OCT prognostically and therapeutically. Localization and diagnosis of a particular lesion still depends upon data derived from the history, physical examination, visual field, and funduscopic findings.

R. C. Sergott, MD

Vision and Driving in Multiple Sclerosis

Schultheis MT, Manning K, Weisser V, et al (Drexel Univ, Philadelphia, PA; et al)

Arch Phys Med Rehabil 91:315-317, 2010

Objective.—To examine the relationship between measures of visual dysfunction and driving performance in persons with multiple sclerosis (MS).

Design.—Between-group comparison.

Setting.—All data were collected in an outpatient research setting.

Participants.—Persons (N = 66) with MS of the relapsing remitting type (26 self-reporting visual difficulties; 40 self-reporting no visual difficulties) and 26 age- and sex-matched healthy controls.

Interventions.—Not applicable.

Main Outcome Measures.—Measures of vision included visual acuity, depth perception, and color perception. Driving was measured using documented accident/violation rate and self-reported driving behaviors.

Results.—Quantitative analysis only revealed that MS persons with self-reported visual difficulties performed significantly worse than healthy controls on color perception (Kruskal-Wallis; $\chi^2_2 = 8.89$, $P = .01$). There were no group differences on driving behaviors, and correlational analysis revealed a lack of relationship between the selected visual (visual acuity, depth perception, color perception) and driving performance measures (documented accident/violation rate and self-limiting driving behaviors).

Conclusions.—Persons with MS who self-reported difficulties with vision had acceptable visual acuity, despite demonstrating impairment in color perception. The fact that visual acuity remains the most common measure for visual fitness to drive remains problematic. There is a need to further define measures of visual dysfunction relevant to driving among this clinical population.

▶ This article highlights the importance of developing assessments for the impact of various visual disorders upon the visual quality of life. Certainly, standard Snellen visual acuity and various perimetry techniques do not capture that information. Multiple sclerosis (MS) is especially challenging because it also affects speed of the eye movements as well as coordination and cognitive function. Any programs designed to help the driving performance of patients with MS must also address these issues.

R. C. Sergott, MD

9 Imaging

Conventional MRI and magnetisation transfer imaging of the brain and optic pathway in primary open-angle glaucoma
Kitsos G, Zikou AK, Bagli E, et al (Univ of Ioannina, Greece)
Br J Radiol 82:896-900, 2009

Neuropathological studies in experimental and human glaucoma have shown degenerative changes in the optic pathway. The purpose of the study was to evaluate, with conventional MRI and magnetisation transfer imaging, the brain and the optic pathway of patients with primary open-angle glaucoma (POAG). 26 patients, aged 67.4 ± 8.6 years, and 26 control subjects were studied. The presence of white matter hyperintensities (WMH) was evaluated on fluid-attenuated inversion recovery images of the brain. The area of the optic nerves was assessed on coronal short tau inversion recovery images. Magnetisation transfer ratio (MTR) was measured in the chiasm and in the grey and white matter (CGM and CWM) of the calcarine fissure. More WMH were observed in patients (total 261, mean 10.8, standard deviation 12.7) than in control subjects (total 127, mean 4.7, standard deviation 5.7; $p<0.001$). The area (mm^2) of optic nerves (10.7 ± 5.7) and the MTR (%) of the chiasm (53.7 ± 8.4), the CWM (60.9 ± 4.2) and the CGM (53.6 ± 5.6) were all lower in patients than in control subjects (13.6 ± 4.3, 62.1 ± 6.2, 67.6 ± 8.6 and 57.0 ± 4.6, respectively; $p<0.05$). The area of optic nerves showed significant correlation with the MTR of the chiasm ($R = 0.41$), the MTR of the CGM ($R = 0.33$), the MTR of the CWM ($R = 0.34$) and the cup to disc ratio ($R = -0.46$). POAG leads to optic nerve atrophy and degeneration of the optic pathway. The finding of an increase in the number of WMH suggests that cerebrovascular disease may play a role in the pathogenesis of POAG.

► Glaucoma is the second most common cause of blindness in the world. In most cases the disease is insidious progressive, causing no obvious symptoms until optic disc damage is advanced. Glaucoma causes damage to retinal ganglion cells, the lateral geniculate nucleus of the thalamus, and the primary visual cortex. Neuronal degeneration of the optic nerve, the lateral geniculate nucleus, and the visual cortex has also been observed in postmortem studies of patients with glaucoma. Previous reports suggest that by the time symptoms become evident, there has been a loss of nearly half of the complement of retinal ganglion cells. Therefore, early detection of physiologic or structural changes of the optic pathway could prove advantageous in evaluating patients at risk and to monitor progression/stabilization of disease for patients undergoing therapy.

The authors of this article use another well-known physiologic adjunct to magnetic resonance imaging (MRI) known as magnetization transfer imaging (MTI). Rather than providing a discrete image, MTI values represent a relative quantification of large macromolecules and their contribution to the overall signal. Because MTI results in a quantifiable value, it can be used as an indirect measure of macromolecular content in a tissue volume. These quantities are consistent and reproducible in normal gray and white matter. In certain disease states, alterations in magnetization transfer (MT) values are reported even when the tissue appears normal on conventional MRI. The prototypical example is in multiple sclerosis in which measures of MT normal appearing white matter deviate markedly from normal. These observed MT changes are attributed to real degradation of myelin components that are not yet visible on standard MRI.

The authors used MRI and MTI to evaluate 26 patients with bilateral high-tension primary open angle glaucoma (POAG) and compared the imaging results with 24 age- and sex-matched controls. Intraocular pressures for the study group were in excess of 21 mm Hg. Patients with POAG had a significantly smaller cross-sectional area of the optic nerves (Fig 2 in the original article) relative to controls. MT ratios (MTR) measured in the chiasm, cerebral white matter, (Fig 4 in the original article) and gray matter were lower in POAG patients compared with controls. There was a positive correlation between the area of the optic nerves and the MTR values of the chiasm. In addition, the patient subgroup showed a significantly higher number of white matter lesions compared with controls, suggesting some association between POAG and cerebral microvascular disease.

Lowering intraocular pressure is not always sufficient in preventing further axonal and ganglion loss in glaucoma. Therefore, other noninvasive measures are needed to monitor this disease and to assess whether the integrity of the optic pathway could prove invaluable in assessing stability of the disease and monitoring effects of therapy. Other investigators have shown supplemental value in other physiology MR techniques, such as functional MRI (fMRI) and diffusion tensor imaging (DTI) in the assessment of the optic pathways in glaucoma. Of all of these techniques MTI is probably the easiest method to perform on standard clinical equipment. If proven to be reliable and reproducible, MTI could prove invaluable in the serial assessment of patients with glaucoma.

A. E. Flanders, MD

Is CT Still Useful in the Study Protocol of Retinoblastoma?

Galluzzi P, Hadjistilianou T, Cerase A, et al (Azienda Ospedaliera Universitaria Senese, Siena, Italy; Univ of Siena, Italy)

AJNR Am J Neuroradiol 30:1760-1765, 2009

Background and Purpose.—Intralesional calcium deposition is considered a key element for differentiating retinoblastoma from simulating lesions. Our aim was to assess whether MR imaging associated with ophthalmologic investigations (ophthalmoscopy and ultrasonography) could replace CT in the detection of diagnostic intralesional calcifications in retinoblastoma.

Materials and Methods.—Ophthalmoscopic findings, MR images, CT scans, and histologic examination of 28 retinoblastomas from 23 consecutive children (11 males, 12 females; age range at admission, 1–35 months; mean age, 11 months; median age, 9 months) were retrospectively evaluated. Ultrasonography was performed in 18 patients with 21 retinoblastomas. MR imaging included T2-weighted spin-echo and gradient-echo images, fluid-attenuated inversion recovery images, and T1-weighted spin-echo images with and without contrast enhancement. Clinical data were integrated with MR imaging data to evaluate the utility of both approaches to discover calcifications; particularly, a correlation between intralesional signal-intensity void spots on MR imaging and hyperattenuating areas on CT scans was performed.

Results.—Ophthalmoscopy detected calcifications in 12 of 28 eyes (42.85%). Ultrasonography detected calcifications in 20 of 21 eyes (95.23%). CT showed hyperattenuating intralesional areas consistent with calcifications in 27 of 28 eyes (96.42%). MR imaging showed intralesional signalintensity void spots in 25 of 28 eyes (89.28%). All spots detected with MR imaging matched the presence of calcifications on CT scans. Gradient-echo T2*-weighted and fast spin-echo T2-weighted images showed the highest degree of correlation with CT. When we put together ophthalmoscopy, ultrasonography, and MR imaging data, no calcifications detected on CT were missed, and the differential diagnosis was thorough.

Conclusions.—A combination of clinical data and MR images may remove potentially harmful ionizing radiation from the study protocol of retinoblastoma.

▶ CT and MR imaging represent the principle modalities for visual-pathway imaging in children, although MR imaging is preferred due to the lack of ionizing radiation and the excellent depiction of soft-tissue contrast. Although MR imaging is the optimal method for depicting ocular lesions, CT has a higher specificity for identifying microcalcifications within lesions. The disadvantages of CT are reduced contrast resolution compared with MR imaging, and the potential risk of direct radiation exposure and iodinated contrast agents. Moreover, the subgroup of patients with hereditary form of retinoblastoma has inherent radiosensitivity and could benefit from alternative imaging methods, thus avoiding direct exposure to ionizing radiation.

The authors assessed the ability to detect intrinsic calcifications within 28 intraocular lesions. Twenty-seven of the 28 eyes had histologically confirmed calcifications within the lesions (Table 1 in the original article). The method with the lowest rate of detection was ophthalmoscopy (42.9%), whereas ultrasonography had a reasonably high rate of detection (95.2%), as did CT (96.4%). While MRI is considered relatively insensitive to discriminating calcium from surrounding soft tissue, certain complexes of calcium are known to produce characteristic appearances on specific pulse sequences. As the authors noted, high-resolution 3-dimensional (3D) fast spin echo/transverse turbo spin echo (FSE/TSE) and 3D gradient echo sequences exhibited perfect (100%) specificity in discriminating calcium from surrounding tissue matrix (Fig 2 in the original article). Specificity decreased to 87.5% when thicker (lower resolution) 2-dimensional (2D) gradient echo images were used. However, the 3 techniques combined yielded a 100% correspondence to calcifications identified on corresponding CT images. While larger aggregate calcifications were identified on MRI, small punctate calcifications were also readily visible with the 3D techniques (Fig 5 in the original article).

The authors conclude that the combination of ultrasonography and high-resolution MR imaging can obviate the need to use CT to document the presence of intralesional calcification in retinoblastoma. The only potential pitfall to their observations in this subgroup of patients is that particular stages of hemorrhage (eg, deoxyhemoglobin and hemosiderin) can also produce areas of low signal intensity on gradient echo and T2-weighted images and, thereby, mimic calcification on MRI. Hemorrhage would not create characteristic shadowing on ultrasonography. Moreover, as the authors point out, intralesional hemorrhage is relatively uncommon with retinoblastoma and should normally not provide a diagnostic dilemma.

A. E. Flanders, MD

Lack of Correlation between the Histologic and Magnetic Resonance Imaging Results of Optic Nerve Involvement in Eyes Primarily Enucleated for Retinoblastoma

Wilson MW, Rodriguez-Galindo C, Billups C, et al (Univ of Tennessee Health Science Ctr, Memphis, TN; St Jude Children's Res Hosp, Memphis, TN)
Ophthalmology 116:1558-1563, 2009

Purpose.—To correlate the histologic and magnetic resonance imaging results of the optic nerve in eyes primarily enucleated for retinoblastoma.

Design.—Retrospective, clinicopathologic correlation.

Participants.—Sixty-seven consecutive patients with retinoblastoma who underwent primary enucleation.

Methods.—The histologic results of 67 eyes from 67 patients with retinoblastoma who underwent primary enucleation between March 1997 and January 2008 were studied for evidence of optic nerve invasion.

Two neuroradiologists independently reviewed available preoperative magnetic resonance imaging studies with special emphasis on nonenhanced T2-weighted and gadolinium-enhanced T1-weighted imaging for evidence of optic nerve invasion. A weighted κ statistic was used to assess agreement between observers.

Main Outcome Measures.—Correlation between neuroradiologists and histologic results

Results.—Of the 67 eyes studied, 60 had preoperative magnetic resonance images, 58 of which were deemed appropriate for review by both neuroradiologists. Review of the histologic results showed optic nerve involvement in 62 (93%) of 67 eyes: 28 prelaminar (42%), 24 laminar (36%), and 10 postlaminar (15%). On review of the magnetic resonance scans, the first neuroradiologist identified optic nerve involvement in 57 (95%) of 60 eyes: 26 prelaminar (43%), 10 laminar (17%), and 11 postlaminar (18%). The second neuroradiologist identified optic nerve involvement in 46 (77%) of 60 eyes: 33 prelaminar (55%), 9 laminar (15%), and 4 postlaminar (7%). Moderate agreement existed between neuroradiologists (κ, 0.55). Poor and fair agreement existed between each of the 2 neuroradiologists and histologic results, respectively (κ, 0.29 and 0.17). Exophytic tumors showed the greatest disparity (κ, −0.20 and −0.13) between magnetic resonance imaging and histologic results.

Conclusions.—Limited correlation was found between magnetic resonance imaging and histologic results in assessing optic nerve invasion in eyes with retinoblastoma. Magnetic resonance imaging using routine imaging technologies, although useful in the evaluation of retinoblastoma, has limited usefulness in assessing the exact extent of optic nerve invasion; high-risk features of retinoblastoma such as postlaminar invasion remain best defined by histologic analysis. This study demonstrates that the interpretation of optic nerve involvement by a radiologist should not be the determining factor to defer enucleation in favor of neoadjuvant therapy.

▶ This study shows the limitations of MRI in evaluating the extent of optic nerve invasion in retinoblastoma. Accurate identification of optic nerve invasion has significant implications in guiding postoperative therapy with radiation or chemotherapy. Some oncologists advocate use of neoadjuvant chemotherapy before enucleation if optic nerve invasion is identified preoperatively.

Two neuroradiologists retrospectively evaluated the preoperative diagnostic orbital MR studies of 67 patients with retinoblastoma, rating each for the absence and presence of optic nerve invasion and stratifying the invasion as prelaminar, laminar, or postlaminar. Overall, the cohort had minimal histologically proved invasion of the optic nerve that undoubtedly served to push the limits of the imaging techniques, which typically have a slice resolution of approximately 3 mm. The median depth of laminar invasion in this cohort was 0.5 and 2.5 mm for postlaminar invasion. Previous imaging publications have indicated that even postlaminar involvement may be difficult to recognize without associated dilatation of the optic nerve. The inability to demonstrate a good to a very good correlation between MRI and histologic results when the optic nerve was involved underscores the limitations of current mainstream imaging methods. Moreover, agreement between the 2 neuroradiologists in discriminating the extent of invasion was poor with the tendency to overclassify (Fig 1 in the original article) the extent of invasion. This result is not surprising, given the minimum size differential between classes of invasion. However, there was excellent agreement between MRI interpretation and histology when no invasion of any kind was present. This suggests that MRI still may have a predictive role in this subclass of patients and still may be valuable in determining when invasion is present.

A. E. Flanders, MD

Optic Nerve and Optic Radiation Neurodegeneration in Patients with Glaucoma: In Vivo Analysis with 3-T Diffusion-Tensor MR Imaging

Garaci FG, Bolacchi F, Cerulli A, et al (Interventional Radiology and Radiotherapy, Rome, Italy; Univ Hosp Tor Vergata, Rome, Italy)
Radiology 252:496-501, 2009

Purpose.—To evaluate, with high-field-strength diffusion-tensor (DT) magnetic resonance (MR) imaging, the axonal architecture of the optic nerves and optic radiations in patients with glaucoma and determine whether DT MR imaging–derived parameters correlate with disease severity.

Materials and Methods.—The study was approved by the institutional review board. All participants provided written informed consent. Sixteen patients with primary open-angle glaucoma were examined. Glaucoma severity was clinically assessed with use of a six-stage system based on static threshold visual field parameters. Ten healthy individuals served as control subjects. DT MR imaging was performed with a 3-T MR unit. Mean diffusivity (MD) and fractional anisotropy (FA) maps were automatically created. Regions of interest were positioned on the MD and FA maps, and mean MD and mean FA values were calculated for each optic nerve and each optic radiation.

Results.—The optic radiations and optic nerves of patients with glaucoma, as compared with control subjects, had significantly higher MD and significantly lower FA. The mean MD values for the optic nerves and the glaucoma stages varied consistently ($r = 0.8087$, $P < .0001$). A negative correlation between mean FA for the optic nerves and glaucoma stage ($r = -0.7464$, $P < .0001$) was observed.

Conclusion.—Glaucoma is a complex neurologic disease that affects optic nerves and optic radiations. The finding that DT MR imaging–derived MD and FA in the optic nerves correlate with glaucoma severity suggests that these parameters could serve as complementary indicators of disease severity.

▶ Glaucoma is responsible for approximately 10% of blindness worldwide. It is the third leading cause of blindness. Formerly, elevated intraocular pressure was thought to be the inciting element leading to the characteristic retinal ganglion cell degeneration of glaucoma, however, it is now recognized that glaucoma is a primary neural degenerative condition that can involve all parts of the optic pathways. Clinical deterioration of the visual pathways is usually confirmed via serial formal visual field evaluation.

This article is the first imaging study to demonstrate the progressive deterioration of the visual white matter tracts in glaucoma using diffusion tensor (DT) MR imaging. Using a small cohort of patients and controls, the authors have been able to discriminate various clinical grades of glaucoma based on the diffusion characteristics in the white matter. Measurements of free water diffusion (mean diffusivity [MD] and fractional anisotropy [FA]) were taken along the course of the optic nerves and tracts (Fig 1 in the original article). Comparison of these diffusion parameters with the clinical stage of glaucoma showed significant differences in these physiologic values for each clinical stage (Fig 3 in the original article).

While MRI is the most sensitive imaging test for identifying structural abnormalities in the central nervous system, the advanced MR technique of DT imaging (DTI) has the capability of revealing when there is physiologic damage to the white matter even when no structural lesions are visible. This is because destruction or loss of myelin results in measurable perturbations in free water diffusion within axons. Alterations in diffusivity characteristics have been reported in normal appearing white matter of patients with multiple sclerosis. The metrics that were evaluated in this study, MD and FA, reflects the rate of diffusion and directionality of the diffusion, respectively. Damaged white matter characteristically exhibits both elevation in MD and loss of directionality (decrease in anisotropy). It has been suggested that DTI values offer an objective measure of axon and myelin integrity and therefore could be used as a surrogate for assessing clinical deficit and responses to neuroprotective therapies.

In this example, the authors have demonstrated that DTI of the optic radiations and visual pathways could serve as a robust surrogate for evaluating the integrity of vision in patients with glaucoma. It could be used as a biomarker for detecting early degeneration of the pathways before the clinical manifestations become evident, and it could serve as an adjunct in cases where formal visual fields prove inaccurate or impractical. In addition, DTI could be used to monitor the effects of neuroprotective therapies that promote remyelination of damaged axons.

A. E. Flanders, MD

10 Ocular Oncology

I-125 Brachytherapy for Choroidal Melanoma: Photographic and Angiographic Abnormalities: The Collaborative Ocular Melanoma Study: COMS Report No. 30

Boldt HC, Melia BM, Liu JC, et al (Univ of Iowa Hosps and Clinics; Johns Hopkins univ, Baltimore, MD)

Ophthalmology 116:106-115, 2009

Objectives.—(1) To summarize the protocol used for grading features of postradiation abnormalities from fundus photographs and fluorescein angiograms of patients enrolled in the Collaborative Ocular Melanoma Study (COMS); (2) to document the prevalence of features of interest in the posterior pole of these eyes during 8 years of follow-up; and (3) to investigate baseline patient, tumor, and treatment characteristics associated with posterior pole features.

Design.—Observational case series within a randomized, multicenter clinical trial.

Participants.—We evaluated 650 patients who were assigned to and received iodine-125 brachytherapy in the COMS for medium-sized tumors.

Methods.—Color fundus photographs and fluorescein angiograms were taken at baseline and 2, 5, and 8 years; 30 features were graded according to a standard protocol.

Main Outcome Measures.—Prevalence at selected time intervals of fundus photographic features associated with retinopathy and optic neuropathy.

Results.—The percentage of patients with ≥1 feature of interest was 49.2% at baseline, 84.4% at 2 years, 91.2% at 5 years, and 90.7% at 8 years. The most frequent findings across all follow-up examinations were macular microaneurysms (75.6% of examinations), macular angiographic leakage (75.1%), and optic disc hyperfluorescence (62.8%). The median number of features present increased significantly with each follow-up to a maximum of 7 features at 8 years. The prevalence of neovascularization of the disc at 5 years was 5.2%. The prevalence of optic neuropathy at 5 years was 27.4%. Prognostic factors for more prevalent and severe posterior pole abnormalities were diabetes, tumor location close to both optic nerve and foveal avascular zone, and greater dose of radiation to the foveola and optic nerve head.

Conclusions.—The amount and severity of retinopathy and optic neuropathy after iodine-125 brachytherapy increased through 8 years of follow-up. Assessment of photographs and angiograms taken in accord with a standard protocol provided reliable estimates of rates of development of features of retinopathy and optic neuropathy in eyes treated using the COMS brachytherapy protocol. Our findings support earlier reports that tumor factors in addition to radiation treatment may contribute to posterior pole abnormalities.

▶ Brachytherapy, otherwise referred to as plaque radiotherapy, is the application of a radiation device that delivers direct, short term, short penetration to an organ or site. In the eye, brachytherapy is used mostly for tumors, particularly choroidal melanoma, and the most common isotope is iodine 125. This therapy provides excellent control of 88% per the Collaborative Ocular Melanoma Study and 97% of patients per our analysis from the Ocular Oncology Service at Wills Eye Institute.[1] Precision in tumor measurement, plaque design, and plaque placement are critical to excellent tumor control.

One of the most bothersome problems with ocular radiation is the list of complications. According to this report, the list of macular complications at 8 years included retinal hemorrhage (40%), retinal nerve fiber layer infarcts (7%), microaneurysms (90%), capillary nonperfusion (74%), and macular hyperfluorescence on fluorescein angiography (90%). So, by definition, at least 90% of patients had radiation maculopathy. The list of optic disc complications at 8 years included optic disc hyperfluorescence on angiography (68%) and optic disc pallor (13%).

These lists of complications are a trade-off for good tumor control. And these complications do not necessarily mean poor visual acuity. In an analysis of visual acuity of more than 1100 patients managed on the Ocular Oncology Service at Wills Eye Institute, poor visual acuity of 20/200 or worse was found in 24% of eyes with small melanoma, 30% with medium melanoma, and 64% with large melanoma.[2] Currently, we are investigating newer plaque designs with better protection of the macula and optic disc in an attempt to minimize complications. Additionally, interventions with medications to protect the eye from retinal vascular leakage are being investigated.

C. L. Shields, MD

References

1. Shields CL, Cater J, Shields JA, et al. Combined plaque radiotherapy and transpupillary thermotherapy for choroidal melanoma in 270 consecutive patients. *Arch Ophthalmol.* 2002;120:933-940.
2. Shields CL, Shields JA, Cater J, et al. Plaque radiotherapy for uveal melanoma. Long-term visual outcome in 1106 patients. *Arch Ophthalmol.* 2000;118:1219-1228.

Prospective Clinical Trial Evaluating the Efficacy of Photodynamic Therapy for Symptomatic Circumscribed Choroidal Hemangioma

Boixadera A, García-Arumí J, Martínez-Castillo V, et al (Hosp Vall d'Hebron, Barcelona, Spain)

Ophthalmology 116:100-105, 2009

Purpose.—To evaluate photodynamic therapy (PDT) for symptomatic circumscribed choroidal hemangioma (CCH).

Design.—Prospective, multicenter, nonrandomized clinical trial.

Participants.—Thirty-one eyes of 31 patients with posterior pole CCH and symptoms caused by exudation into the macular area.

Intervention.—Photodynamic therapy was applied by Zeiss laser. Intravenous verteporfin at 6 mg/m^2 body surface was administered before treatment, and light emitted at 689 nm for photosensitization. The treatment spot diameter was calculated on early-phase frames of pretreatment indocyanine green angiography. Fifteen minutes after starting the verteporfin infusion, the laser beam was applied to the retina at radiant exposure 50 J/cm^2 and exposure time 83 seconds. One to 4 treatments were applied at 12-week intervals over 1 year. Standardized evaluation was performed before and at 4-week intervals after each treatment, and at 3, 6, 9, and 12 months. All patients were followed for ≥12 months.

Main Outcome Measures.—The primary outcome measure was the absence of exudative retinal detachment at the 12-month follow-up visit on ophthalmoscopy, fluorescein angiography, and optical coherence tomography. Secondary measures were the visual acuity outcome, with best-corrected visual acuity determined by the Early Treatment for Diabetic Retinopathy Study chart, tumor thickness decrease on B-scan ultrasonography, and adverse events.

Results.—Among the total, 82.8% of patients required 1, 13.8% 2, and 3.4% 3 PDTs to eliminate exudative retinal detachment. Visual acuity increased from a mean of 20/60 to 20/35 (P<0.001). Sixty-nine percent of patients demonstrated visual recovery (P<0.001). Cystoid macular edema regressed in all cases and exudative macular detachment disappeared in all but 2 cases. The CCH thickness decreased in all cases from a mean of 3.0 to 1.7 mm, with the most intense effect seen after 4 weeks of treatment (P<0.001). Visual fields showed resolution of central scotomas. There were no severe adverse events.

Conclusions.—Combining PDT with the standard age-related macular degeneration protocol is an effective treatment for CCH in terms of resolution of exudative subretinal fluid and recovery of VA.

▶ Circumscribed choroidal hemangioma is a benign vascular tumor that classically occurs in the posterior pole of the eye. The tumor is an average of 6 mm in base and 3 mm in thickness, appears orange in color, shows acoustic solidity on ultrasound, and typically produces chronic subretinal fluid with eventual macular edema. Based on a natural history report in the era before photodynamic therapy (PDT), poor visual acuity of 20/200 or worse is found in about 50% of cases.[1] With the introduction of PDT, it is anticipated that long-term visual acuity will be much better.

Vision loss from choroidal hemangioma can result from subretinal fluid, cystoid and noncystoid macular edema, retinal atrophy, and often-overlooked causes like refractive error (induced hyperopia from the foveal elevation) and amblyopia (because it is believed that these tumors are present early in life). Asymptomatic tumors are generally observed. There are several treatment options for symptomatic choroidal hemangioma, including methods of laser photocoagulation with argon and diode, transpupillary thermotherapy, PDT, plaque radiotherapy, and external beam radiotherapy.

These authors prospectively evaluated PDT for 31 cases of circumscribed choroidal hemangioma. Most patients responded to 1 (83%) or 2 (14%) PDTs with complete resolution of the subretinal fluid. Visual acuity was improved in 69%, stable in 28%, and decreased in 3%. There was no damage to the overlying retinal vessels. Our personal experience with nearly 50 cases of choroidal hemangioma treated with PDT is similar to this with excellent tumor control. However, it should be realized that complications of this technique can include choroidal ischemia, choroidal neovascular membrane, subretinal hemorrhage, exudative choroidal or retinal detachment, and visual loss. Based on these observations, PDT appears to be a safe and effective treatment for symptomatic circumscribed choroidal hemangioma.

C. L. Shields, MD

Reference

1. Shields CL, Honavar SG, Shields JA, Cater J, Demirci H. Circumscribed choroidal hemangioma. Clinical manifestations and factors predictive of visual outcome in 200 consecutive cases. *Ophthalmology.* 2001;108:2237-2248.

Clinical Trials – More Than an Assessment of Treatment Effect: LXV Edward Jackson Memorial Lecture

Ferris FL (Natl Eye Inst, Bethesda, MD)
Am J Ophthalmol 147:22-32, 2009

Purpose.—To review the development of clinical trials and demonstrate their value beyond the assessment of the treatment effect.

Design.—Retrospective literature review.

Methods.—Retrospective literature review.

Results.—There has been a rapid increase in the number of clinical trials in ophthalmology as assessed by the number of ophthalmic publications and the number of ongoing National Eye Institute-(NEI) sponsored clinical trials over the last four decades. The public health significance of the results of these NEI clinical trials goes beyond the demonstration of treatment effects and side effects. From these trials, we learn about the clinical course and risk factors of disease, allowing us to better determine who and when to treat. Furthermore, the collaboration of investigators, as they develop and carry out protocols, facilitates incorporation of new ideas into the practice of medicine.

Conclusions.—The practice of medicine is increasingly dependent on the results of carefully designed clinical trials. The determination as to whether a new treatment is safe and effective is important, but the additional information we can obtain regarding natural history, risk factors, and patient satisfaction adds immeasurably to our ability to care for our patients.

▶ Clinical trials have evolved over many years to be the gold standard by which therapies are judged. There is much more that we gather from clinical trials over and above therapeutic effect. This information includes the clinical course or natural history of a disease, identification of high risk patients who might benefit from treatment, and low risk patients who can defer treatment, and perhaps most importantly, the patient's assessment of a treatment.

Clinical trials, in some way, shape, or form, originated in Biblical days with a question on the true benefit of eating royal food to achieve good health versus nuts and vegetables to reach the same endpoint. In the end, nuts and vegetables won. One of the most famous clinical trials was in 1747 in the study of the effects of limes on scurvy among British sailors. Even though these early trials were slipshod and poorly organized, their value was eventually realized. Limes were put aboard ships 42 years later to prevent scurvy.

The first randomized trial in ophthalmology dates to 1952 regarding oxygen treatment for retinopathy of prematurity. Since then, this approach to answer clinical questions has rapidly progressed. The exponential growth of clinical trial reports is evident in the Cochrane Eyes and Vision Group report that identified the number of published Medline studies at about 300 in the 1970s and 3000 in the 2000s. The tremendous increase in knowledge of eye disease is outstanding but needs to be balanced with the expense of the investigation. Most trials run about $10 000 to $50 000 per patient per year, and some cost more. In the long run, cost-benefit analyses often show that the patient gains improvement in disease, and the government, insurance company, or patient does benefit and saves money based on the trial result.

Some trials are tedious to follow and understand. One example is the Age Related Eye Disease Study (AREDS) where results were accurate and detailed for clinical research, but were difficult for the practicing clinician to swallow and digest. Dr Ferris simplified the details to a practical age-related macular degeneration (AMD) scale with 5 grades of severity from 0 to 4, with each adding risk for progression to advanced AMD. He emphasized that collaboration is the best direction for the future to solve more difficult ophthalmologic problems.

C. L. Shields, MD

Corneoscleral necrosis after episcleral Au-198 brachytherapy of uveal melanoma

Chaudhry IA, Liu M, Shamsi FA, et al (King Khaled Eye Specialist Hosp, Riyadh, Saudi Arabia; Cullen Eye Inst, Houston, TX)

Retina 29:73-79, 2009

Purpose.—To describe the risk factors for the development of corneoscleral necrosis (CSN) and its management in patients with primary choroidal or ciliochoroidal melanoma who underwent episcleral Au-198 brachytherapy.

Methods.—Clinical records of patients with symptoms of dry eye, foreign body sensation, pain, and evidence of CSN after Au-198 brachytherapy for uveal melanoma treated over a 22-year period were reviewed retrospectively. Risk factors for the development of CSN were identified and various methods of management were evaluated. The data were analyzed using multivariant analysis. A $P < 0.05$ was taken as a level of statistical significance.

Results.—Of the 202 eyes of 202 patients treated with Au-198 radioactive plaque, 15 (7.4%) patients with symptomatic complaints of dry eye and pain showed evidence of CSN. First signs were noted as early as 1 month to as late as 5 years (median time 5 months) after the treatment. Risk factors for the development of CSN included tumor thickness greater than 6 mm and ciliary body involvement ($P < 0.05$). Associated risk factor included intraocular pressure greater than 21 mmHg. Four patients required conservative management, 11 patients required scleral patch and/or conjunctival flaps, and 6 eyes eventually required enucleation. Eyes which developed CSN were more likely to undergo enucleation compared with eyes having no evidence of CSN ($P < 0.05$). None of the eyes with CSN, which required enucleation because of the failed treatment, had histopathologic evidence of recurrent tumor or tumor invading sclera.

Conclusion.—Corneoscleral necrosis may occur soon or several years after Au-198 brachytherapy for uveal melanoma. Risk factors for CSN include tumor thickness greater than 6 mm, ciliary body involvement, and intraocular pressure >21 mmHg. Closer follow-up, early recognition, and timely intervention may avert serious consequences.

▶ There are several isotopes available for plaque radiotherapy of intraocular tumors, including cobalt 60, iodine 125, iridium 192, ruthenium 106, palladium 103, and gold 198. Early and late complications have been reported with these devices, including dry eye, cataract, retinopathy, papillopathy, neovascular glaucoma, vitreous hemorrhage, and scleral necrosis. Scleral necrosis tends to be found more often with ruthenium 106 plaque radiotherapy as the dose to the melanoma base is over 100 000 cGy to achieve an apex dose of 8000 cGy compared to 30 000 cGy basal dose for iodine 125 with same apex dose. It is also recognized that thicker tumors and those in the ciliary body region where a rectus muscle might be temporarily disinserted for plaque placement are also factors to consider in the development of scleral necrosis. In this analysis, Chaudry found tumors > 6 mm in thickness to be at higher risk than those < 6 mm for eventual scleral necrosis from gold 198 plaque treatment.

Gold 198 plaque radiotherapy is rarely used for ocular radiotherapy. The most commonly used isotopes include iodine 125 and ruthenium 106. The Collaborative Ocular Melanoma Study used iodine 125 radiotherapy. Our preference is iodine radiotherapy, as it can be custom-fit to treat a specific tumor to a specific depth, avoiding visually sensitive structures such as the disc and macula. Other plaques, such as cobalt and ruthenium, are not quite as custom-designed, so the same plaque is used over and over for one or many years without a specific tumor fit. However, each iodine plaque is tediously redesigned per individual tumor features.

The most important fact about scleral necrosis is to be able to recognize it as a thinning of the sclera and not to panic about fear of tumor recurrence. Necrosis is usually recognized several months to years after radiotherapy and starts as a small black thinning of the sclera, evolves over a few months to nearly the size of the plaque, and stabilizes. It is very rare for perforation to occur. These authors did not comment on the speed of evolution of the necrosis nor did they indicate perforation.

The management of scleral necrosis following plaque radiotherapy involves either observation with topical lubrication versus patch graft. We came to realize that a scleral patch was not always necessary. Currently, we prefer cautious observation and have not scleral patched a patient for more than 8 years.

C. L. Shields, MD

The value of screening in melanoma

Stratigos AJ, Katsambas AD (Univ of Athens Med School, Greece)
Clin Dermatol 27:10-25, 2009

The incidence of cutaneous melanoma has increased substantially in most white populations during the past several decades. Despite improvements in the early recognition of melanoma and the use of novel diagnostic techniques that enhance our diagnostic capabilities, disease-related mortality remains a significant public health issue. In the absence of effective treatment approaches for advanced disease, the best means for reducing deaths by melanoma are screening as well as professional and public education. The role of population-or community-based screening remains controversial, but evidence from self-selected screening campaigns, health care professional surveillance, and specialized pigmented lesions clinics underscores the value of screening and early detection programs, particularly in high-risk groups. Annual screening campaigns coupled with intense media promotion have become commonplace in many countries, and despite their low yield of melanoma detection, the dissemination of educational material and information to the public during these events is important in increasing public awareness. Future directions should include using screening campaigns to target middle-aged and older men and persons of lower socioeconomic status, who suffer most from the burden of the disease and its associated mortality. On a worldwide scale, comprehensive educational and screening campaigns should be implemented or intensified in underserved areas and geographic regions with lower survival rates, such as Eastern European countries. A better understanding of the biology of the disease, already occurring with notable strides, will help us to define better those individuals who will benefit most from screening and early detection efforts. Technologic advances and new diagnostic modalities will afford a more reliable and vigilant surveillance of high-risk individuals, whereas the wide use of the Internet will enhance the distribution of relevant information to the public with the ultimate goal of achieving a better control of melanoma.

► According to these authors, cutaneous melanoma is considered a preventable and curable disease. In the United States, there are about 60 000 new cases of skin melanoma per year and 8000 deaths from skin melanoma metastasis. It is projected that 1 in 52 men and 1 in 77 women will develop these cancers during their lifetime. Despite these grim figures, the overall survival from melanoma has improved to over 90% at 5 years in the United States, but remains low (60%) in less medically developed countries such as the Czech Republic and Slovenia. It is presumed that this difference was related to the lack of prevention, education and early detection in those countries.

Screening is a strategy that uses visual examination in a population to detect disease without signs or symptoms. In the 1970s there was a rise in the incidence and mortality of melanoma, so several investigators started melanoma screening programs so that tumors could be detected in a prognostically favorable stage. This screening strategy has been found statistically beneficial for other cancers, such as breast cancer, with improvement in mortality and colon cancer with 30% mortality benefit. Some data suggest similar benefit for skin melanoma. The American Academy of Dermatology noted that 240 000 screenings during 1992-1994 yielded 363 melanomas, 98% of which were stage 1 and 90% of which were in situ or thin. The acronym HARMM—representing history of previous melanoma, age > 50 years, regular dermatologist absent, male gender, and mole changing—was used to identify the high-risk persons.

These authors state, "In the absence of effective treatment approaches for advanced disease, the best means for reducing deaths by melanoma are screening as well as profession and public education." This has been clearly shown with breast cancer and colon cancer, and is now evident with skin melanoma.

C. L. Shields, MD

Ocular melanoma: relatively rare but requiring respect

Shields CL, Shields JA (Wills Eye Inst, Philadelphia, PA)

Clin Dermatol 27:122-133, 2009

Primary ocular melanoma can involve the uveal tract, conjunctiva, eyelid, or orbit. Uveal melanoma is the most common ocular melanoma and carries a serious prognosis, especially if the tumor is medium or large in size. Conjunctival melanoma manifests on the surface of the eye and has been increasing in incidence. Eyelid and primary orbital melanoma are the least common variants. Early diagnosis from annual ocular examination by an experienced ophthalmologist and treatment strategies are reviewed.

▶ In this review, the authors lead off with "ocular melanoma is uncommon but deadly." They describe the clinical features of uveal, conjunctival, eyelid, and orbital melanoma. In the United States, uveal melanoma affects approximately 2500 patients per year and conjunctival melanoma occurs in about 200 patients per year. Eyelid and orbital melanomas are less common with only few case series published.

Regarding uveal melanoma, the incidence is quoted at 6 per million per year in the United States, and the most important factors for the development of this malignancy is the presence of congenital ocular melanocytosis and choroidal nevus. Melanocytosis carries a 1/400 risk for melanoma, and nevus shows 1/8845 risk for transformation to melanoma. Risk factors for growth of nevus into melanoma include thickness >2 mm, subretinal fluid, symptoms, orange pigment, and margin touching the optic disc. Patients with 3 features have a 53% chance for transformation, and the riskiest combination of factors was thickness >2 mm, margin touching disc, and symptoms which showed nearly 70% transformation. The most common methods for treatment of melanoma include radiotherapy or enucleation. Unfortunately, systemic therapy adds little to improve prognosis. Survival depends primarily on tumor thickness, and at 5 years is 84% for small melanoma (<3 mm thickness), 68% for medium melanoma (3-8 mm thickness), and 47% for large melanoma (>8 mm thickness).

Regarding conjunctival melanoma, the most common source is primary acquired melanosis. This tumor appears as a slightly thickened brown or pink mass on the surface of the eye. The initial therapy is of utmost importance in the patient's long-term care as "no touch" surgery under dry conditions to avoid tumor seeding is advised. Recurrence and multiple surgeries continue to plague the patient. At 10 years follow-up of 150 consecutive cases, exenteration was necessary in 16%, metastasis occurred in 26%, and death in 13%.

The threat of ocular melanoma is real. Despite its rarity, this malignancy is deadly. The authors encourage efforts for early detection and prompt referral for therapy to improve the patient's life prognosis.

C. L. Shields, MD

Positive Interaction Between Light Iris Color and Ultraviolet Radiation in Relation to the Risk of Uveal Melanoma: A Case-Control Study

Schmidt-Pokrzywniak A, Jöckel KH, Bornfeld N, et al (Univ of Halle-Wittenberg, Germany; Univ of Duisburg-Essen, Germany; Univ of Duisburg-Essen, Germany)

Ophthalmology 116:340-348, 2009

Purpose.—To examine the association among phenotypic characteristics, chronic and intermittent ultraviolet (UV) radiation, and the risk of uveal melanoma.

Design.—Case-control study.

Participants.—Overall, between September of 2002 and March of 2005, 1677 eligible subjects (age range: 20–74 years, living in Germany) participated. Interviews were conducted with 459 incident uveal melanoma cases (response proportion 94%), 827 population controls (55%), 180 ophthalmologist controls (52%), and 187 sibling controls (57%).

Methods.—Data on phenotypic characteristics and chronic and intermittent UV radiation exposure were obtained from a self-administered postal questionnaire and computer-assisted telephone interview. We used conditional logistic regression to estimate odds ratios adjusting for the matching factors. Furthermore, we studied the presence of synergy (super additive of risk or relative excess risk due to interaction) between light iris color and several UV radiation exposures.

Main Outcome Measures.—Hair color at age 20 years, eye color, untanned skin color, ability to tan, propensity to burn on exposure, freckling, occupational sun exposure, artificial UV radiation, burns to the eyes.

Results.—In all 3 control groups, fair skin color, freckling as a child, nevi on the upper arms, burns to the eyes, use of sunlamps, and ever worked outside for 4 or more hours per day were positively associated with uveal melanoma. The association with eye color was apparent only in population controls (odds ratio = 1.9; 95% confidence interval [CI], 1.4 –5.2), resulting in a relative excess risk due to interaction of 0.9 (95% CI, −0.6 –2.3) for light iris color and more than 5 eye burns (UV-related keratitis) and 0.6 (95% CI, −0.3 to 1.5) for light iris color and eye protection.

Conclusions.—Our interaction analyses suggest that there is an etiologic synergism between light iris color and the exposure of UV radiation. People with light iris color may have an especially increased risk for uveal melanoma if they are exposed to UV radiation.

▶ Does sun exposure lead to skin melanoma? Yes, there is unequivocal evidence to indicate the strong relationship of ultraviolet light exposure with the development of cutaneous melanoma. Patients at the highest risk have light skin color, propensity to sunburn, and intermittent periodic intensive exposure to sunlight like long-anticipated, well-earned vacations to sunny Caribbean beaches.

Does sun exposure lead to uveal melanoma? Well, there are studies that suggest a relationship and others that refute it. Li and associates found a higher rate of melanoma occurrence toward the macula in patients with light eye color.[1] Animal studies have shown that melanomas can develop with 475 nm wavelength light exposure.[2]

Light iris color is a potent risk factor for the development of uveal melanoma. Weis and coworkers performed a meta-analysis of 113 published reports and found that light iris color, light skin color, and inability to tan were host factors at risk for uveal melanoma.[3] Shah and associates performed a similar meta-analysis and found that environmental risk factors included exposure to ultraviolet light in welding and a borderline risk for chronic sunlight exposure.[4] There have been 2 reports to attribute melanoma development to sunlamp use.[5,6]

In this report, the authors interviewed and compared 459 affected patients against 827 population controls, 180 ophthalmologist controls, and 187 sibling controls. In comparison with all 3 control groups, they found that light skin color, childhood freckling, and upper arm nevi were associated with increased risk of uveal melanoma. Light iris color was a risk factor for melanoma in comparison with the population controls. Furthermore, a synergistic effect was found between light iris color and multiple episodes (>5) of keratitis from snow blindness, welder's flash, or sunburn. In addition, there was a synergy for melanoma in light iris color and lack of eye protection from the sun (sunglasses or hat) and regular sunlamp use at a young age.

So, we have learned from this well-designed study that patients with light iris are at particular risk for the development of uveal melanoma. An effort should be made to protect these patients with sun hats or sunglasses, and they should be advised against using sun lamps.

C. L. Shields, MD

References

1. Li W, Judge H, Gragoudas ES, Seddon JM, Egan KM. Patterns of tumor initiation in chroidal melanoma. *Cancer Res.* 2000;60:3757-3760.
2. Manning WS Jr, Greenlee PG, Norton JN. Ocular melanoma in a long Evans rat. *Contemp Top Lab Anim Sci.* 2004;43:44-46.
3. Weis E, Shah CP, Lajous M, Shields JA, Shields CL. The association between host susceptibility factors and uveal melanoma: a metaanalysis. *Arch Ophthalmol.* 2006;124:54-60.
4. Shah CP, Weis E, Lajous M, Shields JA, Shields CL. Intermittent and chronic ultraviolet light exposure and uveal melanoma: a meta-analysis. *Ophthalmology.* 2005; 112:1599-1607.
5. Seddon JM, Gragoudas ES, Glynn RJ, Egan KM, Albert DM, Blitzer PH. Host factors, UV radiation, and risk of uveal melanoma: a case-control study. *Arch Ophthalmol.* 1990;108:1274-1280.
6. Tucker MA, Shields JA, Hartge P, Augsburger J, Hoover RN, Fraumeni JF Jr. Sunlight exposure as a risk factor for intraocular malignant melanoma. *N Engl J Med.* 1985;313:789-792.

Anterior Segment Optical Coherence Tomography and Ultrasound Biomicroscopy in the Imaging of Anterior Segment Tumors

Pavlin CJ, Vásquez LM, Lee R, et al (Univ of Toronto, Ontario, Canada; et al)

Am J Ophthalmol 147:214-219, 2009

Purpose.—To evaluate the utility of anterior segment optical coherence tomography (OCT) in the imaging of anterior segment tumors and compare the images to ultrasound biomicroscopy (UBM).

Design.—Prospective observational case series.

Methods.—Eighteen eyes of 18 patients with anterior segment tumors were evaluated at Princess Margaret Hospital. The evaluation included clinical examination, clinical photography, anterior segment OCT, and UBM. Comparison of images obtained by both methods was done.

Results.—Anterior segment OCT imaged small hypopigmented tumors with complete penetration. Cysts were incompletely imaged behind the iris pigment epithelium. Highly pigmented tumors, large tumors, and ciliary body tumors were incompletely penetrated. Even without complete penetration it was possible to differentiate cystic lesions from solid lesions. UBM penetrated all tumors completely.

Conclusions.—Anterior segment OCT can penetrate small hypopigmented tumors and supply some information on internal characteristics of other tumors. UBM is preferable for clinical anterior tumor assessment and follow-up because of its superior ability to penetrate large tumors, highly pigmented tumors, and ciliary body tumors.

▶ There are several ways to image the anterior segment of the eye, including methods of external and slit lamp photography, fluorescein angiography, and ultrasonography. Despite the excellent depiction of the posterior segment of the eye on standard B-scan ultrasonography, the anterior segment of the eye is poorly imaged. Historically, this was improved with the placement of a water bath directly on the open globe and with topical anesthesia. Even this technique led to only minimal improvement in imaging and overall poor resolution. Two methods have been developed over the past 20 years to improve imaging of the anterior segment of the eye. Ultrasound biomicroscopy (UBM) was introduced in 1990 as a method of high-resolution cross-sectional sound wave imaging, and later anterior segment optical coherence tomography (OCT) was commercially available in 2001 for similar light wave imaging of the anterior segment of the eye.

UBM is a near-contact system whereby a 50-MHz transducer is brought close to the corneal surface and imaged through coupling gel of 1% methylcellulose. The transducer has a moving device that scans back and forth over the ocular surface. UBM generally takes about 10 to 15 minutes to perform the test and organize the results with a printed hard copy. Anterior segment OCT is a noncontact system whereby the patient rests his or her chin on a chinrest and focuses on a target at which time a scan is taken in 20 seconds or more from a machine that is about 6 inches or more from the face. This device performs 250 A scans in 125 milliseconds for a low-resolution image and

512 A scans in 250 milliseconds for a high-resolution image. With anterior segment OCT, resolution to 18 microns axially, 60 microns laterally, and depth of 3- to 6-mm penetration is achieved. OCT takes about 2 minutes to perform the test, organize the results, and print a hard copy.

The main difference between UBM and anterior segment OCT is that the former uses sound waves, whereas the latter uses light waves for image capture. In this report the authors examined 18 patients with various tumors and cysts of the anterior segment and found that UBM provided more complete information on the tumor configuration, extent, and internal characteristics than did OCT. UBM showed better penetration and visualization of the entire mass, whereas OCT often only showed the anterior portion of the mass and the posterior portion was shadowed. This observation occurs because anterior segment OCT light waves are diminished with pigmented interfaces like nevus and pigmented cyst wall.

There are, however, advantages of anterior segment OCT over UBM. OCT is a noncontact technology, performed with the patient casual and upright in a chair and comfortable with minimal fear of the test. UBM is near-contact, performed with the patient reclined and perhaps anxious, and the eye is held open with an open bottom eye cup filled with gel and a probe moving within 1 inch of the cornea. There is a large difference in patient comfort and time consumption between the two techniques. I foresee that with improved light penetration with OCT, the depth of penetration and overall resolution will improve and this, coupled with the important patient comfort factor, will perpetuate this technique for the assessment of anterior segment lesions.

C. L. Shields, MD

Imaging the Infant Retina with a Hand-held Spectral-Domain Optical Coherence Tomography Device

Scott AW, Farsiu S, Enyedi LB, et al (Duke Univ Med Ctr, Durham, NC)
Am J Ophthalmol 147:364-373, 2009

Purpose.—To evaluate and treat infant retina through the use of a hand-held spectral-domain optical coherence tomography (SD OCT) device in selected cases of Shaken Baby syndrome (SBS).

Design.—Observational case series.

Methods.—A novel SD OCT system was optimized and evaluated for infant imaging. An adult eye was imaged with both a standard clinical SD OCT system and the hand-held system. Four eyes of two infants with a history of SBS were imaged with the hand-held system. One infant was imaged again during follow-up examinations. Robust image processing algorithms were developed to create high-quality images. Images were assessed for usefulness in demonstrating pertinent morphologic features.

Results.—The novel SD OCT unit proved effective for data acquisition and comparable with conventional chinrest SD OCT. Rapid data acquisition limited motion artifact within the B-scan, although there was slight motion between B scans. The SD OCT images provided previously unseen details with regard to the morphologic features of retinal lesions in these infant eyes. This information influenced prognosis and management.

Conclusions.—As with adults, the hand-held customized SD OCT proved to be an invaluable tool in the differentiation of disease processes or injury in these eyes under study. SD OCT imaging systems may be considered a useful adjunct to RetCam fundus photography for assessment and clinical management in cases of SBS.

▶ Optical coherence tomography (OCT) is an imaging tool based on the principles of light wave reflection on tissues, and has been used for several years to depict the adult retina. To perform this test, a patient must place his or her chin on a chinrest, resting upright in a chair and remaining still without movement for a few minutes. This technique has been used in children as young as 4 years old, particularly if cooperative.[1] Younger children cannot be imaged because of their movement during testing. In this report, the authors discuss a recently developed handheld OCT device that can be used in the operating room on children while under anesthesia.

There are two types of OCT, the time domain (TD) and the spectral domain (SD) formats, based on different principles of physics. TD-OCT was the first generation of imaging with approximately 8- to 10-micron resolution; it was shown useful in children, but was only available in the upright, sitting, nonportable format. Some attempted to adapt the TD-OCT to children under anesthesia using various novel suspensions of the machine, but this was difficult. SD-OCT is the second-generation model, and provides 5-micron resolution with 2-dimensional (2D) and 3-dimensional (3D) imaging at a speed 40 times faster than TD-OCT. In this report, the authors adapted a research handheld SD-OCT to image the infant retina during examination under anesthesia in cases of shaken baby syndrome.

They first compared the device in a cooperative adult comparing the traditional upright TD-OCT and upright SD-OCT to a reclined handheld SD-OCT. They found that the handheld SD-OCT was superior to the upright TD-OCT and equivalent to the upright SD-OCT. Next, they evaluated 4 children with shaken baby syndrome and found high-resolution retinal OCT images of intraretinal hemorrhages, retinal schisis, and macular hole with this novel device. They concluded that it was safe and effective for infant use. I will further suggest that this device be used in the assessment of certain adult patients who cannot sit still at the upright device, such as elderly or noncooperative adults, or comatose or bed-ridden patients. OCT is an extremely valuable tool in the assessment of retinal anatomy.

C. L. Shields, MD

Reference

1. Shields CL, Mashayekhi A, Luo CK, Materin MA, Shields JA. Optical coherence tomography in children. Analysis of 44 eyes with intraocular tumors and simulating conditions. *J Pediatr Ophthalmol Strabismus*. 2004;41:338-344.

Complex Palpebral Odontogenic Choristoma: A Reappraisal of the Origin of Teeth-Bearing Periocular Lesions

Jakobiec FA, Nguyen J, Mandell K, et al (Harvard Med School, Boston, MA)

Am J Ophthalmol 147:531-543, 2009

Purpose.—To describe the findings observed in a congenital ectopic tooth of the lower inner eyelid and explain its origin.

Design.—Retrospective and interventional clinicopathologic study.

Methods.—Histopathologic evaluation of sequentially excised specimens over 4 years and radiographic study of any associated dental abnormalities, compared with critical reevaluation of similar reported cases in the literature.

Results.—The ectopic eyelid tooth clinically created a dome-shaped mass and microscopically displayed advanced cytodifferentiation but incomplete morphogenesis with clearly identifiable ameloblasts, enamel, odontoblasts, and dentin, surrounded by an intact dental sac. Swollen oral mucosal epithelium with associated sebaceous Fordyce nodules, residual ciliated odontogenic epithelium, embryonic epithelial rests, and accessory mucinous and sero-mucinous accessory salivary glands were discovered in place of normal conjunctiva. The tarsus with meibomian glands was absent but islands of cartilage were present.

Conclusions.—Because of the variety of the ectopic tissues that were exhibited, a causative displacement of oral embryonic epithelium with extensive differentiating potentialities is posited. Two previously reported palpebral dental choristomas also had identical locations in the inferomedial eyelid. This is the site where the phakomatous choristoma may be encountered, but this unencapsulated mass creates an eyelid thickening without a globoid configuration and infiltrates the inferior orbit. After a careful re-appraisal of published reports of orbital cysts bearing a tooth that were formerly diagnosed as "teratomas," we have concluded that they developed from similar embryonic oral (buccal) epithelial displacements rather than from aberrant germ cells, based on the cysts' linings and the associated accessory salivary glands in their walls. This view is further supported by the absence of heterologous teratomatous elements of endodermal or neuroectodermal derivation. A clinical and surgical approach to management and a new diagnostic schema for odontogenic choristomas are proposed.

▶ The most common congenital tumor of the orbit region is the dermoid cyst. This tumor classically occurs superotemporally at the zygomaticofrontal suture and can enlarge within the orbit producing proptosis, within the bone producing a bony canal, or within the temporal fossa producing fullness. Rupture of the congenital dermoid cyst could lead to chronic and repetitive inflammation, fistula formation, scarring and eyelid retraction, and cosmetic deformation. Despite its benign pathology, serious consequences can ensue.

There are other less common congenital tumors of the eye and orbit, including choristomas, such as the limbal dermoid comprising skin tissue in the conjunctiva and cornea most often at the inferotemporal limbus, lipodermoid comprising skin tissue in the superotemporal fornix and orbit, epibulbar osseous choristoma made of pure bone on the episcleral superotemporally, lacrimal choristoma made of ectopic lacrimal gland in the conjunctiva or orbit, phakomatous choristoma comprising ectopic lens classically in the inferonasal eyelid or conjunctiva, and complex choristoma and teratoma made of combination of several tissues in the epibulbar and orbital regions. Many of these choristomas have a "most common" location related to their morphogenesis in embryologic development. In this report, the authors describe an extremely rare odontogenic choristoma comprising an ectopic tooth.

There are only 2 other reports in the literature on this subject, and the tumor in all cases has been located inferomedially in the eyelid, similar to phakomatous choristoma. Additionally, all 3 cases had a normal complement of teeth by examination and panoramic radiography, indicating that there was no tooth missing in the mouth. It is speculated that the misplaced tooth was supernumerary.

The authors further explored the literature on teratomas, which occasionally sport a tooth. Teratomas are most often found in the ovaries and less commonly in the brain and orbit. Teratomas are composed of all 3 germ layers. Teeth have been encountered in 22% to 56% of mature benign cystic teratomas of the ovary, and one unusual case had more than 300 teeth, most of which were poorly developed. Orbital teratomas rarely display teeth. In one series of 60 orbital teratomas and another of 76 orbital teratomas, there were a total of 4 teeth. In summary, the author provided a remarkably illustrated and colorfully descriptive report on an interesting but rare finding, the odontogenic choristoma.

C. L. Shields, MD

11 Pathology

Frequent somatic mutations of *GNAQ* in uveal melanoma and blue naevi

Van Raamsdonk CD, Bezrookove V, Green G, et al (Univ of British Columbia, Vancouver, Canada; Univ of California, San Francisco; et al)

Nature 457:599-602, 2009

BRAF and *NRAS* are common targets for somatic mutations in benign and malignant neoplasms that arise from melanocytes situated in epithelial structures, and lead to constitutive activation of the mitogen-activated protein (MAP) kinase pathway. However, *BRAF* and *NRAS* mutations are absent in a number of other melanocytic neoplasms in which the equivalent oncogenic events are currently unknown. Here we report frequent somatic mutations in the heterotrimeric G protein α-subunit, *GNAQ*, in blue naevi (83%) and ocular melanoma of the uvea (46%). The mutations occur exclusively in codon 209 in the Ras-like domain and result in constitutive activation, turning *GNAQ* into a dominant acting oncogene. Our results demonstrate an alternative route to MAP kinase activation in melanocytic neoplasia, providing new opportunities for therapeutic intervention (Table 1).

▶ The oncogenic events involved in pathogenesis of cutaneous melanoma have been well-described, and include components mitogen-activated protein (MAP) kinase pathway, in particular *BRAF* and *NRAS* oncogenes. However, mutations in these genes are rare in uveal melanoma. Until recently, the early/initiating oncogenic events in uveal melanoma have been unknown. A recent study by Onken et al[1] has shown that G protein α-subunit (*GNAQ*) gene is mutated in approximately half of uveal melanomas at all stages of malignant progression, suggesting that *GNAQ* mutation is an early event in pathogenesis of uveal melanoma.

GNAQ gene encodes for α-subunit of q class of heterotrimeric guanosine triphosphate (GTP) binding protein (Gq). *GNAQ* couples G-protein-coupled receptor signaling to the RAF/MEK/ERF and other intracellular pathways through protein kinase C, activated by stimulation of β phospholipase C. *GNAQ* is involved in endothelin signaling, which is essential for melanocyte survival early in development. The reported mutations of *GNAQ* gene occur in codon 209 in the ras-like domain and lead to constitutive activation, likely through loss of GTPase activity. Genetic, biochemical, and biological studies have shown that *GNAQ* behaves as a dominant oncogene.

Several recent studies yielded additional data on *GNAQ* and its role in uveal melanoma.[2] Van Raamsdonk et al conducted an elegant study which demonstrated that *GNAQ* mutations provide an alternative route to MAP kinase

TABLE 1.—Frequency of *GNAQ* Mutations in Melanocytic Neoplasms

Neoplasm Type and Diagnosis	Mutant (%)	*n*
Cutaneous and mucosal melanomas		
Melanoma on skin without chronic sun-induced damage[22]	0	15
Melanoma on skin with chronic sun-induced damage[22]	4	27
Acral melanoma	0	15
Mucosal melanoma	0	14
'Malignant blue naevus'	50	2
Melanoma arising in congenital naevus	0	3
Spitzoid melanoma	0	2
Total	-	78
Naevi		
Blue naevus	83	29
Naevus of Ota	6	17
Congenital naevus	0	7
Deep penetrating naevus	0	16
Proliferating nodule in giant congenital naevus	0	7
Spitz naevus	0	8
Total	-	84
Ocular melanomas		
Uveal melanoma	46	48
Uveal melanoma cell line	27	15
Conjunctival melanoma	0	11
Total	-	74
Grand total	-	236

Editor's Note: Please check the original article for full references.
The number and type of samples analysed is shown.

activation in melanocytic neoplasia in uveal melanoma and blue nevi. The researchers sequenced entire coding regions of *GNAQ* in broad spectrum of benign and malignant melanocytic neoplasms, and found mutations in *GNAQ* in 83% of blue nevi, 50% of malignant blue nevi, 46% of uveal melanomas, and 6% of nevi of Ota. They found that all *GNAQ* mutations were somatically acquired and occurred exclusively at codon 209. To determine the cellular and molecular events that are induced by *GNAQ* mutation, the authors conducted a series of transfection experiments. They found that transfection with mutant *GNAQ* induced neoplastic transformation of human melanocytes in vitro and also induced formation of atypical blue nevi/pigmented epithelioid melanocytomas at the injection site in vivo in the murine model. Van Raamsdonk et al also confirmed that mutant *GNAQ* contributes to MAP kinase pathway activation in cultured human melanocytes and uveal melanoma cells. This study not only identified *GNAQ* as the most common oncogenic mutation in uveal melanoma and provided evidence regarding its mechanism of induction of melanocytic neoplasia, but also identified *GNAQ* as a genetic link between nevus of Ota and uveal melanoma, and helped explain why nevi of Ota are a risk factor for uveal melanoma.

A later study by Küsters-Vandevelde et al[3] has demonstrated an identical *GNAQ* mutation in primary melanocytic neoplasms of central nervous system

(CNS) (melanocytomas and melanomas), also confirming a genetic link between the cellular blue nevi, primary orbital, and CNS melanoma and uveal melanoma.

T. Milman, MD

References

1. Onken MD, Worley LA, Long MD, et al. Oncogenic mutations in GNAQ occur early in uveal melanoma. *Invest Ophthalmol Vis Sci.* 2008;49:5230-5234.
2. Lamba S, Felicioni L, Buttitta F, et al. Mutational profile of GNAQ in human tumors. *PLoS ONE.* 2009;4:e6833.
3. Küsters-Vandevelde HV, Küsters B, Groenen PJ, et al. Activating mutations of theGNAQ gene: a frequent event in primary melanocytic neoplasms of the central nervous system. [published online ahead of print November 22, 2009]. Acta Neuropathol. doi:10.1007/s00401-009-0611-3.

Oncogenic *GNAQ* mutations are not correlated with disease-free survival in uveal melanoma

Bauer J, Kilic E, Vaarwater J, et al (Univ of Tübingen Med Ctr, Germany; Univ Med Ctr, Rotterdam, The Netherlands; et al)

Br J Cancer 101:813-815, 2009

Background.—Recently, oncogenic G protein alpha subunit q (*GNAQ*) mutations have been described in about 50% of uveal melanomas and in the blue nevi of the skin.

Methods.—*GNAQ* exon 5 was amplified from 75 ciliary body and choroidal melanoma DNAs and sequenced directly. *GNAQ* mutation status was correlated with disease-free survival (DFS), as well as other clinical and histopathological factors, and with chromosomal variations detected by FISH and CGH.

Results.—Of the 75 tumour DNA samples analysed, 40 (53.3%) harboured oncogenic mutations in *GNAQ* codon 209. Univariate and multivariate analysis showed that *GNAQ* mutation status was not significantly correlated with DFS.

Conclusion.—The *GNAQ* mutation status is not suitable to predict DFS. However, the high frequency of *GNAQ* mutations may render it a promising target for therapeutic intervention.

▶ The study by Bauer et al has confirmed that G protein alpha subunit q (*GNAQ*) mutations occurred in half (53%) of the eyes with uveal melanoma and provided additional data regarding an effect of *GNAQ* mutations on patient survival. The authors found no correlation between the disease-free survival and *GNAQ* mutations in their cohort of 75 patients with uveal melanoma. They, however, noted a better prognosis in patients with 2 copies of chromosome 3 irrespective of *GNAQ* status, although these results were not statistically significant, possibly due to a small sample size. These findings are consistent with observations by Onken et al,[1] who found that *GNAQ* mutations are early oncogenic events in uveal melanoma and are independent of tumor stage and chromosomal aberrations. While the results of Bauer et al suggest that screening for *GNAQ* mutations in uveal melanoma will not yield prognostically significant information, they confirmed that *GNAQ* may be a potential target for uveal melanoma therapy.

For further reading on this subject I suggest an article by Raamsdonk et al.[2]

T. Milman, MD

References

1. Onken MD, Worley LA, Long MD, et al. Oncogenic mutations in GNAQ occur early in uveal melanoma. *Invest Ophthalmol Vis Sci.* 2008; 2008;5230-5234.
2. Van Raamsdonk CD, Bezrookove V, Green G, et al. Frequent somatic mutations of GNAQ in uveal melanoma and blue naevi. *Nature.* 2009;457:599-603.

High-Risk Features and Tumor Differentiation in Retinoblastoma: A Retrospective Histopathologic Study

Eagle RC Jr (Wills Eye Inst, Philadelphia, PA)

Arch Pathol Lab Med 133:1203-1209, 2009

Context.—Certain histopathologic risk factors in enucleated eyes are important indicators for adjuvant chemotherapy in patients with retinoblastoma.

Objectives.—To determine the frequency of histopathologic risk factors in a large series of retinoblastomas treated by enucleation on file in the pathology laboratory of a large American eye hospital, assess the relationship between tumor differentiation and age at enucleation, and investigate the frequency of photoreceptor differentiation and the role of retinoma/retinocytoma as retinoblastoma precursor.

Design.—Retrospective histopathologic review of 387 eyes with retinoblastoma treated by enucleation including 297 with no prior treatment.

Results.—Fifty-five of 297 untreated eyes (18.5%) had high-risk features. Retrolaminar optic nerve invasion was present in 31 (10.4%), and 24 (8.1%) had massive uveal invasion (defined as >3 mm in diameter). Of the high-risk eyes, 70.9% had iris neovascularization and 60% had neovascular glaucoma. There was a statistically significant inverse relationship between age at enucleation and the degree of tumor differentiation, evidenced by the presence of rosettes. Tumors in older children tended to be poorly differentiated, while rosettes were often numerous in the tumors of younger infants. In all, 20.4% of tumors contained foci of photoreceptor differentiation, which localized in the base of a predominantly endophytic tumor in about one-fourth. Lack of correlation between photoreceptor differentiation and age at enucleation is consistent with early or prenatal malignant transformation. Both preceding observations provide evidence for the hypothetical role of retinoma as a retinoblastoma precursor.

Conclusions.—Slightly less than 1 in 5 infants with retinoblastoma treated by enucleation at a large American eye hospital would require

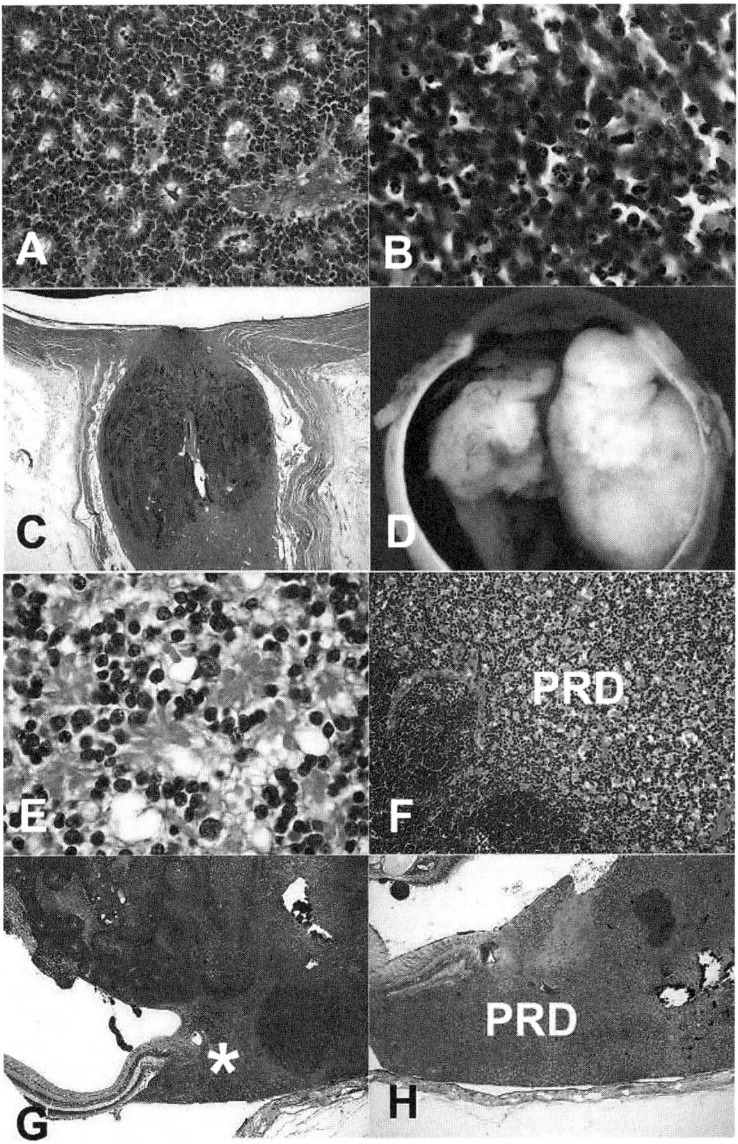

FIGURE.—A, Well-differentiated retinoblastoma from 8-month-old infant contains numerous Flexner-Wintersteiner rosettes. B, Poorly differentiated tumor from 30-month-old child is composed of mitotically active cells with scant cytoplasm. C, Retrolaminar optic nerve invasion. D, Gross photograph showing massive focus of uveal invasion involving ciliary body and choroid. E, Paucicellular focus of photoreceptor differentiation contains bouquetlike aggregates of eosinophilic photoreceptors called fleurettes. Nuclei are bland and mitoses are absent. F, Viable area of photoreceptor differentiation (PRD) is relatively eosinophilic compared to basophilic retinoblastoma at bottom left. G, Sleeves and cuffs of basophilic retinoblastoma (above) bury smaller eosinophilic focus of basal photoreceptor differentiation (star). H, Massive basal focus of PRD rests on inner surface of choroid and surrounds small basophilic focus of retinoblastoma (hematoxylin-eosin [A through C and E through H], original magnifications ×100 [A], ×250 [B and E], ×10 [C, G, and H] ×25 [F]). (Reprinted from Eagle RC Jr. High-risk features and tumor differentiation in retinoblastoma: a retrospective histopathologic study. *Arch Pathol Lab Med.* 2009;133:1203-1209.)

adjuvant chemotherapy on the basis of existing high-risk histopathologic features. Retinoblastomas become progressively less differentiated with time and may be spawned by precursor retinomas (Fig).

▶ This is an exquisitely illustrated and detailed clinicopathologic study of 387 enucleated eyes with retinoblastoma. Some of the epidemiologic observations in this study are consistent with previous large studies on retinoblastoma, such as ratios of sporadic, germline, and familial tumors, and the corresponding average age at presentation. The author found that 18.5% of untreated eyes harbored high-risk histopathologic features (Fig). This figure is similar to recent observations from 2 other major United States institutions, but it is lower than reported in less developed countries and in older American literature, perhaps reflecting delay in diagnosis and/or different biological behavior of the tumors. Eagle noted a strong association between iris neovascularization and neovascular glaucoma and the presence of high-risk features. Thus, iris neovascularization in retinoblastoma may be an important indicator of potential high-risk histopathologic characteristics. The author has also provided data that may shed light on biologic behavior of retinoblastoma. His observation of photoreceptor differentiation in 20.4% of all tumors (Fig), and the inverse relationship between the tumor differentiation and the patient age is consistent with the hypothesis that retinocytoma is a precursor lesion of retinoblastoma.

For further reading on this subject I suggest articles by Uusitan et al,[1] Biswas et al,[2] Dimaras et al,[3] and Gallie et al.[4]

T. Milman, MD

References

1. Uusitan MS, Van Quill KR, Scott IU, Matthay KK, Murray TG, O'Brien JM. Evaluation of chemoprophylaxis in patients with unilateral retinoblastoma with high-risk features on histopathologic examination. *Arch Ophthalmol.* 2001;119: 41-48.
2. Biswas J, Das D, Krishnakumar S, Shanmugam MP. Histopathologic analysis of 232 eyes with retinoblastoma conducted in an Indian tertiary-care ophthalmic center. *J Pediatr Ophthalmol Strabismus.* 2003;40:265-267.
3. Dimaras H, Khetan V, Halliday W, et al. Loss of RB1 induces non-proliferative retinoma: increasing genomic instability correlates with progression to retinoblastoma. *Hum Mol Genet.* 2008;17:1363-1372.
4. Gallie BL, Campbell C, Devlin H, Duckett A, Squire JA. Developmental basis of retinal-specific induction of cancer by RB mutation. *Cancer Res.* 1999;59: 1731s-1735s.

Lack of Correlation between the Histologic and Magnetic Resonance Imaging Results of Optic Nerve Involvement in Eyes Primarily Enucleated for Retinoblastoma

Wilson MW, Rodriguez-Galindo C, Billups C, et al (Univ of Tennessee Health Science Ctr, Memphis; St Jude Children's Res Hosp, Memphis, TN)

Ophthalmology 116:1558-1563, 2009

Purpose.—To correlate the histologic and magnetic resonance imaging results of the optic nerve in eyes primarily enucleated for retinoblastoma.

Design.—Retrospective, clinicopathologic correlation.

Participants.—Sixty-seven consecutive patients with retinoblastoma who underwent primary enucleation.

Methods.—The histologic results of 67 eyes from 67 patients with retinoblastoma who underwent primary enucleation between March 1997 and January 2008 were studied for evidence of optic nerve invasion. Two neuroradiologists independently reviewed available preoperative magnetic resonance imaging studies with special emphasis on nonenhanced T2-weighted and gadolinium-enhanced T1-weighted imaging for evidence of optic nerve invasion. A weighted κ statistic was used to assess agreement between observers.

Main Outcome Measures.—Correlation between neuroradiologists and histologic results.

Results.—Of the 67 eyes studied, 60 had preoperative magnetic resonance images, 58 of which were deemed appropriate for review by both neuroradiologists. Review of the histologic results showed optic nerve involvement in 62 (93%) of 67 eyes: 28 prelaminar (42%), 24 laminar (36%), and 10 postlaminar (15%). On review of the magnetic resonance scans, the first neuroradiologist identified optic nerve involvement in 57 (95%) of 60 eyes: 26 prelaminar (43%), 10 laminar (17%), and 11 postlaminar (18%). The second neuroradiologist identified optic nerve involvement in 46 (77%) of 60 eyes: 33 prelaminar (55%), 9 laminar (15%), and 4 postlaminar (7%). Moderate agreement existed between neuroradiologists (κ, 0.55). Poor and fair agreement existed between each of the 2 neuroradiologists and histologic results, respectively (κ, 0.29 and 0.17). Exophytic tumors showed the greatest disparity (κ, −0.20 and −0.13) between magnetic resonance imaging and histologic results.

Conclusions.—Limited correlation was found between magnetic resonance imaging and histologic results in assessing optic nerve invasion in eyes with retinoblastoma. Magnetic resonance imaging using routine imaging technologies, although useful in the evaluation of retinoblastoma, has limited usefulness in assessing the exact extent of optic nerve invasion; high-risk features of retinoblastoma such as postlaminar invasion remain best defined by histologic analysis. This study demonstrates that the interpretation of optic nerve involvement by a radiologist should not be the determining factor to defer enucleation in favor of neoadjuvant therapy.

▶ MRI has become the most widely used method for the pretreatment imaging work-up and staging in retinoblastoma patients because of its superior soft-tissue contrast resolution and absence of ionizing radiation, which may induce secondary malignancy. Unfortunately, the title of this article says it all. While neuroradiologists were able to correctly interpret lack of optic nerve invasion in retinoblastoma, they were not accurate in assessing the extent of optic nerve invasion by the tumor. This trend held even with the most technologically advanced imaging modalities. Currently, histology remains the gold-standard for identification of high-risk characteristics in retinoblastoma.

T. Milman, MD

Inadvertent Evisceration of Eyes Containing Uveal Melanoma

Eagle RC Jr, Grossniklaus HE, Syed N, et al (Thomas Jefferson Univ, Philadelphia, PA; Emory Univ, Atlanta, GA; Univ of Iowa; et al)

Arch Ophthalmol 127:141-145, 2009

Objectives.—To report an important complication of ocular evisceration therapy for blind, painful eyes that has been unreported in the literature, and to stress the need for careful preoperative evaluation to exclude occult neoplasms prior to therapy.

Design.—Multicenter, retrospective, nonrandomized clinicopathological case series of patients found to have previously unsuspected uveal malignant melanoma during histopathological examination of blind, painful eyes treated by evisceration.

Results.—Histopathological examination of evisceration specimens disclosed previously unsuspected uveal melanoma in 7 patients who were treated for blind, painful eyes. Inflammation caused by necrosis of the tumor and other ocular tissues led to misdiagnosis as endophthalmitis, orbital cellulitis, or idiopathic orbital inflammation in several cases. Preoperative imaging was not performed in 3 cases and failed to detect tumors in the remaining 4 cases. Failure of necrotic tumors to enhance contributed to misdiagnosis.

Conclusions.—The presence of a malignant intraocular neoplasm should be excluded prior to evisceration of any blind eye or blind, painful eye, particularly with opaque media. Necrosis-related inflammation can confound the clinical diagnosis of occult lesions, as can failure of necrotic tumors to enhance on imaging studies.

▶ This controversial article has generated quite a stir in the ophthalmic community, as manifested by an accompanying editorial and 3 comments in the following issue of the *Archives*. The authors caution ophthalmologists against evisceration of blind eyes with opaque media and suboptimal work-up (failure to take thorough clinical and ophthalmic history, inadequate eye exam, and failure to obtain ancillary imaging studies), because such eyes can harbor an unsuspected intraocular tumor (Fig 1 in the original article).

The opponents of this viewpoint state that none of the 7 reported patients had well-documented morbidity from inadvertent evisceration of uveal melanoma. They also note that preoperative imaging may not detect a necrotic or hemorrhagic tumor, as was the case with all 4 reported patients who underwent preoperative imaging studies. They argue that the benefits of evisceration over enucleation (improved cosmesis, decreased likelihood of prosthesis-related complications, shorter and simpler procedure, and maintenance of barrier function of the sclera) outweigh the risks posed by evisceration of intraocular melanoma.

Both sides have a point. In my personal experience with 2 cases of necrotic/hemorrhagic melanoma, the tumors were not picked up on ultrasonography performed by retina specialists. The tumors were diagnosed incidentally in routine vitrectomy specimens, bearing diagnoses of "vitreous hemorrhage" and "retinal detachment/suprachoroidal hemorrhage." These 2 cases illustrate inadequacy of currently available imaging techniques in diagnosing necrotic and hemorrhagic uveal melanoma. Since the long-term benefit of enucleation over evisceration for intraocular melanoma is not clear, and even the most careful evaluation may fail to diagnose this tumor, it seems to me that the main implication of the article by Eagle et al is the potential for medicolegal consequences of eviscerating an unsuspected neoplasm. As the authors state in reply to comments, "Failure to diagnose is a major cause of malpractice litigation." Undoubtedly, careful history, ophthalmic exam, and work-up with appropriate imaging studies are a must in all blind and painful eyes with opaque media. In addition, preoperative patient counseling about the possibility of unsuspected intraocular malignancy is prudent, regardless of the ultimate surgical procedure.

For further reading on this subject I suggest articles by Brown,[1] Rosner,[2] and Perry et al.[3]

T. Milman, MD

References

1. Brown SM. Evisceration of blind, painful eyes with occult uveal melanoma not a crime. *Arch Ophthalmol.* 2009;127:1228-1229.
2. Rosner M. Blind eye with occult malignant melanoma. *Arch Ophthalmol.* 2009; 127:1228-1229.
3. Perry JD, Lewis CD, Levine M. Evisceration after complete evaluation an acceptable option. *Arch Ophthalmol.* 2009;127:1228-1229.

Immunohistochemical Studies of Atypical Conjunctival Melanocytic Nevi

Jakobiec FA, Colby K, Bajart AM, et al (Massachusetts Eye and Ear Infirmary and Harvard Med School, Boston; Ophthalmic Consultants of Boston; et al)
Arch Ophthalmol 127:970-980, 2009

Objective.—To evaluate with immunohistochemical methods 5 atypical melanocytic conjunctival lesions.

Methods.—This was a retrospective clinicoimmunopathologic study. Routine histochemical staining was performed with multiparametric immunohistochemical analysis with monoclonal antibodies immunoreacted on paraffin sections to identify the following cell antigens: S-100, MART-1, HMB-45, CD45, CD68, CD1a, lysozyme, and Ki-67 (nuclear proliferation protein).

Results.—A unique granular cell nevus contained periodic acid–Schiff–positive, diastase-resistant granules and immunoreacted with monoclonal antibodies against S-100 protein and melanocytic-associated antigens MART-1 and HMB-45. Results for CD45, CD1a, CD68, and lysozyme immunostaining of the granular cells were negative. Two epithelioid cell (clonal or inverted) nevi exhibited an identical immunohistochemical profile. Only the balloon cell nevus was MART-1–positive and HMB-45–negative. The granular cell and blue nevi immunoreacted negligibly with Ki-67 (approximately 1% of cells).

Conclusions.—S100 and MART-1 reliably immunostained all nevocytic morphologic variants. HMB-45 immunoreactivity of the granular, epithelioid/clonal, and blue nevi did not indicate a more active or proliferative lesion but instead suggested abnormal melanogenesis. Ki-67 was the most valuable immunohistochemical adjunct to morphology for the diagnosis of these benign variant conjunctival nevi, because melanomas display a much higher proliferation index (>10% nuclear positivity among all cells counted) than the current nevi (approximately 1%).

▶ Melanocytic lesions of the conjunctiva can present a diagnostic dilemma, even to an experienced pathologist. Quoting the words of one of the leading experts in the field of eye pathology: "The more of these conjunctival melanocytic lesions I see, the more difficult they get...." This statement by a wise and experienced observer highlights the diagnostic pitfalls inherent to the pathologic evaluation of melanocytic tumors of the conjunctiva. In the Transactions of the American Ophthalmologic Society of 1999, Hans E. Grossniklaus presented his work, entitled "Indeterminate melanocytic proliferations of the conjunctiva." He concluded that a subset of melanocytic lesions of conjunctiva cannot be reproducibly classified by pathologists as benign or malignant, and a diagnosis of "indeterminate" or "borderline" should be given to such lesions. Despite this observation, neither a physician nor a patient appreciates an "indeterminate" diagnosis; thus, a quest for markers that enable the distinction of benign from malignant conjunctival melanocytic proliferations has been ongoing.

Two recent articles by Furusato et al and Jakobiec et al attempted to provide some data that may facilitate the distinction of benign conjunctival melanocytic lesions from malignant. Furosato and colleagues found that HMB-45 and *WT1* were helpful in distinguishing conjunctival nevi from melanoma, mostly by observation of stratification of immunostaining in nevi, consistent with their maturation. Jakobiec, however, in his study of unusual conjunctival nevi did not find HMB-45 marker useful, noting significant overlap between nevi and melanomas in HMB-45 expression. He noted, however, that Ki-67 proliferation marker was helpful to distinguish the mitotically inactive nevi from melanomas.

Although these 2 studies provide us with some answers regarding how to approach challenging melanocytic conjunctival lesions, they also highlight inadequacy of our current diagnostic methods. At present, careful histopathologic evaluation and a detailed clinicopathologic correlation carry much more weight than any of the immunohistochemical markers in our arsenal.

T. Milman, MD

WT1 and Bcl2 Expression in Melanocytic Lesions of the Conjunctiva: An Immunohistochemical Study of 123 Cases

Furusato E, Hidayat AA, Man Y-G, et al (Inst of Pathology, WA)
Arch Ophthalmol 127:964-969, 2009

Objective.—Recent studies indicate that *WT1* and Bcl2 protein are detected in melanocytic lesions of the skin. We examined, for the first time, *WT1* and Bcl2 expression in a variety of conjunctival melanocytic lesions to evaluate their diagnostic utility compared with other melanocytic markers.

Methods.—Protein expression and localization of *WT1* and Bcl2 were studied by means of immunolabeling and semiquantification in 123 conjunctival melanocytic lesions (71 benign nevi, 21 atypical nevi, 11 primary acquired melanosis, and 20 malignant melanomas). Ancillary immunohistochemical studies were performed with Bcl2, S100, HMB45, and Melan A antibodies.

Results.—*WT1* showed a graded increase in expression in lesions with increasing atypia. Higher mean numbers of *WT1*-positive cells correlated with increasing atypia in melanocytes. In all cases, Bcl2 expression was positive and more robust than was S100, HMB45, or Melan A expression. *WT1* and HMB45 frequently showed diffuse and strong staining in atypical nevi, primary acquired melanosis with atypia, and malignant melanomas compared with benign lesions.

Conclusions.—Bcl2 is a highly sensitive immunohistochemical marker for melanocytic tumors of the conjunctiva; HMB45 and *WT1* staining distinguishes benign from malignant lesions.

Clinical Relevance.—Our results show that HMB45 and WT1 immunolabeling is helpful in the evaluation of conjunctival melanocytic lesions.

Accordingly, we recommend the development of an immunohistochemical panel to classify these lesions.

▶ Melanocytic lesions of the conjunctiva can present a diagnostic dilemma even to an experienced pathologist. Quoting the words of one of the leading experts in the field of eye pathology: "The more of these conjunctival melanocytic lesions I see, the more difficult they get...." This statement by a wise and experienced observer highlights the diagnostic pitfalls inherent to the pathologic evaluation of melanocytic tumors of the conjunctiva. In the Transactions of the American Ophthalmologic Society of 1999, Hans E. Grossniklaus[1] has presented his work entitled "Indeterminate melanocytic proliferations of the conjunctiva." He concluded that a subset of melanocytic lesions of conjunctiva cannot be reproducibly classified by pathologists as benign or malignant, and a diagnosis of "indeterminate" or "borderline" should be given to such lesions. Despite this observation, neither a physician nor a patient appreciates an "indeterminate" diagnosis; thus, a quest for markers, which would enable the distinction of benign from malignant conjunctival melanocytic proliferations has been ongoing.

Two recent articles by Furusato et al and Jakobiec et al attempted to provide some data that may facilitate the distinction of benign conjunctival melanocytic lesions from malignant. Furusato and colleagues found that HMB45 and *WT1* were helpful in distinguishing conjunctival nevi from melanoma, mostly by observation of stratification of immunostaining in nevi, consistent with their maturation. Jakobiec, however, in his study of unusual conjunctival nevi did not find HMB45 marker useful, noting significant overlap between nevi and melanomas in HMB45 expression. He noted, however, that Ki-67 proliferation marker was helpful to distinguish the mitotically inactive nevi from melanomas.

Although these 2 studies provide us with some answers on how to approach challenging melanocytic conjunctival lesions, they also highlight inadequacy of our current diagnostic methods. At present, careful histopathologic evaluation and a detailed clinicopathologic correlation carry much more weight than any of the immunohistochemical markers in our arsenal.

T. Milman, MD

Reference

1. Grossniklaus HE, Margo CE, Solomon AR. Indeterminate melanocytic proliferations of the conjunctiva. *Trans Am Ophthalmol Soc.* 1999;XCVII:157-170.

Excision of Periocular Basal Cell Carcinoma With Stereoscopic Microdissection of Surgical Margins for Frozen-Section Control: Report of 200 Cases

Levin F, Khalil M, McCormick SA, et al (Columbia Univ Med Ctr, NY; The New York Eye and Ear Infirmary; et al)
Arch Ophthalmol 127:1011-1015, 2009

Objective.—To report our experience with 200 cases of basal cell carcinoma (BCC) in 192 patients treated with an enhanced frozen-section control (FSC) technique using stereoscopic microdissection of surgical margins.

Methods.—Retrospective series of 192 patients with 200 lesions diagnosed as BCC of the periocular region. All were excised en bloc with 1-mm margins beyond the clinically apparent tumor and examined using an enhanced FSC technique with stereoscopic microdissection of the surgical margins.

Results.—Of 200 malignant BCCs, 93.0% represented primary tumors. The overall recurrence rate was 1.0%, with a mean follow-up of 4 years. In patients with primary lesions, the overall recurrence rate was 1.1%, with a mean follow-up of 3.9 years. There were no recurrences in the secondary tumor group after a mean follow-up of 4.8 years. Of the 200 lesions, 66.0% lesions required a single en bloc resection to achieve tumor-free margins.

Conclusions.—An enhanced FSC technique using stereoscopic microdissection of the surgical margins permits greater conservation of healthy tissue and yields cure rates comparable to those of the standard FSC technique and Mohs micrographic surgery. We believe that this enhanced FSC technique is a highly effective method for resection of periocular BCC.

▶ The objectives of management of periocular basal cell carcinoma (BCC) are 2-fold: complete tumor excision and maximal sparing of tissue for optimal cosmesis and functionality. Various treatment modalities have been advocated to achieve these goals including, but not limited to, surgical resection with frozen section control of margins and Mohs micrographic surgery (MMS). Despite a plethora of publications on this topic, the evidence for the "absolute best" treatment approach is conflicting. The proponents of MMS state that this procedure is more cost-effective than surgical excision and provides lower recurrence rates, averaging at 1%. The proponents of surgical excision argue the difference in recurrence rates between the 2 procedures is negligible, and does not justify the higher costs of MMS. Both sides feel that their method allows for better tissue preservation.

A recent study by Auw-Haedrich has focused on the recurrence rates of periocular BCC removed with a small surgical safety margin (2-3 mm for nodular BCC and 5 mm for infiltrative BCC), followed by histologic margin evaluation. The authors found that approximately one-third of all tumors removed had histologically positive margin, and that the recurrence rates for such lesions is approximately 30%. The recurrence rates for BCC excised with histologic safety margin of <0.1 mm and >0.2 mm were 15% and 1.7%, respectively. The recurrence rates were higher for infiltrating BCC. The authors concluded that a complete surgical excision with >0.2 mm histologic margin clearance provides good long-term tumor control.

This study by Levin et al has described a technique for management of periocular BCC that provides even better tumor control (1% overall recurrence rate) while maximizing tissue sparing. This technique involves excising tumor en bloc with 1 mm surgical margin and using a grossing microscope at frozen section area to microdissect surgical margins for frozen-section analysis (Figs 1-4 in the original article). The authors noted that two-thirds of tumors removed with a single en block excision had histologically negative margins. They advocate that the en block excision with stereoscopic microdissection of margins for frozen section control yields recurrence rates comparable with MMS, yet maximizes tissue preservation and cost-effectiveness.

It is useful to add this well-illustrated technique to the armamentarium of treatment modalities for periocular BCC. Ultimately, the management of BCC in this location rests on the surgeon's experience with specific treatment method, the availability of ancillary resources needed for implementation of a specific treatment method, and on patient-specific considerations.

For further reading on this subject I suggest articles by Tierney et al,[1] Mosterd et al,[2] and Auw-Haedrich et al.[3]

T. Milman, MD

References

1. Tierney EP, Hanke CV. Cost effectiveness of Mohs micrographic surgery: review of the literature. *J Drugs Dermatol.* 2009;8:914-922.
2. Mosterd K, Krekels GAM, Nieman FHM, et al. Surgical excision versus Mohs' micrographic surgery for primary and recurrent basal cell carcinoma of the face: a prospective randomized controlled trial with 5-years' follow-up. *Lancet oncol.* 2008;9:1149-1156.
3. Auw-Haedrich C, Frick S, Boehringer D, Mittelviefhaus H. Histologic safety margin in basal cell carcinoma of the eyelid. Correlation with recurrence rate. *Ophthalmology.* 2009;116:802-806.

Changes in the 7th Edition of the AJCC TNM Classification and Recommendations for Pathologic Analysis of Lacrimal Gland Tumors

Rootman J, White VA (Univ of British Columbia and Vancouver General Hosp, Canada)

Arch Pathol Lab Med 133:1268-1271, 2009

In our recent work to update the American Joint Committee on Cancer's *AJCC Cancer Staging Manual,* we brought the staging system in line with that of salivary gland malignancies to better describe the range of these tumors. In addition, we have suggested that information be collected on biomarkers and clinical and histologic data points. This revised staging, along with careful histologic analysis and patient follow-up, may provide

TABLE 1.—Definition[a]

	Primary Tumor (T)
TX	Primary tumor cannot be assessed
T0	No evidence of primary tumor
T1	Tumor 2 cm or smaller in greatest dimension, with or without extraglandular extension into the orbital soft tissue
T2	Tumor larger than 2 cm but not larger than 4 cm in greatest dimension[b]
T3	Tumor larger than 4 cm in greatest dimension[b]
T4	Tumor invades periosteum or orbital bone or adjacent structures
T4a	Tumor invades periosteum
T4b	Tumor invades orbital bone
T4c	Tumor invades adjacent structures (brain, sinus, pterygoid fossa, temporal fossa)
	Regional lymph nodes (N)
NX	Regional lymph nodes cannot be assessed
N0	No regional lymph node metastasis
N1	Regional lymph node metastasis
	Distant metastasis (M)
MX	Distant metastasis cannot be assessed
M0	No distant metastasis
M1	Distant metastasis

[a]Used with the permission of the American Joint Committee on Cancer (AJCC), Chicago, Illinois. The original source for this material is the *AJCC Cancer Staging Manual*, Seventh Edition (2009) published by Springer Science and Business Media LLC, www.springerlink.com.
[b]Because the maximum size of the lacrimal gland is 2 cm, T2 and greater tumors will usually extend into the orbital soft tissue.

information that helps develop more targeted management for these lesions (Tables 1 and 2).

▶ The new 7th edition of the American Joint Committee on Cancer (AJCC) staging system incorporates clinically relevant, site-specific, tumor node metastasis (TNM) classification system for primary cancers of the eye, orbit, and ocular adnexa. The uniform use of this staging system will hopefully allow us to compare prognosis and treatments on equivalently sized and staged tumors, and will allow for further refinement of staging of eye cancers. The revised staging system is particularly useful in management of lacrimal gland tumors. Rootman and White refined the TNM classification of lacrimal gland tumors to bring it in line with that of salivary gland malignancies, which shows a good separation in outcome from T1 to T4. They approached the site-specific aspect of lacrimal gland tumor staging by distinguishing between periosteal and bony involvement, and by creating a category of unresectable disease (Table 1). Rootman and White also have expanded the histologic classification of lacrimal gland tumors on the basis of the World Health Organization classification of salivary gland tumors (Table 2). As the authors note: "Hopefully, careful histologic analysis, use of the 7th edition of the AJCC Cancer Staging Manual, and

TABLE 2.—Histopathologic Type[a]

Major malignant primary epithelial tumors
Low grade
Carcinoma ex pleomorphic adenoma
Polymorphous low-grade carcinoma
Mucoepidermoid carcinoma, grades 1 and 2
Epithelial-myoepithelial carcinoma
Cystadenocarcinoma and papillary cystadenocarcinoma
Acinic cell carcinoma
Basal cell adenocarcinoma
Mucinous adenocarcinoma
High grade
Carcinoma ex pleomorphic adenoma (malignant mixed tumor) that includes adenocarcinoma and adenoid cystic carcinoma arising in a pleomorphic adenoma
Adenoid cystic carcinoma, not otherwise specified
Adenocarcinoma, not otherwise specified
Mucoepidermoid carcinoma, grade 3
Ductal adenocarcinoma
Squamous cell carcinoma
Sebaceous adenocarcinoma
Myoepithelial carcinoma
Lymphoepithelial carcinoma
Other rare and unclassifiable carcinomas

[a]Used with the permission of the American Joint Committee on Cancer (AJCC), Chicago, Illinois. The original source for this material is the *AJCC Cancer Staging Manual*, Seventh Edition (2009) published by Springer Science and Business Media LLC, www.springerlink.com.

long-term follow-up will allow us to develop more specific and rational management of these difficult tumors and enable us to decrease the sometimes dismal morbidity and mortality of lacrimal epithelial tumors."

For further reading on this subject I suggest articles by Finger[1] and Weis et al.[2]

T. Milman, MD

References

1. Finger PT. The 7th edition AJCC staging system for eye cancer. An international language for ophthalmic oncology. *Arch Pathol Lab Med.* 2009;133:1197-1198.
2. Weis E, Rootman J, Joly TJ, et al. Epithelial lacrimal gland tumors. Pathologic classification and current understanding. *Arch Ophthalmol.* 2009;127:1016-1028.

Epithelial Lacrimal Gland Tumors: Pathologic Classification and Current Understanding

Weis E, Rootman J, Joly TJ, et al (Univ of Alberta, Edmonton, Canada; Vancouver General Hosp and the Univ of British Columbia, Canada; et al)
Arch Ophthalmol 127:1016-1028, 2009

Objective.—To apply the updated epithelial salivary gland classification scheme to a large cohort of lacrimal gland tumors so as to provide an updated lacrimal gland tumor classification scheme.

Methods.—A retrospective multicenter cohort study of 118 cases of epithelial neoplasia was undertaken. Main outcome measures included pathologic analysis, subtyping, and survival.

Results.—Of 118 cases, 17 (14%) were reclassified using the proposed expanded classification scheme based on the current World Health Organization classification of salivary gland tumors. The most frequent neoplasms were pleomorphic adenoma and adenoid cystic carcinoma, of which we highlight more unusual histologic features. Three tumors were found to be unclassifiable with the updated scheme, with 2 having histologically malignant features. Deficiencies and variations in pathologic assessment were noted. Variation in the histologic findings of pleomorphic adenoma and assessment of the extent of invasion of carcinoma ex pleomorphic adenoma were highlighted.

Conclusions.—The use of the more histologically diverse classification of salivary gland tumors can be successfully applied to the epithelial lacrimal gland neoplasms. This expanded classification system led to reclassifying 14% of cases. Currently, there are no consistent pathologic standards for processing and evaluating these lesions.

▶ Understanding that the lacrimal gland tumors compare with the more common counterparts of the major salivary gland has made it imperative to adapt WHO's classification of salivary gland tumors to the lacrimal gland pathology. This comprehensive approach to the epithelial tumors of the lacrimal gland has been reflected in the 2006 Armed Forces Institute of Pathology (AFIP) monograph on lacrimal gland tumors, and in the studies by Shields et al[2] and Bernardini et al.[1] The most recent work by Weis and colleagues reviews the standards of histologic analysis of epithelial lacrimal gland neoplasms based on the updated epithelial salivary gland classification scheme, and proposes an updated classification system for epithelial lacrimal gland tumors. This is a comprehensive, detailed, and beautifully illustrated article that sets the guidelines for histopathologic subtyping of primary epithelial malignancies of the lacrimal gland. Accurate diagnosis of these lesions is an important step in development of the consistent pathologic standards for their processing and evaluation.

For further reading on this subject I suggest an article by Font et al.[3]

T. Milman, MD

References

1. Bernardini FP, Devoto MH, Croxatto JO. Epithelial tumors of the lacrimal gland: an update. *Curr Opin Ophthalmol.* 2008;19:409-413.
2. Shields JA, Shields CL, Epstein JA, Scartozzi R, Eagle RC Jr. Review: primary epithelial malignancies of the lacrimal gland: the 2003 Ramon L. Font lecture. *Ophthal Plast Reconstr Surg.* 2004;20:10-21.
3. Font RL, Croxatto JO, Rao N. *Tumors of the Eye and Ocular Adnexa.* 2006;. 5th ed.5. Washington, DC: American Registry of Pathology and Armed Forces Institute of Pathology; 2006.

Clinical and Histopathologic Features of Failed Descemet Stripping Automated Endothelial Keratoplasty Grafts

Lee JA, Djalilian AR, Riaz KM, et al (Univ of Illinois at Chicago; et al)
Cornea 28:530-535, 2009

Purpose.—To study the histopathologic features of Descemet stripping automated endothelial keratoplasty (DSAEK) grafts removed after graft failure and to correlate with relevant clinical features.

Methods.—Retrospective study of 8 cases in 7 patients who experienced DSAEK graft failure during the surgeons' learning phase. Perioperative clinical findings were correlated with pathologic findings of the explanted graft specimens. Imaging software was used to measure the central and peripheral thickness of each graft.

Results.—Graft failure occurred in association with graft detachment or excessive surgical manipulation. In 4 cases, the donor tissue detached, including 2 cases with routes for bubble escape. In 3 cases, the graft remained attached but failed to clear. The mean preoperative DSAEK button thickness was 205 ± 61.8 μm. Average death to preservation time was 8 hours 47 minutes, and average preservation to surgery time was 2 days 22 hours. By light microscopy, explanted donor tissue showed varying degrees of keratocyte degeneration and marked endothelial cell loss. Two specimens with bubble escape had less endothelial loss, and 1 specimen showed epithelial ingrowth at the interface. Repeat keratoplasty (5 DSAEK, 2 penetrating keratoplasty) was successful in 6 of 7 cases.

Conclusions.—This series correlates factors that may play a role in DSAEK failure with histopathologic features of explanted DSAEK lenticules. Marked endothelial loss was common in cases with surgical trauma but was less in cases with bubble escape. One specimen showed an epithelial membrane on the stromal interface. Outcomes of repeat DSAEK in these patients seem promising (Fig 1).

▶ Endothelial keratoplasty has evolved into an alternative to traditional penetrating keratoplasty in corneas with disease limited to the endothelium. Descemet stripping automated endothelial keratoplasty (DSAEK) is currently the most popular technique for endothelial transplantation, which involves stripping of Descemet's membrane without host posterior stroma and placement of donor button, comprising posterior stroma, Descemet's membrane, and endothelium,

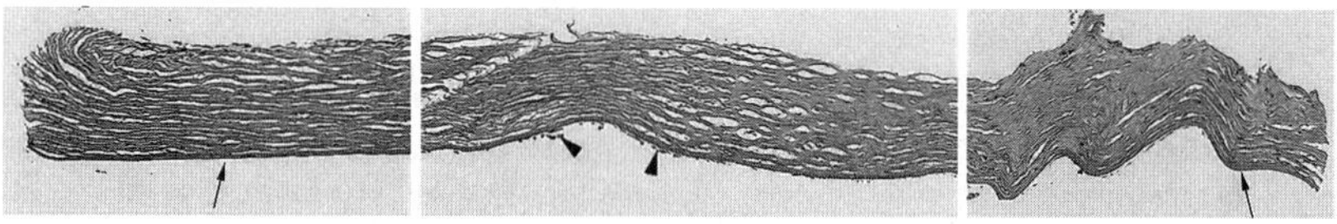

FIGURE 1.—Composite histology of explanted lenticule from patient 1. Periphery of the lenticule demonstrates nearly complete loss of endothelium (arrows). Centrally, there is some preservation of endothelium (arrowheads). (Reprinted from Lee JA, Djalilian AR, Riaz KM, et al. Clinical and histopathologic features of failed Descemet stripping automated endothelial keratoplasty grafts. *Cornea*. 2009;28: 530-535.)

onto the posterior surface of the cornea through a small incision. The donor tissue is held in place by a temporary intracameral air-bubble tamponade.

Several recent clinicopathologic case series have addressed the histopathology of failed DSAEK grafts. Of particular interest are the 2 studies by Suh et al and Lee et al.

Suh et al described histopathologic features of 19 failed DSAEK grafts and noted endothelial attenuation or absence in 84% of cases with either persistent lenticle detachment or primary graft failure. Fibrocellular tissue on stromal surface was observed in 58% of failed DSAEK grafts. The authors hypothesized that retained foreign material at the interface may stimulate fibroblast activation. Another recent study by Shulman et al[1] has shown that stromal inflammation may also play a role in fibroblast activation and fibrocellular membrane formation. Retained Descemet's membrane on stromal surface was observed in 26% of failed DSAEKs. Decentered graft with retention of full-thickness cornea at 1 edge of the graft was observed in 21% of cases. All eccentric lenticle trephinations were complicated by epithelial ingrowth. The authors concluded that the most common complication causing DSAEK failure was endothelial cell loss related to intraoperative and postoperative lenticle manipulation, and that the stromal interface membranes may have contributed to graft dislocation.

Lee et al studied histopathology of 8 failed DSAEK grafts. The authors similarly observed that endothelial cell loss was the major histopathologic finding in the failed grafts, while interface fibrocellular and epithelial membranes were less frequently encountered. Interestingly, Lee et al noted greater endothelial cell loss in the periphery of DSAEK lenticle (Fig 1), and suggested that this differential loss of peripheral endothelium could be secondary to rubbing of the exposed endothelial surface in a 60/40 taco fold during insertion, or due to increased wrinkling of the graft periphery during insertion, or related to forceps-induced trauma of peripheral tissue. In addition to excessive manipulation and bubble escape leading to endothelial cell loss, Lee et al noted that longer preservation interval of donor tissue may have contributed to endothelial cell loss and to graft dislocation.

The observations from these clinicopathologic studies of failed DSAEK grafts will help guide the modifications in surgical technique and postoperative management of endothelial keratoplasty.

For further reading on this subject I suggest articles by Shulman et al[1] and Oster et al.[2]

T. Milman, MD

References

1. Shulman J, Kropinak M, Ritterband DC, et al. Failed Descemet-stripping automated keratoplasty grafts: a clinicopathologic analysis. *Am J Ophthalmol.* 2009; 148:752-759.
2. Oster SF, Ebrahimi KB, Eberhart CG, Schein OD, Stark WJ, Jun AS. A clinicopathologic series of primary graft failure after Descemet's stripping and automated endothelial keratoplasty. *Ophthalmology.* 2009;116:609-614.

Histopathologic Examination of Failed Grafts in Descemet's Stripping with Automated Endothelial Keratoplasty

Suh LH, Dawson DG, Mutapcic L, et al (Univ of Miami, FL; et al)

Ophthalmology 116:603-608, 2009

Purpose.—To study the histopathologic features of 19 corneal posterior lamellar grafts in eyes for which Descemet's stripping with automated endothelial keratoplasty (DSAEK) has failed.

Design.—Retrospective case series with clinicopathologic correlation.

Participants.—Nineteen cases of DSAEK failures undergoing repeat DSAEK or penetrating keratoplasty.

Methods.—The histopathologic results of posterior lamellar grafts (also termed *DSAEK grafts*), recipient corneas, or both from 19 cases of failed DSAEK were examined.

Main Outcome Measures.—Abnormalities in the DSAEK graft and in the interface between the recipient cornea and the DSAEK graft were assessed.

Results.—Histopathologic features in 19 failed DSAEK grafts revealed attenuation of endothelial cells (16 cases) and presence in the graft–host interface of fibrocellular tissue (11 cases), retained Descemet's membrane (5 cases), epithelial ingrowth (4 cases), or a combination thereof. Four DSAEK grafts had full-thickness corneal layers at 1 edge.

Conclusions.—Presence of interface material, such as fibrocellular tissue, retained Descemet's membrane, and epithelial ingrowth, are potential causes of dislocation. Endothelial attenuation was the most common finding in failed grafts. Decentered DSAEK grafts with full-thickness

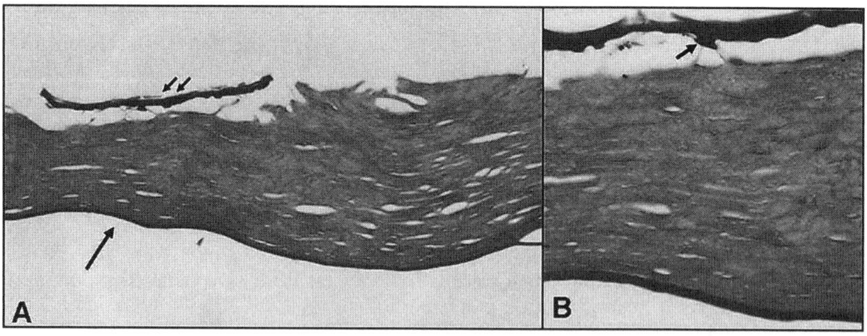

FIGURE 1.—A, Photomicrograph showing a lack of corneal endothelial cells in the Descemet's membrane portion of a failed posterior lamellar graft (single arrow) and a portion of the host Descemet's membrane (double arrows; stain, periodic acid–Schiff; original magnification, ×100). **B**, Photomicrograph showing posterior nodular excrescences present in the host Descemet's membrane representing Fuchs' endothelial dystrophy (arrow; stain, periodic acid–Schiff; original magnification, ×400). (Reprinted from Suh LH, Dawson DG, Mutapcic L, et al. Histopathologic examination of failed grafts in Descemet's stripping with automated endothelial keratoplasty. *Ophthalmology.* 2009;116:603-608, with permission from the American Academy of Ophthalmology.)

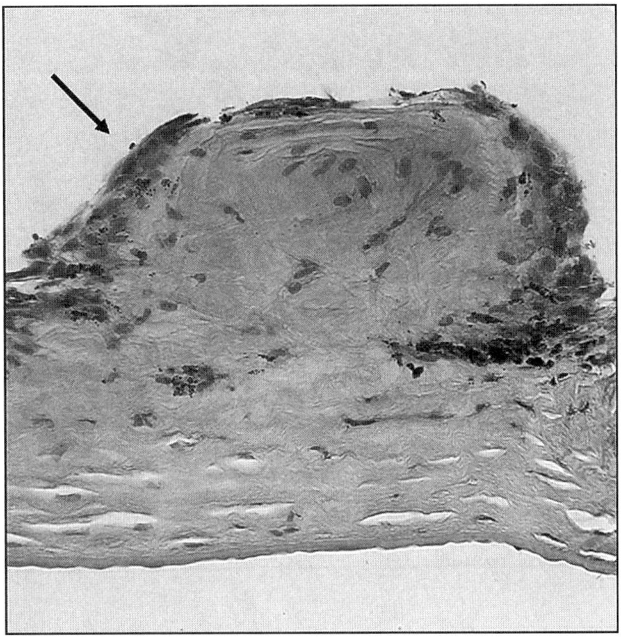

FIGURE 2.—Photomicrograph showing fibrocellular tissue on the anterior stromal surface (arrow) of a failed posterior lamellar graft (stain, hematoxylin–eosin; original magnification, ×200). (Reprinted from Suh LH, Dawson DG, Mutapcic L, et al. Histopathologic examination of failed grafts in Descemet's stripping with automated endothelial keratoplasty. *Ophthalmology.* 2009;116:603-608, with permission from the American Academy of Ophthalmology.)

corneal layers at 1 edge are a potential cause for epithelial ingrowth (Figs 1-4).

▶ Endothelial keratoplasty has evolved into an alternative to traditional penetrating keratoplasty in corneas with disease limited to the endothelium. Descemet's stripping automated endothelial keratoplasty (DSAEK) is currently the most popular technique for endothelial transplantation, and involves stripping of Descemet's membrane without host posterior stroma and placement of donor button, comprising posterior stroma, Descemet's membrane, and endothelium, onto the posterior surface of the cornea through a small incision. The donor tissue is held in place by a temporary intracameral air-bubble tamponade.

Several recent clinicopathologic case series have addressed the histopathology of failed DSAEK grafts. Of particular interest are the 2 studies by Suh et al and Lee et al.

Suh et al described histopathologic features of 19 failed DSAEK grafts and noted endothelial attenuation or absence in 84% of cases with either persistent lenticle detachment or primary graft failure (Fig 1). Fibrocellular tissue on stromal surface was observed in 58% of failed DSAEK grafts (Fig 2). The authors hypothesized that retained foreign material at the interface may

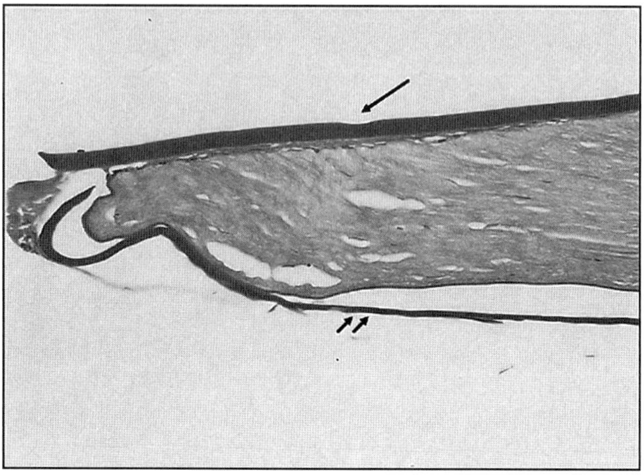

FIGURE 3.—Photomicrograph showing retained Descemet's membrane on the stromal surface of a failed posterior lamellar graft (arrow) and donor Descemet's membrane of graft tissue (double arrows; stain, periodic acid–Schiff; original magnification, ×200). (Reprinted from Suh LH, Dawson DG, Mutapcic L, et al. Histopathologic examination of failed grafts in Descemet's stripping with automated endothelial keratoplasty. *Ophthalmology*. 2009;116:603-608, with permission from the American Academy of Ophthalmology.)

stimulate fibroblast activation. Another recent study by Shulman et al has shown that stromal inflammation may also play a role in fibroblast activation and fibrocellular membrane formation. Retained Descemet's membrane on stromal surface was observed in 26% of failed DSAEKs (Fig 3). Decentered graft with retention of full-thickness cornea at 1 edge of the graft was observed in 21% of cases. All eccentric lenticle trephinations were complicated by epithelial ingrowth (Fig 4). The authors concluded that the most common complication causing DSAEK failure was endothelial cell loss related to intraoperative and postoperative lenticle manipulation, and that the stromal interface membranes may have contributed to graft dislocation.

Lee et al studied histopathology of 8 failed DSAEK grafts. The authors similarly observed that endothelial cell loss was the major histopathologic finding in the failed grafts, while interface fibrocellular and epithelial membranes were less frequently encountered. Interestingly, Lee et al noted greater endothelial cell loss in the periphery of DSAEK lenticle (Fig 1), and suggested that this differential loss of peripheral endothelium could be secondary to rubbing of the exposed endothelial surface in a 60/40 taco fold during insertion, or due to increased wrinkling of the graft periphery during insertion, or related to forceps-induced trauma of peripheral tissue. In addition to excessive manipulation and bubble escape leading to endothelial cell loss, Lee et al noted that longer preservation interval of donor tissue may have contributed to endothelial cell loss and to graft dislocation.

The observations from these clinicopathologic studies of failed DSAEK grafts will help guide the modifications in surgical technique and postoperative management of endothelial keratoplasty.

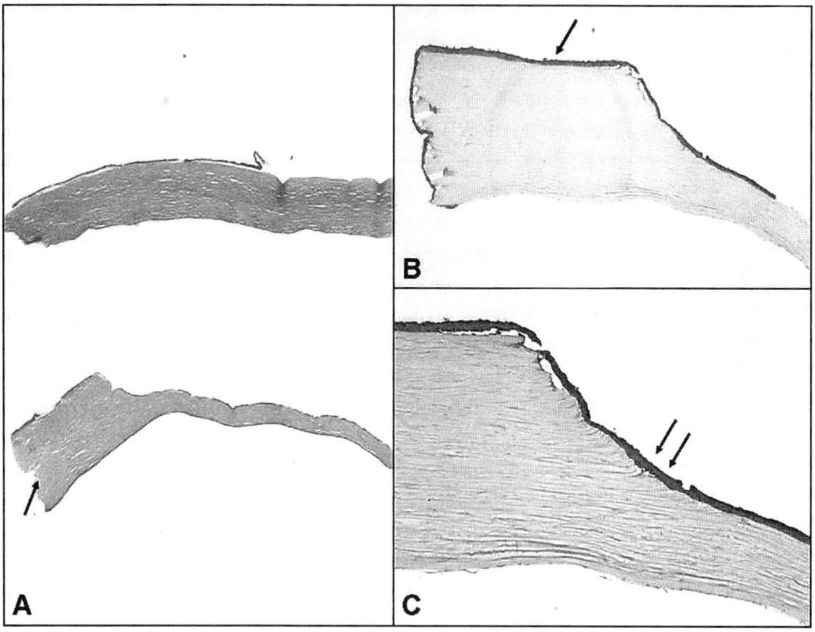

FIGURE 4.—A, Photomicrograph showing recipient cornea and the posterior lamellar graft. One edge of the posterior lamellar graft has a full-thickness cornea (arrow; stain, periodic acid–Schiff; original magnification, ×20). B, Photomicrograph showing the epithelial surface of the full-thickness portion of the graft (arrow; stain, anticytokeratin CAM 5.2; original magnification, ×40). C, Photomicrograph showing epithelial ingrowth on the stromal surface of the posterior lamellar graft contiguous with the epithelium of the full-thickness portion of the graft (double arrows; stain, anticytokeratin CAM 5.2; original magnification, ×100). (Reprinted from Suh LH, Dawson DG, Mutapcic L, et al. Histopathologic examination of failed grafts in Descemet's stripping with automated endothelial keratoplasty. *Ophthalmology.* 2009;116:603-608, with permission from the American Academy of Ophthalmology.)

For further reading on this subject I suggest articles by Shulman et al[1] and Oster et al[2]

T. Milman, MD

References

1. Shulman J, Kropinak M, Ritterband DC, et al. Failed Descemet-stripping automated keratoplasty grafts: a clinicopathologic analysis. *Am J Ophthalmol.* 2009; 148:752-759.
2. Oster SF, Ebrahimi KB, Eberhart CG, Schein OD, Stark WJ, Jun AS. A clinicopathologic series of primary graft failure after Descemet's stripping and automated endothelial keratoplasty. *Ophthalmology.* 2009;116:609-614.

Corneal Ectasia After Excimer Laser Keratorefractive Surgery: Histopathology, Ultrastructure, and Pathophysiology

Dawson DG, Randleman JB, Grossniklaus HE, et al (Emory Univ School of Medicine, Atlanta, GA; et al)
Ophthalmology 115:2181-2191, 2008

Purpose.—To evaluate the histopathology and ultrastructure of corneas developing ectasia after LASIK or photorefractive keratectomy (PRK).

Design.—Retrospective case series.

Participants.—Thirteen specimens from 12 patients undergoing corneal transplantation for progressive ectasia after LASIK (12 specimens) or PRK (1 specimen) were obtained for histopathologic and ultrastructural evaluation.

Methods.—All 13 ectatic corneas were submitted in formalin for light microscopy. Nine specimens were bisected, and the second half was placed in 2.5% glutaraldehyde for transmission electron microscopy (TEM).

Main Outcome Measures.—Corneal histopathology, ultrastructure, and pathophysiology.

Results.—Light microscopy of the post-LASIK specimens showed corneal epithelial hypoplasia and occasional foci of epithelial hyperplasia, Bowman's layer breaks, a normal stromal thickness of the LASIK flap, a normal thickness of the hypocellular primitive stromal scar, a thinned residual stromal bed (RSB), and larger than normal artifacteous interlamellar clefts in the RSB of the ectatic region. The post-PRK specimen showed similar findings with the addition of a thinned hypercellular fibrotic stromal scar. TEM showed thinning of the collagen lamellae and loss of lamellar number in the RSB of post-LASIK ectasia corneas or throughout the entire corneal stromal bed in the post-PRK ectasia cornea, with the posterior aspect of the corneal stroma being most affected.

Conclusions.—Histopathologic and ultrastructural studies suggest that interlamellar and interfibrillar biomechanical slippage occurs when the cornea becomes ectatic after LASIK or PRK in the postoperative stress-bearing regions of the corneal stroma. This 2-phase chronic biomechanical failure process is similar to that seen in keratoconus. Composite sciences classify this chronic biomechanical failure process as interfiber fracture (Figs 1-5).

▶ The 2 articles by Meghpara et al and Dawson et al highlight the recent advances in understanding of the biochemical and biomechanical mechanisms that may be at play in pathogenesis of keratoectatic disorders.

The study by Meghpara and colleagues confirms the previously demonstrated presence of biochemical alterations in keratoconus, such as decreased expression of α1-proteinase inhibitor and upregulation of Sp1 and matrix metalloproteinases. The authors found similar biochemical alterations in keratoglobus, providing further evidence for common pathogenic pathways in both of these keratoectasias.

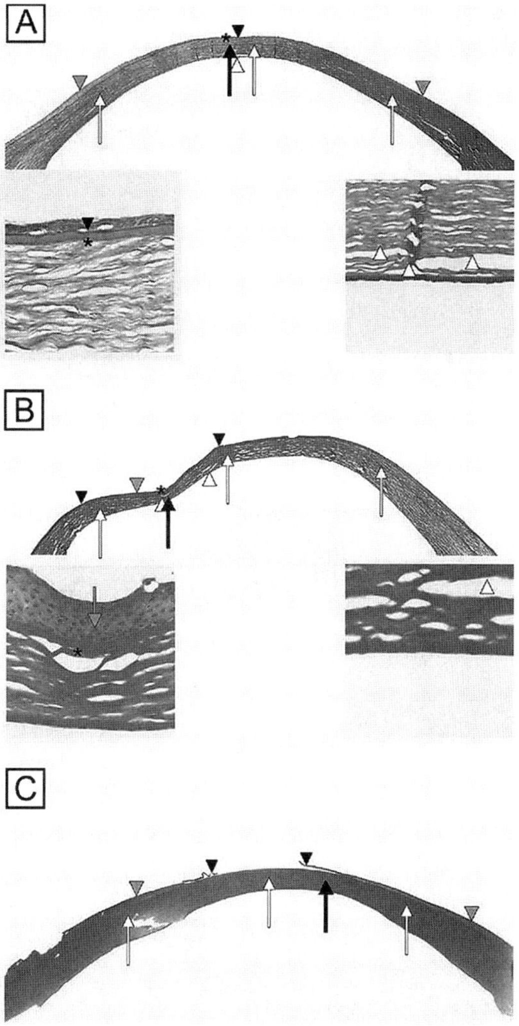

FIGURE 1.—Representative light photomicrographs of human post-LASIK corneal buttons with ectasia. **A,** Case 11 shows epithelial hypoplasia (*black arrowhead*) over an ectatic region and peripheral epithelial hyperplasia (*grey arrowheads*). In addition to epithelial hypoplasia, ectatic regions commonly displayed Bowman's layer breaks (*black asterisk*) and larger than normal artifacteous interlamellar clefts (*white arrowhead*), particularly in the posterior-most region of the RSB. The insets show higher magnification views demonstrating epithelial hypoplasia, Bowman's layer breaks, and larger than normal artifacteous clefting. **B,** Case 10 had the thinnest total corneal thickness (152 μm) and thinnest residual stroma bed (31 μm). Epithelial hyperplasia (*grey arrowhead*), a Bowman's layer break (*black asterisk*), and larger than normal artifacteous clefting (*white arrowhead*) were present in the thinnest area of this cornea. The insets show higher magnification views of the epithelial hyperplasia, Bowman's layer break, and larger than normal artifacteous clefts. **C,** Case 1 was a toluidine blue-stained section of an ectatic post-LASIK cornea similar to (**A**), although Bowman's layer breaks or larger than normal artifacteous clefts were not found in these glutaraldehyde-fixed corneal specimens. LASIK interface wound (*white arrows*). LASIK interface wound at location of thinnest total corneal thickness (*black arrows*). **A** and **B,** Periodic acid-Schiff, $\times$20. **C,** Toluidine blue, $\times$20. Insets: higher magnification views, $\times$400. (Reprinted from Dawson DG, Randleman JB, Grossniklaus HE, et al. Corneal ectasia after excimer laser keratorefractive surgery: histopathology, ultrastructure, and pathophysiology. *Ophthalmology.* 2008;115:2181-2191, with permission from the American Academy of Ophthalmology.)

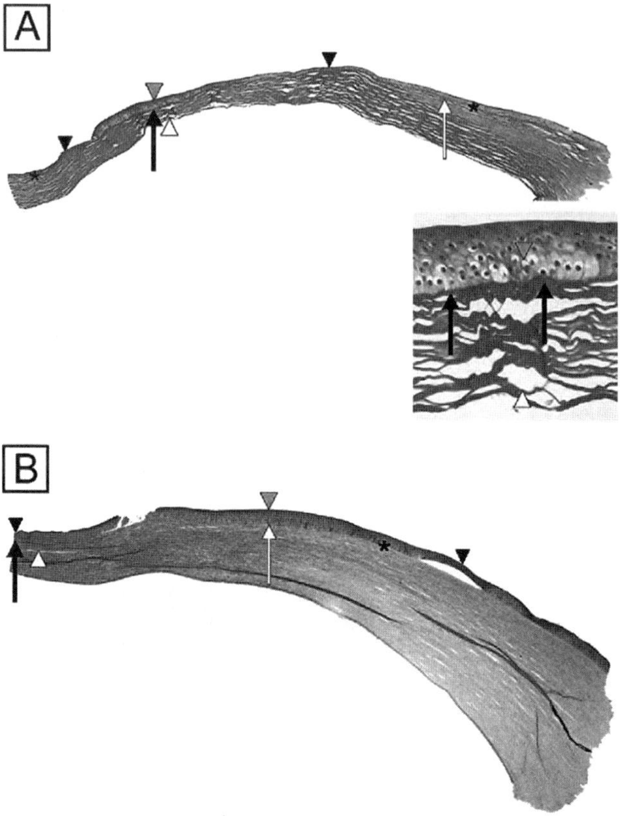

FIGURE 2.—Representative light photomicrographs of the human post-PRK corneal button with ectasia. A, Epithelial hyperplasia (*grey arrowhead*) and hypoplasia (*black arrowhead*) is seen over the ectatic region and peripheral corneal stroma, respectively. Bowman's layer is missing centrally (*black asterisk* marks the ablated ends of Bowman's layer) and a 10-μm–thick subepithelial fibrotic scar (*white arrows*) is present. The ectatic portion of this corneal button shows thinning of the subepithelial fibrotic scar (*black arrows*) and residual stroma, as well as larger than normal artifacteous clefts between lamellae (*white arrowhead*), particularly in the posterior-most region of the RSB. B, The same case is shown with a toluidine blue-stained section used for guiding TEM evaluations. Because this section was obtained from a remelted paraffin-embedded block, it still has some artifacteous clefting present despite subsequent glutaraldehyde fixation. Note again the epithelial hypoplasia over the ectatic region of the cornea (*left black arrowhead*) and peripheral areas of epithelial hyperplasia (*grey arrowhead*) and hypoplasia (*right black arrowhead*), ablated end of Bowman's layer (*black asterisk*), and 10-μm subepithelial fibrotic scar (*white arrows*). In the ectatic portion of this corneal button, the subepithelial fibrotic scar is thinned (*black arrow*), the stromal bed is thinned, and some larger than normal artifacteous clefting occurs between lamellae (*white arrowhead*). A, Periodic acid-Schiff staining, $\times$20. B, Toluidine blue staining, 40$\times$. Inset: higher magnification views, $\times$100. (Reprinted from Dawson DG, Randleman JB, Grossniklaus HE, et al. Corneal ectasia after excimer laser keratorefractive surgery: histopathology, ultrastructure, and pathophysiology. *Ophthalmology.* 2008;115:2181-2191, with permission from the American Academy of Ophthalmology.)

Dawson et al hypothesized that liberation of proteolytic enzymes by degenerated keratocytes may incite interlamellar fracture, the early step in pathogenesis of keratoconus and postexcimer laser keratorefractive surgery-related ectasia. Subsequent interfibrillar disruption of fibril-associated collagens or

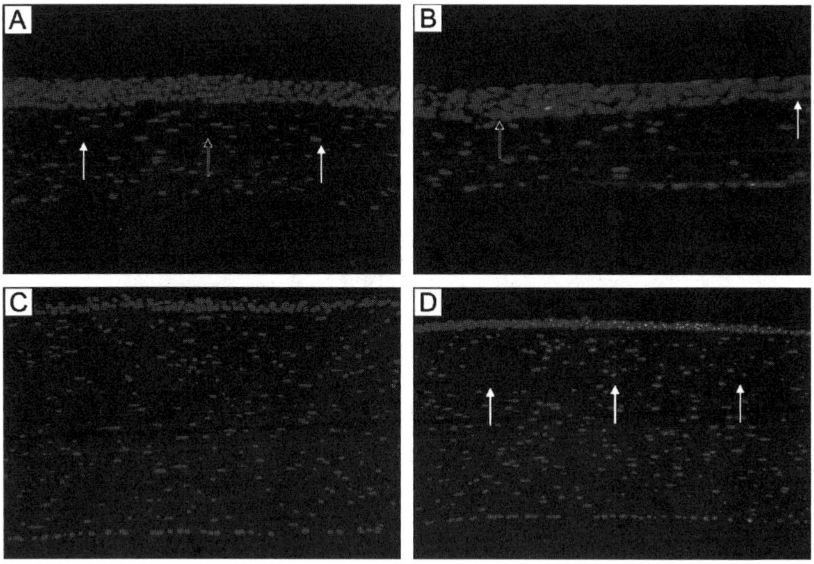

FIGURE 3.—**A,** DAPI-stained immunofluorescence section of post-LASIK ectasia case 5 showing how keratocytes appeared in the ectatic region of the cornea. LASIK interface wound (*white arrows*). LASIK interface wound at location of thinnest total corneal thickness (*black arrow*). **B,** DAPI-stained section of post-PRK ectasia case 1 showing how keratocytes appeared in the ectatic region of the cornea. Subepithelial fibrotic scar (*white arrow*). Subepithelial fibrotic scar at location of thinnest total corneal thickness (*black arrow*). **C,** DAPI-stained section of a normal 51-year-old white female donor cornea. **D,** DAPI-stained section of a 51-year-old white male uncomplicated post-LASIK donor cornea 10 years after surgery. **A–D,** DAPI staining, original magnification ×40. (Reprinted from Dawson DG, Randleman JB, Grossniklaus HE, et al. Corneal ectasia after excimer laser keratorefractive surgery: histopathology, ultrastructure, and pathophysiology. *Ophthalmology.* 2008;115:2181-2191, with permission from the American Academy of Ophthalmology.)

collagen-proteoglycan bonds may lead to the clinical manifestations of keratoectatic disorders (Figs 1-5).

Clearly, the precise mechanisms which lead to keratoectasia are not yet elucidated, but these 2 studies bring us closer to this goal.

T. Milman, MD

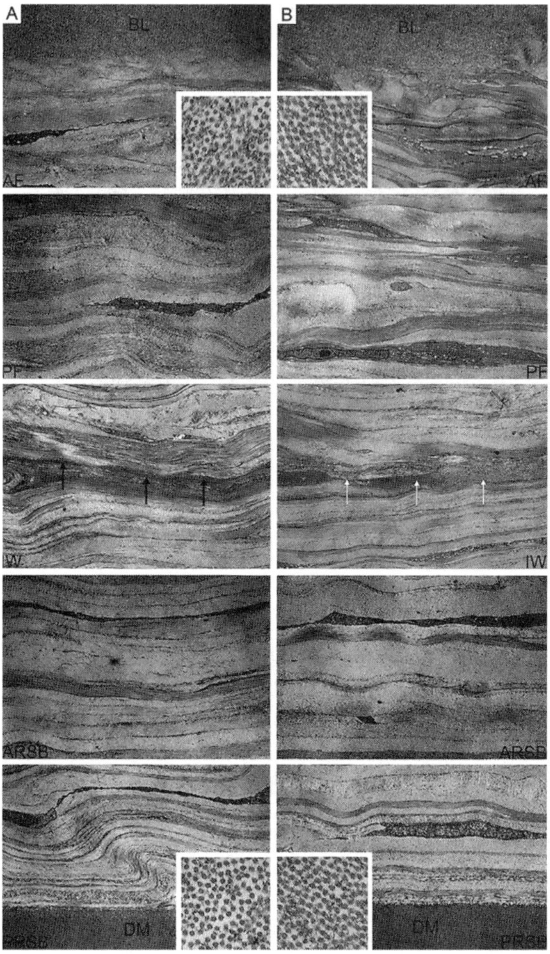

FIGURE 4.—Representative TEM images from post-LASIK ectasia case 1 showing a montage view (anterior to posterior) of the full-thickness cornea in the ectatic region (**A**) compared with a portion of the same corneal button in a non-ectatic region (**B**). The lamellae in the ectatic region of the LASIK flap averaged 0.9 ± 0.2 μm thick (similar to mean lamellar thickness in non-ectatic regions), whereas the lamellae of the RSB were thinner than normal averaging 0.9 ± 0.2 μm (35% thinner than the non-ectatic region). The interface wound is of normal morphology and averaged 1.9 ± 1.1 μm thick (similar in morphology and thickness to non-ectatic regions). By using the stromal thicknesses measured directly from the toluidine blue-stained thick sections, we calculated the number of lamellae in the LASIK flap as 69 lamellae (similar to the number of lamellae in the non-ectatic region) and in the RSB as 99 lamellae (46% reduced in number compared with the non-ectatic region). Insets show higher magnification TEM views where collagen fibril diameters and interfibrillar distances were measured. In the anterior aspect of the LASIK flap, the collagen fibril diameter averaged 25.0 ± 1.1 nm (within normal diameters) and the interfibrillar distance averaged 44.4 ± 1.0 nm (within normal interfibrillar distances). In the posterior aspect of the RSB, the collagen fibril diameter was slightly higher than normal, averaging 27.2 ± 1.1 nm (5% higher than normal), and the interfibrillar distance was also higher than normal, averaging 54.0 ± 6.5 nm (10% higher than normal). Interface wound in ectatic region of corneal button (*black arrows*). Interface wound in non-ectatic region of corneal button (*white arrows*). BL = Bowman's layer; DM = Descemet's membrane; AF = anterior flap; PF = posterior flap; IW = interface wound; ARSB = anterior residual stromal bed; PRSB = posterior residual stromal bed. TEMs, ×4750. Insets: higher magnification views, ×90,000. (Reprinted from Dawson DG, Randleman JB, Grossniklaus HE, et al. Corneal ectasia after excimer laser keratorefractive surgery: histopathology, ultrastructure, and pathophysiology. *Ophthalmology.* 2008;115:2181-2191, with permission from the American Academy of Ophthalmology.)

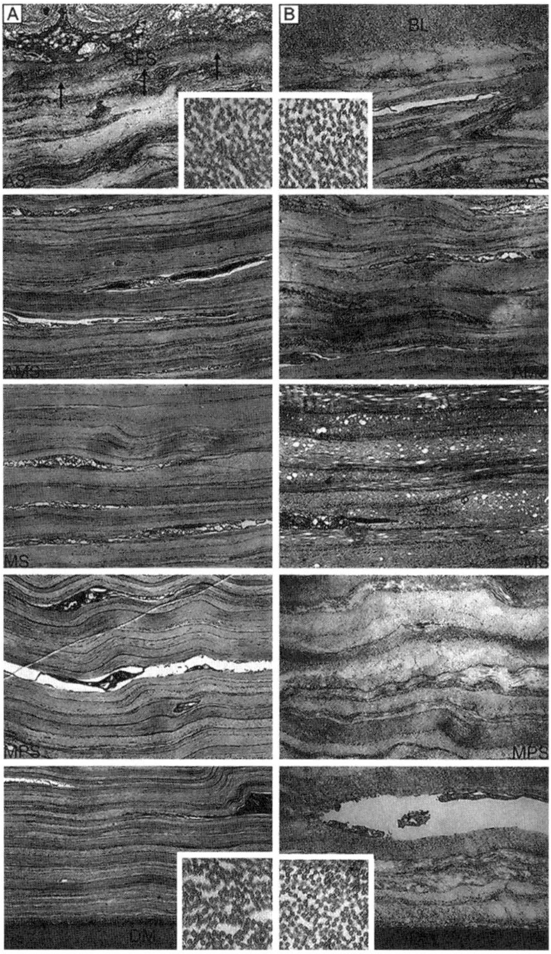

FIGURE 5.—Representative TEM images from post-PRK ectasia case 1 showing a montage view (anterior to posterior) of the full-thickness cornea in the ectatic region (**A**) compared with a portion of the same corneal button that was in a non-ectatic region (**B**). The lamellae in the anterior third of the ectatic region averaged 0.73 ± 0.2 μm thick (14% thinner than the non-ectatic region), the mid-third averaged 0.73 ± 3 μm thick (36% thinner than the non-ectatic region), and the posterior third averaged 0.72 ± 0.2 μm thick (42% thinner than the non-ectatic region). By using the stromal thicknesses measured directly from the toluidine blue-stained thick section, we calculated the number of lamellae in the ectatic region as 197 lamellae (38% reduced in number compared with the non-ectatic region). Insets show higher magnification TEM views where collagen fibril diameter and interfibrillar distance were measured. In the anterior third of the ectatic region, the collagen fibril diameter averaged 25.6 ± 1.9 nm (within normal diameters) and the interfibrillar distance averaged 45.1 ± 5.9 nm (within normal interfibrillar distances). In the posterior third of the ectatic region, the fibril diameter was slightly higher than normal averaging 29.8 ± 1.9 nm (11% higher than normal) and the interfibrillar distance was higher than normal averaging 48.5 ± 3.1 nm (6% higher than normal). Inferior border of subepithelial fibrotic scar and anterior stroma (*black arrows*). SFS = subepithelial fibrotic scar; BL = Bowman's layer; DM = Descemet's membrane; AS = anterior stroma; AMS = anterior mid-stroma; MS = mid-stroma; MPS = mid-posterior stroma; PS = posterior stroma. TEMs, ×4750. Insets: higher magnification views, ×90,000. (Reprinted from Dawson DG, Randleman JB, Grossniklaus HE, et al. Corneal ectasia after excimer laser keratorefractive surgery: histopathology, ultrastructure, and pathophysiology. *Ophthalmology.* 2008;115:2181-2191, with permission from the American Academy of Ophthalmology.)

Histopathologic and Immunohistochemical Studies of Keratoglobus

Meghpara B, Nakamura H, Vemuganti GK, et al (Univ of Illinois at Chicago; Summa Health System, Akron, OH; L. V. Prasad Eye Inst, Hyderabad, India)
Arch Ophthalmol 127:1029-1035, 2009

Objective.—To examine histopathologic and immunohistochemical features of human corneal buttons from patients who developed keratoglobus.

Methods.—Nine corneal buttons were obtained during penetrating keratoplasty from patients with keratoglobus. Histologic features were examined using hematoxylin-eosin–stained sections. Immunohistochemical staining for α1-proteinase inhibitor, Sp1, and matrix metalloproteinases 1, 2, and 3 was performed, with 2 normal and 2 corneal sections with keratoconus as controls.

Results.—Hematoxylin-eosin staining revealed diffuse stromal thinning and focal disruptions in Bowman's layer in all keratoglobus specimens. Similar abnormal immunostaining results for α1-proteinase inhibitor and Sp1 were detected in keratoglobus and keratoconus at their respective active disease sites. Immunostaining for matrix metalloproteinases 1, 2, and 3 was significantly more intense in corneas with keratoglobus than in normal controls. Matrix metalloproteinase staining intensity was especially prominent in areas where the underlying Bowman's layer was disrupted.

Conclusions.—Histological features in our keratoglobus specimens are consistent with previous reports. The similarities in immunohistochemical labeling between keratoglobus and keratoconus suggest that these entities may share common mechanisms that are involved in stromal thinning.

▶ This study by Meghpara et al and another study by Dawson et al,[1] highlight the recent advances in understanding of the biochemical and biomechanical mechanisms, which may be at play in pathogenesis of keratoectatic disorders.

The study by Meghpara and colleagues confirms the previously demonstrated presence of biochemical alterations in keratoconus, such as decreased expression of α1-proteinase inhibitor and upregulation of Sp1 and matrix metalloproteinases. The authors found similar biochemical alterations in keratoglobus, providing further evidence for common pathogenic pathways in both of these keratoectasias (Figs 2-5 in the original article).

Dawson et al hypothesized that liberation of proteolytic enzymes by degenerated keratocytes may incite interlamellar fracture, the early step in pathogenesis of keratoconus and postexcimer laser keratorefractive surgery-related ectasia. Subsequent interfibrillar disruption of fibril-associated collagens or collagen-proteoglycan bonds may lead to the clinical manifestations of keratoectatic disorders.

Clearly, the precise mechanisms which lead to keratoectasia are not yet elucidated, but these 2 studies bring us closer to this goal.

T. Milman, MD

Reference

1. Dawson DG, Randleman JB, Grossniklaus HE, et al. Corneal ectasia after excimer laser keratorefractive surgery: histopathology, ultrastructure, and pathophysiology. *Ophthalmology.* 2008;115:2181-2191.

Clinicopathologic Correlations in Giant Cell Arteritis: A Retrospective Study of 107 Cases

Zhou L, Luneau K, Weyand CM, et al (Emory Univ School of Medicine, Atlanta, GA)

Ophthalmology 116:1574-1580, 2009

Objective.—To correlate the pathologic findings of temporal artery biopsies in patients clinically defined as positive, presumed, or negative for giant cell arteritis (GCA).

Design.—Retrospective case series.

Participants and Controls.—Patients evaluated for GCA.

Methods.—Temporal artery biopsies examined between 1989 and 2007 were studied. Clinical information and residual tissue for immunohistochemical staining was identified in 107 patients. Clinical information was used to make a diagnosis of "positive," "presumed," or "negative" GCA. The biopsies were reviewed in a masked fashion and classified as "positive," "indeterminate," or "negative" based on published, classic pathologic diagnosis (CPD) criteria. All biopsies were immunostained for CD3 and CD68 and graded as "negative," "mildly" (+), "moderately" (++), or "markedly" (+++) positive. Clinical and pathologic results were correlated and a modified pathologic diagnosis classification (MPD) scheme was developed. The modified scheme was compared in a masked fashion with the final clinical diagnosis and positive and negative predictive values (PVs) were calculated.

Main Outcome Measures.—Pathologic diagnosis and final clinical diagnosis.

Results.—Using the MPD classification, there were 25%, 16%, and 61% positive, indeterminate, and negative biopsies, respectively. There was excellent correlation between the modified pathologic criteria and final clinical diagnosis (correlation coefficient 0.997; $P < 0.0001$; $k = 0.81$). The positive PVs for CPD and MPD were 85% and 96%, respectively. The negative PVs for CPD and MPD were 64% and 61%, respectively. Positive and negative biopsies strongly correlated with clinical diagnoses of positive and negative for GCA, respectively, whereas indeterminate cases moderately correlated with presumed GCA. The diagnosis did not change from the original biopsy in 11 patients who had a second biopsy. Immunostaining for CD 68 was helpful in several indeterminate cases.

Conclusions.—We recommend using the modified histologic classification of temporal artery biopsies. There are indeterminate cases that cannot be further defined using current pathologic classification criteria. A second

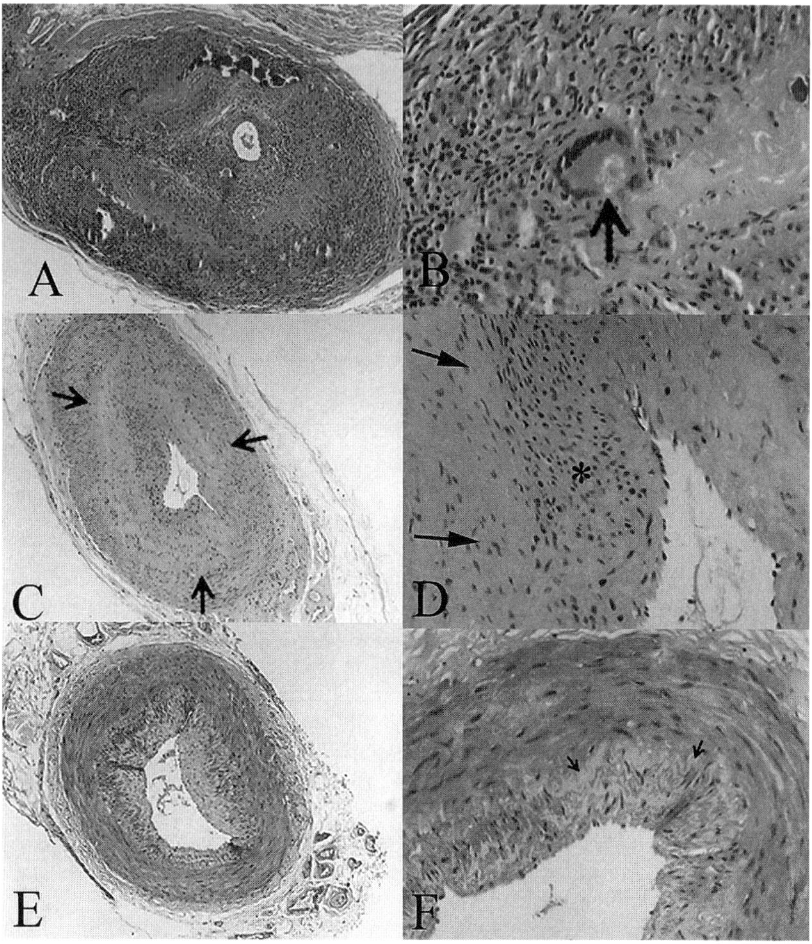

FIGURE 1.—Classic pathologic diagnosis (CPD) criteria. **A**, **B**, CPD positive includes intimal hyperplasia and chronic inflammation in all layers of the artery wall, including in many cases giant cells (arrow). **C**, **D**, CPD indeterminate includes intimal hyperplasia and a concentric scar centered for 360° around the inner elastic lamina (arrows, between brackets) and/or a full-thickness scar in the wall of the artery. There is also fibroplasia of the intima present (*). **E**, **F**, CPD negative shows a normal intima, media, and adventia. The lumen is patent, there is no intimal hyperplasia, and the inner elastic lamina is intact (arrows). Note the intimal hyperplasia and narrowing of the lumen in A to D compared with **E** and **F**. (Hematoxylin and eosin; **A**, **C**, and **E** original magnification, ×25; **B**, **D**, and **F** original magnification, ×100.). (Reprinted from Zhou L, Luneau K, Weyand CM, et al. Clinicopathologic correlations in giant cell arteritis: a retrospective study of 107 cases. *Ophthalmology.* 2009;116:1574-1580, with permission from the American Academy of Ophthalmology.)

biopsy has very limited value. Immunostaining for CD68 may be helpful in indeterminate cases, although the diagnosis in these cases is based on clinical judgment (Figs 1-3).

▶ The histopathologic evaluation of temporal artery biopsies can occasionally present a diagnostic challenge. While most pathologists will readily diagnose

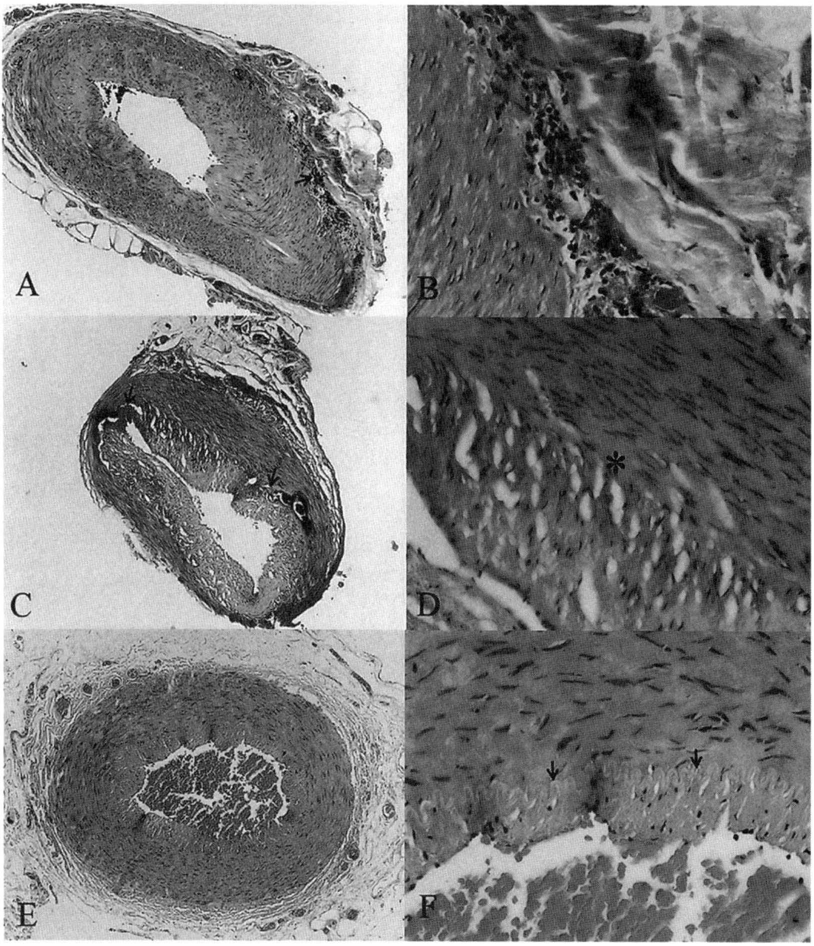

FIGURE 2.—Modified pathologic diagnosis (MPD) criteria. **A, B,** MPD positive includes the same features as for CPD. Additionally, focal chronic inflammation in any layer of the artery wall (arrow), including surrounding vasa vasora, are included. **C, D,** MPD indeterminate includes the same features as for CPD. Additionally, a focal concentric scar around the inner elastic lamina for any number of clock hours (between arrows) with loss of the inner elastic lamina (*) are included. **E, F,** MPD negative is the same as for CPD negative. The inner elastic lamina (arrows) is intact. (Hematoxylin and eosin; **A, C,** and **E** original magnification, ×25; **B, D,** and **F** original magnification, ×100.). (Reprinted from Zhou L, Luneau K, Weyand CM, et al. Clinicopathologic correlations in giant cell arteritis: a retrospective study of 107 cases. *Ophthalmology.* 2009;116:1574-1580, with permission from the American Academy of Ophthalmology.)

the temporal artery biopsies showing intimal hyperplasia and chronic transmural inflammation centered at the level of the internal elastic lamina as positive for giant cell arteritis (GCA) and the biopsies which lack these findings negative, the picture is frequently not as black and white.

The strength of the study by Zhou et al is in its correlation of these "indeterminate" biopsies with experienced clinical judgment of specialists renowned for

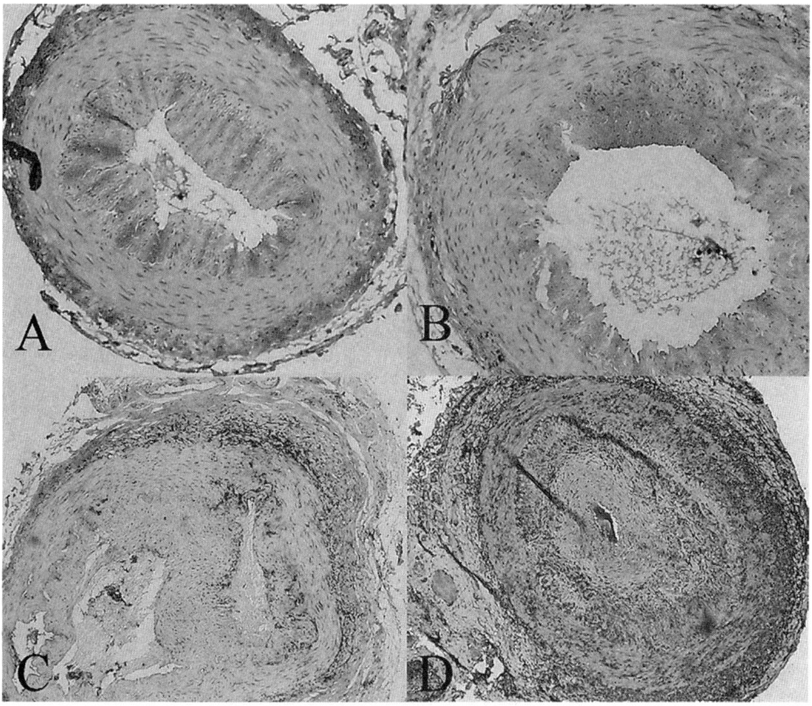

FIGURE 3.—The grading system defined in this study for immunohistochemistry staining in the temporal artery sections. A, $CD68^{-}$; B, $CD68^{+}$; C, $CD68^{++}$; D, $CD68^{+++}$. (Peroxidase antiperoxidase; original magnification ×10.). (Reprinted from Zhou L, Luneau K, Weyand CM, et al. Clinicopathologic correlations in giant cell arteritis: a retrospective study of 107 cases. *Ophthalmology.* 2009;116: 1574-1580, with permission from the American Academy of Ophthalmology.)

their expertise in treatment of GCA This clinicopathologic correlation has allowed the authors to expand the inclusive diagnostic criteria for GCA-positive and GCA-indeterminate/ "healed" temporal artery biopsies. According to these proposed modified diagnostic criteria, temporal artery biopsies with intimal hyperplasia and inflammation of any layer of the vessel wall, including vasa vasora, are GCA-positive. The biopsies with a concentric scar of any length at the level of internal elastic lamina and intimal hyperplasia were diagnosed as indeterminate or "healed" GCA. The authors also noted utility of a macrophage marker, CD68 immunostain, in identifying subtle transmural inflammation, leading to reclassification of indeterminate biopsies into GCA-positive. In our laboratory, we typically use CD45 immunostain (leukocyte common antigen, LCA) for this purpose, because this marker identifies both lymphocytes and macrophages (Figs 1-3).

Of course, it would be too hasty to change the pathologic diagnostic criteria of GCA on the strength of 1 study. However, it may be wise to apply both "classic" and "modified" diagnostic criteria to ambiguous cases and correlate the pathologic diagnosis with clinical impression.

T. Milman, MD

Laboratory Diagnosis of Amoebic Keratitis: Comparison of Four Diagnostic Methods for Different Types of Clinical Specimens

Boggild AK, Martin DS, Lee TY, et al (Toronto General Hosp, Ontario, Canada; Ontario Agency for Health Protection and Promotion, Canada; et al)

J Clin Microbiol 47:1314-1318, 2009

Amoebic keratitis causes significant ocular morbidity in contact lens wearers. Current diagnostic methods for amoebic keratitis are insensitive and labor-intensive and have poor turnaround time. We evaluated four laboratory methods for detection of acanthamoebae in clinical specimens. Deidentified, delinked consecutive specimens from patients with suspected amoebic keratitis were assayed for acanthamoebae by direct smear analysis, culture, and PCR using two different primer sets specific for *Acanthamoeba* ribosomal DNA. The consensus reference standard was considered fulfilled when the results for any two of the four tests were positive, and the outcome measures were sensitivity and specificity. Of 107 specimens assayed over an 18-month period, 20 were positive for acanthamoebae. The sensitivity and specificity of each assay were as follows, respectively: for smear analysis, 55% (95% confidence interval [CI], 33.2 to 76.8%) and 100%; for culture, 73.7% (95% CI, 54.4 to 93.0%) and 100%; for PCR using Nelson primers, 90% (95% CI, 76.9 to 100%) and 90.8% (95% CI, 84.7 to 96.9%); and for PCR using JDP primers, 65% (95% CI, 44.1 to 85.9%) and 100%. Nelson primer PCR demonstrated a single-organism level of analytic sensitivity. The performance characteristics of the assays varied by specimen type, with contact lenses and casings showing the highest rates of detectable acanthamoebae and the highest diagnostic sensitivities for direct smear analysis, culture, and JDP primer PCR, though these results are based on small numbers and should be interpreted cautiously. These findings have important implications for clinicians collecting diagnostic specimens and for diagnostic laboratories, especially in outbreak situations (Tables 1 and 2).

▶ The laboratory diagnosis of *Acanthamoeba* keratitis (AK) remains a challenge. In a review of 72 consecutive cases of AK presenting between

TABLE 1.—Comparison of Four Diagnostic Methods Used for Evaluation of 107 Clinical Specimens from Patients Suspected to have AK[a]

Assay	No. Positive	No. Negative	Sensitivity (%)	Specificity (%)	PPV (%)	NPV (%)
Direct microscopy	11	96	55.0	100	100	90.6
Culture[b]	14	91	73.7	100	100	94.6
PCR						
Nelson primers	26	81	90.0	90.8	69.2	97.5
JDP primers	13	94	65.0	100	100	91.6

[a]PPV, positive predictive value; NPV, negative predictive value.
[b]Two specimens were not set up for culture.

TABLE 2.—Performance Characteristics of Four Methods for Diagnosis of AK Used for Evaluation of 107 Clinical Specimens by Specimen Type

	Value (%) for Specimen Type					
	Corneal Scraping ($n = 81$)		Contact Lens Solution ($n = 17$)		Contact Lenses and Casings ($n = 6$)	
Assay	Sensitivity	Specificity	Sensitivity	Specificity	Sensitivity	Specificity
Direct microscopy	46.2	100.0	50.0	100.0	100.0	100.0
Culture[a]	75.0	100.0	50.0	100.0	100.0	100.0
PCR						
Nelson primers	84.6	91.2	100.0	92.3	100.0	66.7
JDP primers	46.2	100.0	100.0	100.0	100.0	100.0

[a]Two specimens were not set up for culture.

1984 and 1992, Bacon et al[1] demonstrated 71% to 74% sensitivity of corneal culture, and only 54% sensitivity of epithelial biopsy in the diagnosis of *Acanthamoeba* infection. Because corneal culture, the gold standard of laboratory diagnosis of AK, requires specialized technical expertise and a long turnaround time, a search for technically simple, rapid, sensitive, and specific detection method of *Acanthamoeba* infection has been ongoing. In the 1980s, acridine orange, calcofluor white, and fluorescent antibody stains have been advocated for rapid detection of *Acanthamoeba* organisms, but were technically difficult to perform and required fluorescent microscope. Subsequent work by Grossniklaus et al[2] in 2003 has shown superiority of routine hematoxylin and eosin stain to these specialized staining methods in diagnosis of AK in penetrating keratoplasty specimens. The authors concluded that an experienced observer should be able to detect *Acanthamoeba* organisms with high sensitivity and specificity in routinely stained preparations of removed corneal buttons. However, either due to lack of expertise or due to difficulties involved in tissue sampling of corneal epithelial scrapings, the cytopathologic diagnosis of AK remains a challenge.

Two recent studies have focused on developing methods to increase sensitivity of rapid diagnosis of AK. One study by Shiraishi et al has described 100% sensitivity of detection of AK using serial frozen sections of corneal scrapings stained with Fungiflora Y rapid detection method (Table 1, Fig 1 in the original article). Although the authors advocate this detection method as rapid, inexpensive, and easy to perform, it does require equipment and personnel skilled in frozen section preparation and availability of a fluorescent microscope. Thus, although conceptually appealing, this detection method is unlikely to gain a widespread popularity.

The second work by Boggild et al has compared Nelson primer polymerase chain reaction (PCR) and JDP primer PCR with other routine diagnostic methods, such as smears and cultures. The authors found that Nelson primer PCR had a higher sensitivity than culture and direct microscopy (90% vs. 74% and 55%, respectively), but slightly lower specificity than culture and direct microscopy (91% vs. 100% and 100%, respectively) (Tables 1 and 2). The authors concluded that despite slightly lower specificity, Nelson primer PCR can be used as a rapid screening method for AK, particularly in patients with appropriate clinical presentation. The positive results could then be followed by a specific confirmatory test, such as JDP primer PCR. This study paves the way for future work on molecular diagnosis of AK. Unfortunately, until inexpensive and easy-to-use molecular diagnostic methods are developed for AK, we still have to rely on culture and hematoxylin and eosin stains of corneal biopsies.

T. Milman, MD

References

1. Bacon AS, Frazer DG, Dart JK, Matheson M, Ficker LA, Wright P. A review of 72 consecutive cases of Acanthamoeba keratitis, 1984-1992. *Eye (Lond)*. 1993;7: 719-725.
2. Grossniklaus HE, Waring GO 4th, Akor C, Castellano-Sanchez AA, Bennett K. Evaluation of hematoxylin and eosin and special stains for the detection of Acanthamoeba keratitis in penetrating keratoplasties. *Am J Ophthalmol*. 2003; 136:520-526.

Rapid detection of *Acanthamoeba* cysts in frozen sections of corneal scrapings with Fungiflora Y

Shiraishi A, Kobayashi T, Hara Y, et al (Ehime Univ Graduate School of Medicine, Japan)

Br J Ophthalmol 93:1563-1565, 2009

Aims.—To evaluate the usefulness of serial frozen sections of corneal scrapings stained with Fungiflora Y (FFY) to diagnose *Acanthamoeba* keratitis (AK).

Methods.—Eight patients with suspected AK were studied. Serial frozen sections were made from part of the corneal epithelial scrapings and stained with FFY. The remaining corneal epithelial scrapings were submitted for laboratory culture.

Results.—The FFY stained frozen sections were completed within an hour, and *Acanthamoeba* cysts were detected under a fluorescence microscope in all eight patients. The same sections were examined with a light microscope, and *Acanthamoeba* cysts were confirmed to be present from their morphological characteristics. Five of the eight patients had positive laboratory cultures for *Acanthamoeba*.

Conclusion.—FFY staining of frozen sections of corneal scrapings is a rapid and reliable technique which can be used to make an early diagnosis of AK (Fig 1, Table 1).

▶ The laboratory diagnosis of *Acanthamoeba* keratitis (AK) remains a challenge. In a review of 72 consecutive cases of AK presenting between 1984 and 1992, Bacon et al[1] demonstrated 71% to 74% sensitivity of corneal culture, and only 54% sensitivity of epithelial biopsy in the diagnosis of *Acanthamoeba* infection. Because corneal culture, the gold standard of laboratory

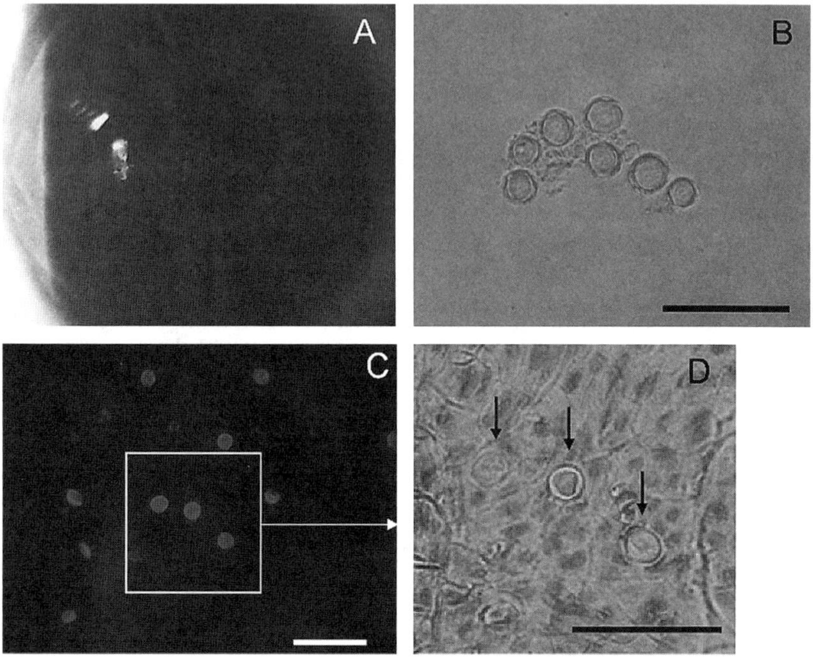

FIGURE 1.—Slit-lamp photograph and histological findings from a patient with *Acanthamoeba* keratitis. (A) Slit-lamp photograph of the cornea of a patient with *Acanthamoeba* keratitis (case 6). Dendriform keratopathy and radial keratoneuritis can be seen. (B) *Acanthamoeba* cysts isolated from the contact lens case of the same patient. (C) FFY staining of frozen sections of corneal scrapings of the same patient showing amebic cysts as bright green circles, while the corneal epithelial cells or inflammatory cells do not fluoresce. (D) Light microscopy showing amoebic cysts in the same section (all bars = 50 μm). (Reprinted from Shiraishi A, Kobayashi T, Hara Y, et al. Rapid detection of *Acanthamoeba* cysts in frozen sections of corneal scrapings with Fungiflora Y. *Br J Ophthalmol.* 2009;93:1563-1565.)

diagnosis of AK, requires specialized technical expertise and a long turnaround time, a search for technically simple, rapid, sensitive, and specific detection method of *Acanthamoeba* infection has been ongoing. In the 1980s, acridine orange, calcofluor white, and fluorescent antibody stains have been advocated for rapid detection of *Acanthamoeba* organisms, but were technically difficult to perform and required fluorescent microscope. Subsequent work by Grossniklaus et al[2] in 2003 has shown superiority of routine hematoxylin and eosin stain to these specialized staining methods in diagnosis of AK in penetrating keratoplasty specimens. The authors concluded that an experienced observer should be able to detect *Acanthamoeba* organisms with high sensitivity and specificity in routinely stained preparations of removed corneal buttons. However, either due to lack of expertise or due to difficulties involved in tissue sampling of corneal epithelial scrapings, the cytopathologic diagnosis of AK remains a challenge.

Two recent studies have focused on developing methods to increase sensitivity of rapid diagnosis of AK. One study by Shiraishi et al has described 100% sensitivity of detection of AK using serial frozen sections of corneal

TABLE 1.—Clinical Details of Each Patient

								Clinical signs				
Patient No	Age	Sex	Best-corrected Visual Acuity Before Treatment (Weeks)	Duration (Weeks) of Symptoms Before Diagnosis of *Acanthamoeba* keratitis	Immunosuppresion Treatment Before Diagnosis	Culture	Fungiflora Y	Dendriform Epitheliopathy	Radial Keratoneuritis	Ring Infiltrate	Best-corrected Visual Acuity After Treatment	Follow-up Period (Months)
1	37	Male	20/125	12	Topical steroid	–	+	+	+	–	20/50	12
2	24	Male	20/40	3	–	+	+	–	+	–	20/16	6
3	25	Female	20/40	3	Topical steroid	+	+	–	+	–	20/16	3
4	35	Male	20/32	3	–	+	+	+	+	–	20/16	6
5	18	Female	20/600	2	Topical steroid	+	+	+	+	–	20/25	3
6	25	Female	20/100	3	Topical steroid	–	+	+	+	–	20/16	3
7	25	Female	20/32	1	Topical steroid	+	+	+	+	–	20/16	5
8	33	Male	1f/counting finger	6	Topical steroid	–	+	–	–	+	20/1000	4

scrapings stained with Fungiflora Y rapid detection method (Table 1, Fig 1). Although the authors advocate this detection method as rapid, inexpensive, and easy to perform, it does require equipment and personnel skilled in frozen section preparation and availability of a fluorescent microscope. Thus, although conceptually appealing, this detection method is unlikely to gain widespread popularity.

The second work by Boggild et al has compared Nelson primer polymerase chain reaction (PCR) and JDP primer PCR with other routine diagnostic methods, such as smears and cultures. The authors found that Nelson primer PCR had a higher sensitivity than culture and direct microscopy (90% vs. 74% and 55%, respectively), but slightly lower specificity than culture and direct microscopy (91% vs. 100% and 100%, respectively). The authors concluded that despite slightly lower specificity, Nelson primer PCR can be used as a rapid screening method for AK, particularly in patients with appropriate clinical presentation. The positive results could then be followed by a specific confirmatory test, such as JDP primer PCR. This study paves the way for future work on molecular diagnosis of AK. Unfortunately, until inexpensive and easy-to-use molecular diagnostic methods are developed for AK, we still have to rely on culture and hematoxylin and eosin stains of corneal biopsies.

T. Milman, MD

References

1. Bacon AS, Frazer DG, Dart JK, Matheson M, Ficker LA, Wright P. A review of 72 consecutive cases of Acanthamoeba keratitis, 1984–1992. *Eye (Lond).* 1993;7: 719-725.
2. Grossniklaus HE, Waring GO 4th, Akor C, Castellano-Sanchez AA, Bennett K. Evaluation of hematoxylin and eosin and special stains for the detection of Acanthamoeba keratitis in penetrating keratoplasties. *Am J Ophthalmol.* 2003; 136:520-526.

12 Socio-Economics

The Physician's Response to Climate Change

Sarfaty M, Abouzaid S (Thomas Jefferson Univ, Philadelphia, PA)

Fam Med 41:358-363, 2009

Climate change will have an effect on the health and well-being of the populations cared for by practicing physicians. The anticipated medical effects include heat- and cold-related deaths, cardiovascular illnesses, injuries and mental harms from extreme weather events, respiratory illnesses caused by poor air quality, infectious diseases that emanate from contaminated food, water, or spread of disease vectors, the injuries caused by natural disasters, and the mental harm associated with social disruption. Within several years, such medical problems are likely to reach the doorsteps of many physicians. In the face of this reality, physicians should assume their traditional roles as medical professionals, health educators, and community leaders. Clinicians provide individual health services to patients, some of whom will be especially vulnerable to the emerging health consequences of global warming. Physicians also work in academic medical institutions and hospitals that educate and provide continuing medical education to students, residents, and practitioners. The institutions also produce a measurable carbon footprint. Societies of physicians at national, state, and local levels can choose to use their well-developed avenues of communication to raise awareness of the key issues that are raised by climate change as well as other environmental concerns that have profound implications for human health and well-being.

▶ This article written by a college friend is an excellent summary of how climate change relates to health and what physicians can do about this issue. Heat waves and floods have a direct negative impact on cardiac, respiratory, and infectious diseases. There are many steps that can be taken to decrease energy use and the carbon footprint of medical offices and hospitals.

Just as there are information technology specialists, it would seem that energy efficiency specialists could help design work places to meet the goal of "2% solution" to decrease the carbon footprint by 40% in 20 years.

E. J. Cohen, MD

Vaccine Refusal, Mandatory Immunization, and the Risks of Vaccine-Preventable Diseases

Omer SB, Salmon DA, Orenstein WA, et al (Emory Univ, Atlanta, GA; Johns Hopkins Bloomberg School of Public Health, Baltimore, MD)

N Engl J Med 360:1981-1988, 2009

Vaccines are among the most effective prevention tools available to clinicians. However, the success of an immunization program depends on high rates of acceptance and coverage. There is evidence of an increase in vaccine refusal in the United States and of geographic clustering of refusals that results in outbreaks. Children with exemptions from school immunization requirements (a measure of vaccine refusal) are at increased risk for measles and pertussis and can infect others who are too young to be vaccinated, cannot be vaccinated for medical reasons, or were vaccinated but did not have a sufficient immunologic response. Clinicians can play a crucial role in parental decision making. Health care providers are cited as the most frequent source of immunization information by parents, including parents of unvaccinated children. Although some clinicians have discontinued or have considered discontinuing their provider relationship with patients who refuse vaccines, the American Academy of Pediatrics Committee on Bioethics advises against this and recommends that clinicians address vaccine refusal by respectfully listening to parental concerns and discussing the risks of nonvaccination.

▶ This article not only discusses the use or refusal of vaccines mostly for preventable, contagious childhood diseases but also the role of physicians in influencing decision making by educating parents/patients about the benefits and risks of vaccines. For some of us, concern about the risks of vaccine is hard to appreciate. We eagerly awaited sufficient effective vaccine against swine flu.

The zoster vaccine is different from vaccines for childhood diseases, including chicken pox caused by the same herpes varicella zoster virus, because it protects the patient from their own latent herpes zoster virus and does not protect others in the community from infection. However, as ophthalmologists we should encourage our patients aged 60 years and above to see their primary care doctor to get the zoster vaccine, which has been proven to both decrease the frequency and severity of shingles. Even patients with a history of shingles should receive this vaccine when they are 60 years old.

E. J. Cohen, MD

Use of Electronic Health Records in U.S. Hospitals

Jha AK, DesRoches CM, Campbell EG, et al (Harvard School of Public Health, Boston, MA; the Inst for Health Policy, Boston, MA; et al)
N Engl J Med 360:1628-1638, 2009

Background.—Despite a consensus that the use of health information technology should lead to more efficient, safer, and higher-quality care, there are no reliable estimates of the prevalence of adoption of electronic health records in U.S. hospitals.

Methods.—We surveyed all acute care hospitals that are members of the American Hospital Association for the presence of specific electronic-record functionalities. Using a definition of electronic health records based on expert consensus, we determined the proportion of hospitals that had such systems in their clinical areas. We also examined the relationship of adoption of electronic health records to specific hospital characteristics and factors that were reported to be barriers to or facilitators of adoption.

Results.—On the basis of responses from 63.1% of hospitals surveyed, only 1.5% of U.S. hospitals have a comprehensive electronic-records system (i.e., present in all clinical units), and an additional 7.6% have a basic system (i.e., present in at least one clinical unit). Computerized provider-order entry for medications has been implemented in only 17% of hospitals. Larger hospitals, those located in urban areas, and teaching hospitals were more likely to have electronic-records systems. Respondents cited capital requirements and high maintenance costs as the primary barriers to implementation, although hospitals with electronic-records systems were less likely to cite these barriers than hospitals without such systems.

Conclusions.—The very low levels of adoption of electronic health records in U.S. hospitals suggest that policymakers face substantial obstacles to the achievement of health care performance goals that depend on health information technology. A policy strategy focused on financial support, interoperability, and training of technical support staff may be necessary to spur adoption of electronic-records systems in U.S. hospitals. (Figs 1 and 2).

▶ This article reports the very low rate (1.5%) of comprehensive electronic medical records (EMRs) in acute care hospitals and the factors associated with this. Inadequate money to invest in EMR was a frequent concern among hospitals with and without EMR. Financial support was identified as something that could facilitate adoption of EMR. EMR systems cost money rather than save money. Physician resistance is much less important according to this study, but concern about decreased clinical productivity is a valid issue. It takes time to create accurate EMRs for each patient encounter, especially for complex patients. Financial support for EMR, necessary staff training, and

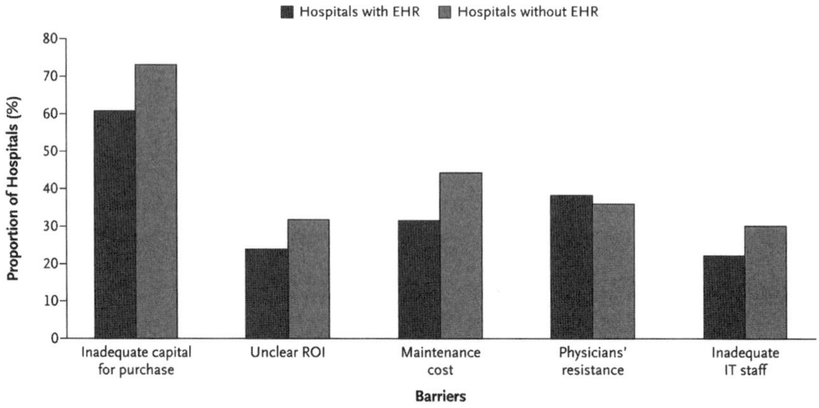

FIGURE 1.—Major perceived barriers to adoption of electronic health records (EHRs) among hospitals with electronic-records systems as compared with hospitals without systems. Hospitals with electronic-records systems include hospitals with a comprehensive electronic-records system and those with a basic electronic-records system that includes functionalities for physicians' notes and nursing assessments. P<0.01 for all comparisons except physicians' resistance (P = 0.20). IT denotes information technology, and ROI return on investment. (Reprinted from Jha AK, DesRoches CM, Campbell EG, et al. Use of electronic health records in U.S. hospitals. *N Engl J Med*. 2009;360:1628-1638, with permission from the Massachusetts Medical Society. All rights reserved.)

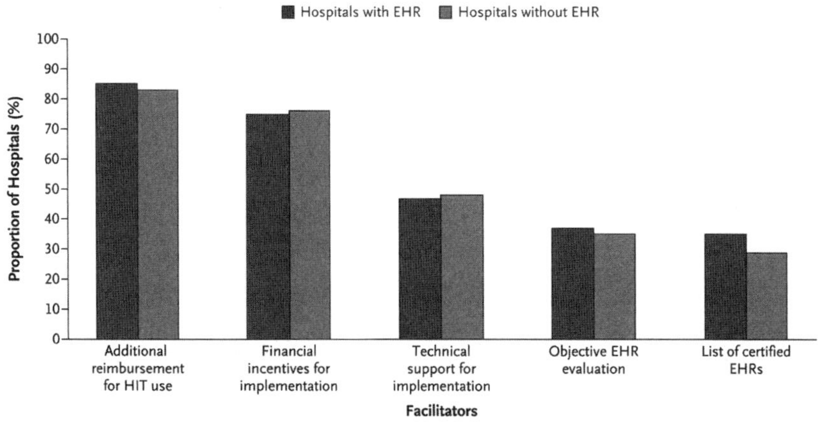

FIGURE 2.—Perceived Facilitators of Adoption of Electronic-Records Systems among Hospitals with Systems as Compared with Hospitals without Systems. Hospitals with electronic-records systems include hospitals with a comprehensive system and those with a basic system that includes functionalities for physicians' notes and nursing assessments. P>0.10 for all comparisons. EHR denotes electronic health record, and HIT health information technology. (Reprinted from Jha AK, DesRoches CM, Campbell EG, et al. Use of electronic health records in U.S. hospitals. *N Engl J Med*. 2009;360:1628-1638, with permission from the Massachusetts Medical Society. All rights reserved.)

necessary steps to enhance widespread adoption of EMR will be welcomed, but who is going to pay?

E. J. Cohen, MD

Reported eye care utilization and health insurance status among US adults

Lee DJ, Lam BL, Arora S, et al (Univ of Miami Miller School of Medicine, Florida)

Arch Ophthalmol 127:303-310, 2009

Objectives.—To estimate prevalence and correlates of eye care utilization by means of data from the National Health Interview Survey.

Methods.—Nearly 290,000 adults 18 years or older participated in the survey from 1997 through 2005. Eye care utilization was based on self-reported contact with an eye care professional in the past year. Participants were classified by level of visual impairment based on response to 2 questions. The survey and logistic regression procedures in SAS statistical software were used to compute 1997 through 2005 pooled eye care utilization rates and to identify correlates of utilization.

Results.—Overall eye care utilization rates were 58.3%, 49.6%, and 33.7%, respectively, for participants with severe, some, and no visual impairment; rates for respondents without health insurance were 35.9%, 23.8%, and 14.3%, respectively. Multivariable logistic regression analyses completed in racial/ethnic and age category subgroups indicated that no reported visual impairment, lack of health insurance, male sex, and low education were associated with low eye care utilization rates.

Conclusions.—Interventions designed to increase eye care utilization rates in select sociodemographic subgroups are needed. Overall utilization rates may also be enhanced if progress is made toward dramatically increasing the number of Americans with health insurance.

▶ It should not be surprising that visual impairment is associated with increased eye care and that lack of insurance decreases eye care significantly. As a consequence, increased insurance coverage will be associated with increased care and cost. Any cost saving associated with greater access to care through universal insurance may occur long term by prevention, early diagnosis, and treatment, but certainly not in the short term. The situation for eye care is probably similar to the situation for health care in general.

In the accompanying editorial there is concern that eye care is not frequent enough among the insured. If educational efforts are successful in encouraging appropriate frequency of care among the insured, medical costs will go up even more. Controlling medical costs is a separate aspect of the problem. Broadening coverage and enhancing usage will certainly make controlling costs even more of a challenge.

E. J. Cohen, MD

A Prospective Randomized Evaluation of Topical Gatifloxacin on Conjunctival Flora in Patients Undergoing Intravitreal Injections

Moss JM, Sanislo SR, Ta CN (Stanford Univ Med Ctr, California)

Ophthalmology 116:1498-1501, 2009

Purpose.—We sought to assess the efficacy of 3-day topical gatifloxacin use in combination with povidoneiodine (PVI) versus PVI alone in eliminating conjunctival bacterial flora in patients scheduled to undergo intravitreal (IVT) injection.

Design.—Prospective, randomized single-blind clinical trial.

Participants.—We included 129 patients scheduled to undergo 273 IVT injections at California Vitreoretinal Center at Stanford University.

Methods.—Study patients were randomized to self-administration of gatifloxacin drops for 3 days before injection, or no pretreatment antibiotics. Cultures were collected from the bulbar conjunctiva at the injection site and at the corresponding location in the fellow eye before PVI preparation. After topical PVI treatment and immediately before injection, a third culture was obtained at the injection site. Additionally, the injection needle was also cultured after the procedure.

Main Outcome Measures.—Incidence of positive bacterial samples collected from injection site conjunctiva and injection needles.

Results.—Three-day gatifloxacin use resulted in a significantly lower rate of SeptiChek (Becton Dickinson, Franklin Lakes, NJ) positive cultures compared with untreated controls (21% vs 48% respectively, $P = 0.005$). After topical PVI, the rate of positive bacterial cultures in gatifloxacin-treated and control eyes were similar (8% and 4%, respectively; $P = 0.324$).

Conclusions.—Although 3-day topical gatifloxacin use is effective in reducing the frequency of conjunctival bacterial growth relative to untreated eyes, antibiotic use confers no additional benefit in combination with PVI than eyes receiving PVI alone. This supports that topical PVI is an effective preinjection monotherapy for infection prophylaxis in the setting of IVT injections (Fig 1).

▶ Topical antibiotics are not approved for prophylaxis, although their use postoperatively is part of standard care. Conjunctival culture data confirm that coagulase-negative staphylococcus is by far the most common conjunctival organism (75% of positive cultures), but *Staphylococcus aureus*, *Streptococcus* species, and gram-negative rods are present in 6% to 7% of positive conjunctival cultures. This article reports that a 3-day course of preoperative topical gatifloxacin is better than nothing in suppressing conjunctival flora, but is no better than preoperative topical povidoneiodine (PVI) alone. Preoperative topical PVI remains the only proven treatment effective in preventing postoperative endophthalmitis as determined by the landmark article by Speaker and Menikoff.[1] Efficacy against coagulase-negative staphylococcus is critical, but other more virulent organisms are also present on the conjunctiva. With

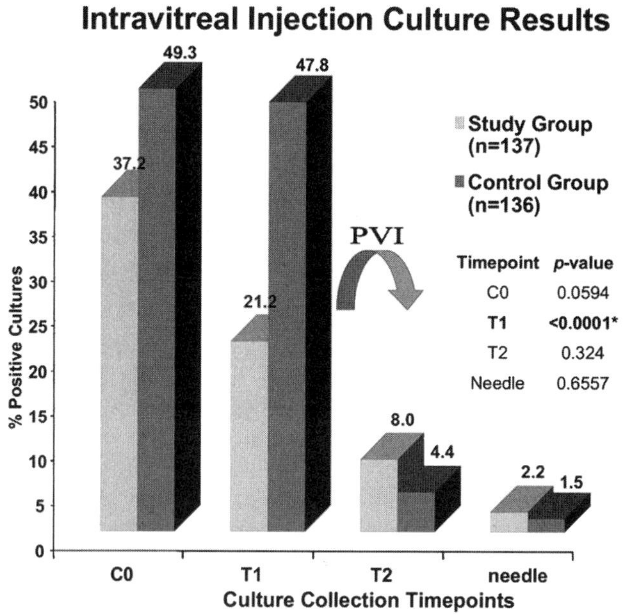

FIGURE 1.—Percentage of positive cultures for SeptiChek broth at each culture collection timepoint. C_0: Anatomically mirrored site 4 mm posterior to the limbus in the inferotemporal quadrant of the contralateral eye on the day of injection where neither group had received antibiotic pretreatment. T_1: Injection site culture collected on day of injection before any dilation drops or povidone-iodine (PVI) preparation from the inferotemporal quadrant of the bulbar conjunctiva 4 mm posterior to the limbus, after 3-day gatifloxacin use in study group participants and no antibiotics in control group patients. T_2: Injection site culture from same site as T_1 immediately before injection and after PVI preparation in all participants. Needle: Injection needle collected for culture immediately after the procedure. (Reprinted from Moss JM, Sanislo SR, Ta CN. A prospective randomized evaluation of topical gatifloxacin on conjunctival flora in patients undergoing intravitreal injections. *Ophthalmology.* 2009;116:1498-1501, with permission from the American Academy of Ophthalmology.)

increasing resistance of *staphylococcus* organisms to fourth generation fluoroquinolones, it is good to know that PVI remains effective.

E. J. Cohen, MD

Reference

1. Speaker MG, Menikoff JA. Prophylaxis of endophthalmitis with topical povidone-iodine. *Ophthalmology.* 1991;98:1769-1775. 10.1016/j.ophtha.2009.02.024.

Patient Knowledge of Physician Responsibilities and Their Preferences for Care in Ophthalmology Teaching Clinics

Guffey R, Juzych N, Juzych M (Wayne State Univ, Detroit, MI; Michigan Public Health Inst, Okemos)

Ophthalmology 116:1610-1614, 2009

Purpose.—To determine how well patients understand the hierarchy of a teaching hospital, what factors influence patient knowledge, and how patients feel about their role in training physicians.

Design.—Prospective cross-sectional survey.

Participants.—A total of 312 patients attending 1 of 3 ophthalmology clinics at the Kresge Eye Institute in July 2006.

Methods.—Survey of knowledge about the training and responsibilities of medical students, residents, and attending physicians was conducted, as well as subjective evaluation regarding patient comfort with treatment by physicians in training. Knowledge Score was correlated with subjective Comfort Score and demographics using analysis of variance.

Main Outcome Measures.—Knowledge Score and subjective Comfort Score.

Results.—A total of 312 surveys were completed. Some 56% of questions were answered correctly. Higher education was the only significant factor for increased Knowledge Score ($P<0.001$). Respondents with a higher Knowledge Score had a correspondingly higher Comfort Score ($P = 0.004$) and are significantly more comfortable with treatment provided by physicians in training (residents). Clinic site ($P = 0.002$) and increasing age ($P = 0.02$) are also significant independent factors for increased comfort with treatment provided by physicians in training.

Conclusions.—Patients have moderate knowledge of the training and hierarchy of medical students, residents, and attending physicians. Increased patient knowledge is a significant independent factor for increased patient comfort with treatment by physicians in training. Clinic site and increased age are also significant factors for comfort with treatment by physicians in training.

▶ Patient care by physicians at various levels of training always raises ethical issues about what patients know and how they would feel if they knew more. This article reports that only 50% of knowledge questions were answered correctly, a level that indicates to me less than moderate knowledge. Not surprisingly, greater education of patients was associated with more knowledge. Importantly, 90% of patients wanted to know the level of training of the doctor. Interestingly, greater knowledge (> 60% scores) was associated with greater comfort with treatment by physicians in training compared with patients with less knowledge (less than 20% scores). So it appears that patients want to know, and knowledge will make them more receptive to care by physicians in training, but knowledge level cut-offs are very low.

The data were obtained in clinical settings but applied to issues related to informed consent for surgical procedures. Despite the findings, it is possible that knowledgeable patients may prefer to have surgery performed by an attending rather than a supervised physician in training.

E. J. Cohen, MD

A perspective on commercial relationships between ophthalmology and industry

Jampol LM, Packer S, Mills RP, et al (Northwestern Univ, Chicago, IL)
Arch Ophthalmol 127:1194-1202, 2009

Relationships between physicians and industry including pharmaceutical companies and device manufacturers are being closely scrutinized by the public and the media. These companies can contribute beneficially to patient outcomes by supporting research that improves eye care. However, ethical issues may arise that affect practicing ophthalmologists, researchers, academic faculty, and ophthalmologic organizations. These topics were discussed at a symposium sponsored by the American Ophthalmological Society in May 2008. After this meeting, the council of the society developed this perspective to clarify some of the issues at the interface of industry and ophthalmology. The perspective is intended to provide some guidance to physicians, researchers, and professional societies and to enhance further dialogue.

▶ This is an article about ethical issues that arise in relationships between ophthalmologists, drug companies, and device manufacturers. As professionals, we have a duty to what is in the vulnerable patient's best interest. By contrast, business aims to maximize profits.

There is a good discussion on many issues raised by the interactions of practicing ophthalmologists with drug representatives. Acceptance of drug samples of new, more expensive medicines may encourage physicians to prescribe them rather than recommend less expensive generic alternatives. Being on a company speaker bureau assumes one will not say negative things about the products and involves using approved slides during speaking engagements, thereby removing control of the speaker over content. Participation on medical advisory boards involves listening to favorable presentations and providing feedback that can help in marketing. Participating in drug studies produces data controlled by the company and takes time away from other activities.

Even unrestricted educational grants for CME courses are considered problematic because industry only gives money to what it has determined causes doctors to prescribe their drugs and use their devices. Similarly, industry fellowship support is also viewed as something that leads to influence and bias. Industry's intention is to create good will and gratitude.

Unfortunately, other sources of support are limited. This article is worth reading. If it makes one uncomfortable, it may enhance our personal commitment to professional behavior.

E. J. Cohen, MD

Analysis of ophthalmology workforce and delivery of emergency department eye care in Florida

Witmer MT, Margo CE (Univ of South Florida, Tampa)

Arch Ophthalmol 127:1522-1527, 2009

Objective.—To measure annual population-based volume of emergency department (ED) eye care and concurrent ophthalmology on-call coverage.

Methods.—Analysis and correlation of the 2006 Florida Agency of Health Care Administration ED and inpatient data sets with the 2007 Florida Physician Workforce Survey.

Results.—The Florida Physician Workforce Survey showed 46.3% of ophthalmologists surveyed took ED call in Florida in 2006. Based on estimates derived from the survey, 462 to 532 ophthalmologists participated in ED coverage that year. The level of workload varied considerably depending on International Classification of Diseases code diagnosis. Annual workload for open wounds to the eye, on average, ranged from 2.7 to 3.1 per ophthalmologist taking ED call.

Conclusions.—Strategic planning for the delivery of ED eye care needs to consider both the number and types of cases presenting to the ED and the availability of ophthalmologists to provide care that other specialists cannot. This preliminary study explores the use of a workload statistic that may help to gauge manpower needs in the future.

▶ This article tries to analyze the workload of ophthalmologists for emergency department eye care in Florida. The annual workload for open globes was determined to be 2.7 to 3.1 cases for ophthalmologists taking call. This understates the workload because emergency room call requires that ophthalmologists be available promptly 24 hours per day, 7 days per week, although the number of actual cases may be low. In addition, most ophthalmologists have already moved away from hospital-based practices, so the burden of call is shifted to those who take call at facilities offering 24/7 ophthalmic care. Emergency department coverage should be shared among a large number of doctors, both to distribute the burden and maintain the skills that ophthalmologists have when they complete training.

E. J. Cohen, MD

Patient-Centered Communication to Assess and Enhance Patient Adherence to Glaucoma Medication

Hahn SR (The Albert Einstein College of Medicine of Yeshiva Univ, Bronx, NY)

Ophthalmology 116:S37-S42, 2009

Topic.—Using an understanding of a patient's difficulty in revealing nonadherence and patient-centered communication skills to identify and address barriers to adherence to glaucoma medication regimens.

TABLE 1.—The Stages of Readiness to Change: Patient Psychology and Recommended Physician Interventions

Stage	Psychology	Intervention	Suggested "First Ask" Statements and Questions
Precontemplation	Lack of concern, ignorance, or denial	Raising concern: educate/address denial	Tell me in your own words about your understanding and concerns about glaucoma. Tell me what your understanding and concerns are about what glaucoma may do to your vision in the future?
Contemplation	Ambivalence	Shift ambivalence to positive action	As above for Precontemplation PLUS: Tell me what concerns you have about taking medication for glaucoma.
Preparation	Decision resolution	Transform into action	What concerns do you have, and how ready are you to start medication for glaucoma? Which of the potential/experienced side effects do you think you'll be able to live with, and which not?
Action	Engage in changing behavior	Help organize activity and provide results	What information do you need and what instruction do you need in the technique of taking eyedrops for you to start the drops?
Maintenance	Integrate new behavior to daily life	Identify barriers and create solutions	How are you going to schedule taking your medications into your daily routine? How can you make sure that you can get refills of medication before you run out?
Relapse*	Demoralized, shame, decreased or loss of self-efficacy	Reenergize behavior change	A lot of patients have trouble taking their drops every day, especially for treatments like this one, which have to be taken for a long time. It's normal to get out of the routine once in a while. What would be a better routine for you to follow, so you can take your drops every day?

*Although Termination is the ideal final stage of change, a more realistic expectation is a lifetime of maintenance marked by relapses.

Clinical Relevance.—In addition to cost and logistical difficulties with obtaining and administering medicine, a patient's adherence to medication is influenced by the balance between the perceived need for medication and concerns about taking medication.

Methods.—This article is based on both the author's clinical experience and peer-reviewed research on effective doctor-patient communication and assessment and management of nonadherence.

Results.—Three strategies have been identified that help physicians to detect and address problems with adherence: (1) a 4-step adherence assessment interview designed to detect nonadherence that decreases patient resistance to revealing nonadherence by applying a shared decision-making process and mitigating social undesirability; (2) asking open-ended questions in ask-tell-ask sequences; and (3) tailoring interventions to the patient's stage of readiness for change.

Conclusions.—Patients conceal nonadherence because they want to be thought of by their physicians as good patients. They are driven to nonadherence by an imbalance between their perceived need for medication and their concerns about taking it. Patient-centered communication techniques can engage the patient in shared decision making about medication, thereby redefining the good patient as someone who works with his or her health care provider to address adherence barriers. Those barriers can be explored with open-ended questions designed to elicit the patient's understanding and concerns, to provide information, and to assess change in the patient's understanding and attitudes. Communication will be more effective if it is based on the patient's stage of readiness to adopt adherent self-management practices (Table 1).

▶ This article is part of a supplement addressing nonadherence of patients with glaucoma with topical medications. It is relevant to doctor/patient communications in general. Nonadherence is a particular problem in treating patients with asymptomatic diseases. Patients do not admit to nonadherence because they do not want their doctors to think that they are bad patients. Doctors should ask patients about their understanding and concerns about their disease, and then tell them what they need to understand better. In the ask-tell-ask dialogue recommended in this article, the doctor asks again to see if the patient's understanding has improved and assesses the patient's motivation to change his or her behavior. Motivation to change habitual behavior has stages that are explained. Patient-centered ask-tell-ask communication helps patients and doctors work together to improve adherence to recommended medication regimens.

E. J. Cohen, MD

Article Index

Chapter 1: Cataract Surgery

Chapter 2: Refractive Surgery

Chapter 3: Glaucoma

Chapter 4: Cornea

Chapter 5: Retina

Chapter 6: Oculoplastic Surgery

Chapter 7: Pediatric Ophthalmology

Chapter 8: Neuro-ophthalmology

Chapter 9: Imaging

Chapter 10: Ocular Oncology

Chapter 11: Pathology

Chapter 12: Socio-Economics

Author Index

A

B

C

D

E

F

G

H

I

J

K

L

M

W

X

Y

Z

Oseledec, V.I., 1968, "A multiplicative ergodic theorem. Ljapunov characteristic numbers for dynamical systems," Trans. Moscow Math. Soc. **19**, 197.

Packard, N.H., 1986,"Lattice models for solidification and aggregation," in [Wolfram 1986].

Parisi, G., 1987, "Facing Complexity," Physica Scripta **35**, 123.

Peacocke, A.R., 1983, *The Physical Chemistry of Biological Organization*, Oxford University Press.

Peebles, P.J.E., 1966, "Primordial helium abundance and primordial fireball," Astrophys. J., **146**, 542.

Prigogine, I., 1980, *From Being to Becoming: time and complexity in the physical sciences*, W.H. Freeman and Company, San Francisco.

Procaccia, I., 1985, "The static and dynamic invariants that characterize chaos and the relations between them in theory and experiments," Physica Scripta **T9**, 40.

Procaccia, I. and Levine, R.D., 1976, "Potential work—statistical-mechanical approach for systems in disequilibrium," J. Chem. Phys. **65**, 3357.

Rant, Z., 1956, "Exergie, ein neues Wort für 'technische Arbeitsfähigkeit'," Forschung auf dem Gebiete des Ingenieurwesens **22**(1), 36.

Redlich, O. and Kwong, J.N.S., 1949, "On the thermodynamics of solutions," Chem. Rev. **44**, 233.

Reid, R.C., Prausnitz, J.M., and Sherwood, T.K., 1977, *The properties of gases and liquids*, 3rd ed., McGraw-Hill, New York.

Reif, F., 1965, *Fundamentals of Statistical and Thermal Physics*, McGraw-Hill, Tokyo.

Rensing, L. and Jaeger, N.I., 1985, *Temporal Order*, Springer-Verlag, Berlin.

Rényi, A., 1970, *Probability Theory*, North-Holland Publishing Company, Amsterdam.

Robinson, J., 1978, *Economic Philosophy*, Penguin Books.

Russell, B. and Whitehead, A.N., 1910-13, *Principia Mathematica*, Vols. I-III, Cambridge University Press.

Salem, J.B. and Wolfram, S., 1986, "Thermodynamics and hydrodynamics of cellular automata" in [Wolfram 1986b].

Samuelson, P.A., 1983, *Foundations of Economic Analysis*, Harvard University Press, Cambridge, Massachusetts (enlarged edition).

Schlögl, F., 1980, "Stochastic measures in nonequilibrium thermodynamics," Physics Reports **62**, 267.

Schrödinger, E, 1944, *What is Life?*, Cambridge University Press.

Schuster, P., 1982, "Stages of emerging life—five principles of early organization," J. Mol. Evol. **19**, 47-61.

Shannon C.E., 1948, "A mathematical theory of communication," Bell System Technical Journal **27**, 379.

Shannon, C.E. and Weaver, W., 1949, *The Mathematical Theory of Communication*, University of Illinois Press, Urbana.

Shaw, R., 1981, "Strange attractors, chaotic behaviour, and information flow," Z. Naturforsch. **36a**, 80.

Smith-Sørensen, T., 1976, Acta Chemica Scandinavia **A30**, 555; **A31**, 347 and 437 (1977).

Snow, C.P., 1964, *The Two Cultures and a Second Look*, Cambridge University Press, Cambridge.

Soave, G., 1972, "Equilibrium constants from a modified Redlich-Kwong equation of state," Chem. Eng. Sci. **27**, 1197.

Steinbeck, J., 1937, *Of Mice and Men*, Viking Press.

Szilard, L., 1929, "Über die Entropiverminderung in einem thermodynamischen System bei Eingriffen intelligenter Wesen," Z. Physik **53**, 840.

Takayama, A., 1974, *Mathematical Economics*, The Dryden Press, Hinsdale, Illinois.
Tolman, R.C., 1934, *Thermodynamics and Cosmology*, Oxford University Press.
Tribus, M., Shannon, P.T., Evans, R.B., 1966, "Why thermodynamics is a logical consequence of information theory," Amer. Inst. Chem. Eng. J. **12**, 244.
Turing, A., 1936-37, "On computable numbers, with an application to the Entscheidungsproblem," Proc. London Math. Soc. **42**, 230; **43**, 544.
Turing, A., 1952, "The chemical basis of morphogenesis," Philos. Trans. R. Soc. London **B273**, 37.
Tyson, J.J., 1976, *The Belousov-Zhabotinskii Reaction*, Lecture Notes in Biomathematics 10, Springer-Verlag, Berlin.
Ulanowicz, R.E., 1981, "A unified theory of self-organization" (paper presented at The International Symposium on Energy and Ecological Modelling, sponsored by the International Society for Ecological Modelling, Louisville, Kentucky, April 1981).
Van Hove, L., 1983, "Non-Equilibrium Processes in Early Cosmology," Preprint no TH.3623-CERN, Geneva.
Vidal, C. and Pacault, A. (eds.), 1981, *Nonlinear Phenomena in Chemical Dynamics*, Springer-Verlag, Berlin.
Vidal, C. and Pacault, A. (eds.), 1984, *Non-Equilibrium Dynamics in Chemical Systems*, Springer-Verlag, Berlin.
Von Neumann, J., 1966, *Theory of Self-Reproducing Automata*, edited by A.W. Burks, University of Illinois, Urbana.
Weidlich, W., 1987, "Quantitative social science," Physica Scripta **35**, 380.
Weidlich, W. and Haag, G., 1983, *Concepts and Models of Quantitative Sociolgy*, Springer-Verlag, Berlin.
Weinberg, S., 1972, *Gravitation and Cosmology: Principles and Applications of the General Theory*, John Wiley & Sons, New York.
Wheeler, J.A. and Zurek, W.H. (eds.), 1983, *Quantum Theory and Measurement*, Princeton University Press.
Willamowski, K.-D. and Rössler, O.E., 1980, "Irregular oscillations in a realistic abstract quadratic mass-action system," Z. Naturforsch. **35a**, 317.
Wilson, A.G., Coelho, J.D., Macgill, S.M., and Williams, H.C.W.L., 1981, *Optimization in Locational and Transport Analysis*, John Wiley & Sons, Chichester.
Winfree, A.T., Winfree, E.M., and Seifert, H., 1985, "Organizing centers in a cellular exitable medium," Physica **17D**, 109.
Wolfram, S., 1983, "Statistical mechanics of cellular automata," Rev. Mod. Phys. **55**, 601.
Wolfram, S., 1984a, "Universality and complexity in cellular automata," Physica **10D**, 1.
Wolfram, S., 1984b, "Computation theory of cellular automata," Commun. Math. Phys. **96**, 15.
Wolfram, S., 1986a, "Random sequence generation by cellular automata," Advances in Applied Mathematics **7**, 123.
Wolfram, S. (ed.), 1986b, *Theory and Applications of Cellular Automata*, World Scientific, Singapore.
Zhvonkin, A.K. and Levin, L.A., 1970, "The complexity of finite objects and the development of the concepts of information and randomness by means of the theory of algorithms," Russian Mathematical Surveys **25**, 83.
Zurek, W.H., 1984, "Reversibility and stability of information processing systems," Phys. Rev. Lett. **53**, 391.